D1558044

Nusten 2½5

The Brugada Syndrome:
From Bench to Bedside

The Brugada Syndrome: From Bench to Bedside

EDITED BY

Charles Antzelevitch, PhD

Masonic Medical Research Laboratory
Utica
NY
USA

WITH ASSOCIATE EDITORS

Pedro Brugada, MD, PhD

Cardiovascular Center
Cardiovascular Research and Teaching Institute
Aalst
Belgium

Josep Brugada, MD

Cardiovascular Institute
Hospital Clinic
University of Barcelona
Spain

Ramon Brugada, MD

Masonic Medical Research Laboratory
Utica
NY
USA

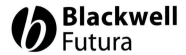

Blackwell
Futura

Blackwell Futura is an imprint of Blackwell Publishing
Blackwell Publishing, Inc., 350 Main Street, Malden, Massachusetts 02148–5020, USA
Blackwell Publishing Ltd, 9600 Garsington Road, Oxford OX4 2DQ, UK
Blackwell Science Asia Pty Ltd, 550 Swanston Street, Carlton, Victoria 3053, Australia

First published 2005

ISBN: 1-4051-2778-3

Library of Congress Cataloging-in-Publication Data

The Brugada syndrome: from bench to bedside / edited by Charles Antzelevitch and Pedro
Brugada.
          p.   ;   cm.
     Includes bibliographical references.
     ISBN 1-4051-2778-3
     1. Brugada syndrome.
     [DNLM: 1. Bundle-Branch Block.   2. Tachycardia, Ventricular. WG 330 B891 2004]
   I. Antzelevitch, Charles.   II. Brugada, Pedro.

     RC685.V43B78   2004
     616.1′23—dc22   2004021201
A catalogue record for this title is available from the British Library

Acquisitions: Steve Korn
Production: Kate Bailey and Katrina Chandler
Set in Minion by 9.5 on 12pt by SNP Best-set Typesetter Ltd., Hong Kong
Printed and bound in India by Gopsons Paper Limited, New Dehli

For further information on Blackwell Publishing, visit our website:
www.blackwellfutura.com

The publisher's policy is to use permanent paper from mills that operate a sustainable forestry
policy, and which has been manufactured from pulp processed using acid-free and elementary
chlorine-free practices. Furthermore, the publisher ensures that the text paper and cover board
used have met acceptable environmental accreditation standards.

Notice: The indications and dosages of all drugs in this book have been recommended in the
medical literature and conform to the practices of the general community. The medications
described do not necessarily have specific approval by the Food and Drug Administration for use
in the diseases and dosages for which they are recommended. The package insert for each drug
should be consulted for use and dosage as approved by the FDA. Because standards for usage
change, it is advisable to keep abreast of revised recommendations, particularly those
concerning new drugs.

Contents

Contributors

Charles Antzelevitch, PhD
Masonic Medical Research Laboratory, Utica, NY, USA

Eduardo Bartholomay, MD
Arrhythmia Section, Cardiovascular Institute, Hospital Clínic, Barcelona, Spain

Cristina Basso, MD, PhD
Department of Cardiology and Pathology, University of Padua Medical School, Padua, Italy

Bernard Belhassen, MD
Department of Cardiology, Tel-Aviv Sourasky Medical Center, and Sackler School of Medicine, Tel-Aviv University, Tel-Aviv, Israel

Preben Bjerregaard, MD
St. Louis University, St. Louis, MO, USA

Martin Borggrefe, MD, PhD
University of Heidelberg, University Hospital of Mannheim, Mannheim, Germany

Günter Breithardt, MD
Department of Cardiology and Angiology, Hospital of the University of Münster, Germany; Institute for Arteriosclerosis Research, University of Münster, Germany

Josep Brugada, MD
Cardiovascular Institute, Hospital Clínic, University of Barcelona, Spain

Pedro Brugada, MD, PhD
Cardiovascular Center, Cardiovascular Research and Teaching Institute, Aalst, Belgium

Ramon Brugada, MD
Masonic Medical Research Laboratory, Utica, NY, USA

Gianfranco Buja, MD
University of Padua Medical School, Padua, Italy

José Angel Cabrera, MD
Fundacion Jiménez Diaz, Madrid, Spain

Bruno Cauchemez, MD
Hôpital Lariboisière, Paris, France

Jacques Clémenty, MD
University of Bordeaux II and Hôpital Cardiologique du Haut-Lévêque, Bordeaux, France

Domenico Corrado, MD, PhD
Division of Cardiology, University of Padua Medical School, Padua, Italy

José M. Di Diego, MD
Masonic Medical Research Laboratory, Utica, NY, USA

Lars Eckardt, MD
Department of Cardiology and Angiology, Hospital of the University of Münster, Germany

Fabrice Extramiana, MD
Hôpital Lariboisière, Paris, France

Celso Ferreira, MD, PhD
ABC Foundation. Santo André — São Paulo, Brazil

Jeffrey M. Fish, DVM
Masonic Medical Research Laboratory, Utica, NY, USA

Fiorenzo Gaita, MD
Ospedale Mauriziano, Torino, Ospedale Civile di Asti, Italy

Stéphane Garrigue, MD
Hôpital Cardiologique du Haut-Lévêque, Bordeaux, France

Ihor Gussak, MD, PhD
eResearch Technology, Inc., Bridgewater, NJ, USA

Michel Haïssaguerre, MD
University of Bordeaux II and Hôpital Cardiologique du Haut-Lévêque, Bordeaux, France

Mélèze Hocini, MD
Hôpital Cardiologique du Haut-Lévêque, Bordeaux, France

Li-Fern Hsu, MBBS
Hôpital Cardiologique du Haut-Lévêque, Bordeaux, France

Pierre Jaïs, MD
Hôpital Cardiologique du Haut-Lévêque, Bordeaux, France

Herve Le Marec, MD, PhD
Clinique Cardiologique et des Maladies Vasculaires, and
INSERM U533 Hôpital G&R Laennec CHU de Nantes,
Nantes, France

Loira Leoni, MD
Department of Cardiology, University of Padova, Italy

Barry Maron, MD
Minneapolis Heart Institute Foundation, Minneapolis, MN,
USA

Philippe Maury, MD
Hôpital de Rangueil, Toulouse, France

Lluís Mont, MD
Arrhythmia Section, Cardiovascular Institute, Hospital
Clínic, Barcelona, Spain

Koonlawee Nademanee, MD
Pacific Rim Cardiac Electrophysiology and Research
Institute, Inglewood, CA, USA

Andrea Nava, MD
University of Padua Medical School, Padua, Italy

Jean-Luc Pasquie, MD, PhD
Hôpital Cardiologique du Haut-Lévêque, Bordeaux,
France

Sabine Pattier
Clinique Cardiologique et des Maladies Vasculaires, and
INSERM U533 Hôpital G&R Laennec CHU de Nantes,
Nantes, France

Matthias Paul, MD
Department of Cardiology and Angiology, Hospital of the
University of Münster, Germany

Antonio Pelliccia, MD
Institute of Sports Science, Italian Olympic Committee,
Rome, Italy

Vincent Probst, MD
Clinique cardiologique et des Maladies Vasculaires, and
INSERM U533 Hôpital G&R Laennec, CHU de Nantes,
Nantes, France

Andrés Ricardo Pérez Riera, MD
Cardiology Division, ABC's Faculty of Medicine, ABC
Foundation, Santo André, São Paulo, Brazil

Martin Rotter, MD
Hôpital Cardiologique du Haut-Lévêque, Bordeaux,
France

Prashanthan Sanders, MBBS, PhD
Hôpital Cardiologique du Haut-Lévêque, Bordeaux, France

Christophe Scavée, MD
Hôpital Cardiologique du Haut-Lévêque, Bordeaux, France

Edgardo Schapachnik, MD
Chagas' Disease Department, Dr. Cosme Argerich Hospital,
Buenos Aires, Argentina

Jean-Jacques Schott, PhD
Clinique Cardiologique et des Maladies Vasculaires, and
INSERM U533 Hôpital G&R Laennec, CHU de Nantes,
Nantes, France

Maurizio Schiavon, MD
Center of Sports Medicine, Padova, Italy

Rainer Schimpf, MD
University of Heidelberg, University Hospital of Mannheim,
Mannheim, Germany

Wataru Shimizu, MD, PhD
National Cardiovascular Center, Suita, Japan

Eric Schulze-Bahr, MD
Department of Cardiology, University of Münster, and
Institute for Arteriosclerosis Research, Münster, Germany

Mark Schwab, MD
Pacific Rim Electrophysiology Research Institute, Inglewood
CA, USA

Jeroen P. P. Smits, MD
Experimental and Molecular Cardiology Group,
Cardiovascular Research Institute Amsterdam, Academic
Medical Center, University of Amsterdam; the Interuniversity
Cardiology Institute, The Netherlands

Yoshihide Takahashi, MD
Hôpital Cardiologique du Haut-Lévêque, Bordeaux,
France

Hanno Tan, MD, PhD
Experimental and Molecular Cardiology Group, Academic
Medical Center, Amsterdam, and the Interuniversity
Cardiology Institute, The Netherlands

Gaetano Thiene, MD
Depts. of Cardiology and Pathology, University of Padua
Medical School, Padua, Italy

Gumpanart Veerakul, MD
Pacific Rim Electrophysiology Research Institute,
Inglewood, CA, USA

Jacques Victor, MD
Centre Hospitalier Universitaire, Angers, France

Sami Viskin, MD
Department of Cardiology, Tel-Aviv Sourasky Medical
Center, and Sackler School of Medicine, Tel-Aviv University,
Tel-Aviv, Israel

Thomas Wichter, MD
Department of Cardiology and Angiology, Hospital of the
University of Münster, Germany

Arthur A. M. Wilde, MD, PhD
Experimental and Molecular Cardiology Group, Academic
Medical Center, Amsterdam, and the Interuniversity
Cardiology Institute, The Netherlands

Christian Wolpert, MD
University of Heidelberg, University Hospital of Mannheim,
Mannheim, Germany

Preface

Since its introduction as a new clinical entity in 1992, the Brugada syndrome has attracted great interest because of its high prevalence in many parts of the world and its association with a high risk of sudden death in young adults and less frequently in infants and children. Recent years have witnessed an exponential rise in the number of reported cases and a striking proliferation of papers serving to define the clinical, genetic, cellular, ionic and molecular aspects of the disease. A consensus report published in 2002 delineated diagnostic criteria for the syndrome. Recent studies have suggested a need for refinement of these criteria and have raised questions regarding the optimal approach to therapy. A second consensus conference was held in September of 2003 in Lake Placid, NY. One result of the conference was a consensus document dealing with diagnostic criteria, risk stratification and approaches to therapy which will be simultaneously published in *Circulation* and the *European Heart Journal* in the latter part of 2004. Another is the formulation of this book, which deals in a very comprehensive manner with the clinical, molecular, genetic and cellular aspects of the Brugada syndrome authored by leading experts in the field.

The Brugada syndrome has its roots in Maastricht, The Netherlands. It was an autumn day in 1986 when an anxious father came from Poland to University Hospital Maastricht. He had lost a two-year-old daughter to sudden cardiac death and was distressed that his three-year-old boy was now experiencing episodes of syncope. The boy was found to have a peculiar ECG, manifesting a coved type ST segment elevation in the right precordial leads, similar to that of his sister before she died. Pedro Brugada moved to Aalst, Belgium and with his brother Josep collected eight similar cases. In 1992 they presented these as a new clinical entity character-

ized by an ST segment elevation in V1–V3, RBBB morphology of the ECG, in association with syncope and sudden cardiac death. A rapid succession of publications followed from investigators throughout the world. A consortium comprised of many of those involved with this book sought to define the clinical characteristics and genetic and cellular basis for the syndrome. With the expertise of Jeff Towbin's group at Baylor College of Medicine, the first gene responsible for the syndrome, *SCN5A*, was identified in 1998. Our understanding of the cellular basis for the syndrome evolved in parallel with the characterization of the clinical phenotype in the early 1990s and was termed Phase 2 Reentry.

The book deals not only with these fundamental aspects of the syndrome, but also examines how the mechanisms involved may serve as a paradigm for our understanding of a wide variety of life-threatening arrhythmia syndromes. Current controversies relative to risk stratification are discussed, as are the indications for ICD therapy. Experts including Michel Haïssaguerre, Bernard Belhassen and Sami Viskin were invited to discuss other experimental approaches to therapy.

The editor and associate editors wish to express their gratitude to all of the authors for their valuable contributions. The book is the product of a collaboration of basic and clinical investigators bringing together their unique skills and perspectives to create a work that truly takes us from the bench to the bedside. We are grateful to Medtronic Inc., Guidant Inc. and St. Jude Medical Inc. for providing unrestricted educational grants in support of the consensus conference from which the concept for this book was derived. We also wish to thank our mentors to whom we are all deeply indebted. We are grateful to our colleagues, fellows, and students for their valuable contributions to the current understanding and appreciation of the syndrome and for stimulating discussions that have served as the basis for innovative ideas and investigations. Finally, we are grateful to all of the families and patients who have participated, and are currently participating, in genetic and clinical studies designed to provide further insights into better diagnosis and management of the Brugada syndrome.

Charles Antzelevitch
Pedro Brugada
Josep Brugada
Ramon Brugada

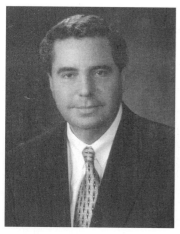

Charles Antzelevitch

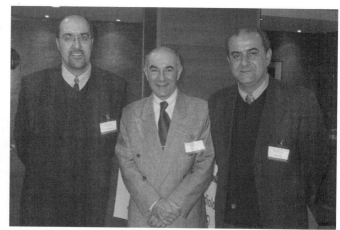

Ramon, Pedro and Josep Brugada

Dedication

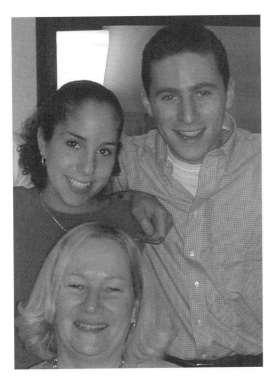

Charles Antzelevitch

To my wife, Brenda, and children, Daniel and Lisa, whose love and support serve as my foundation and daily inspiration and to my parents, Freida and Chaim, brother Morris and sister Debbie and their families for always being by my side. I also dedicate this book to all of my mentors, colleagues, fellows and students, who have contributed importantly to my scientific achievements as well as to the families who found the strength to participate in the studies that form the basis of our present day knowledge of the Brugada syndrome.

CA

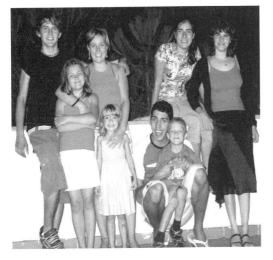

Pedro, Josep and Ramon Brugada

To the patients and families who found the courage to move forward, to give their time to the activities of the Ramon Brugada Sr. Foundation and to participate in research during a very difficult time in their lives. Without them this book would not have been possible. We also dedicate this book to our parents, Ramon and Pepita, truly international grandparents with nine grandchildren born in five different countries. Isabel, Helena, Georgia and Estanis in Spain, Pau in France, Vicky in Holland, Celine in Belgium and Aleix and Claudia in the USA. This was not by chance, but because they pushed us to go farther, to look for better ways of doing things and to be in the best possible place at each moment in time.

PB, JB, RB

CHAPTER 1

Brugada syndrome: overview

C. Antzelevitch, PhD, *et al.*

Introduction

Since its introduction as a new clinical entity in 1992,[1] the Brugada syndrome has attracted great interest because of its high incidence in many parts of the world and its association with high risk for sudden death of young adults and, to a lesser degree, infants and children. Recent years have witnessed an exponential rise in the number of reported cases and a striking proliferation of papers serving to define the clinical, genetic, cellular, ionic, and molecular aspects of the disease.[2] A consensus report published in 2002 delineated diagnostic criteria for the syndrome.[3,4] A second consensus conference was held in September of 2003. This introductory chapter provides an in-depth overview of the clinical, genetic, molecular, and cellular aspects of the Brugada syndrome, incorporating the results of the two consensus conferences and the numerous clinical and basic publications on the subject. The proposed terminology, diagnostic criteria, risk stratification schemes, and device and pharmacologic approach to therapy are based on available clinical and basic studies and should be considered a work in progress that will no doubt require fine tuning as confirmatory data from molecular studies and prospective trials become available.

Clinical characteristics

The Brugada syndrome is characterized by an ST segment elevation in the right precordial ECG leads, V_1–V_3, and a high incidence of sudden death in patients with structurally normal hearts. Although the average age at time of first diagnosis or sudden cardiac death is 40 years, the Brugada phenotype has been reported over a wide range of ages. The youngest patient diagnosed with the syndrome was

2 days of age, and the oldest was 84 years of age. The syndrome is generally thought to be responsible for 4–12% of all sudden deaths and at least 20% of deaths in patients with structurally normal hearts. The incidence of the disease is of the order of 5 per 10 000 inhabitants and, apart from accidents, is the leading cause of death of men under the age of 40 in regions of the world where the syndrome is endemic. Because the ECG is so dynamic and often concealed, it is difficult to estimate the true incidence of the disease in the general population.[5]

The electrocardiographic manifestations of the Brugada syndrome when concealed can be unmasked by sodium channel blockers, a febrile state, or vagotonic agents.[6–9] Three types of repolarization patterns in the right precordial leads are recognized (Table 1.1 and Fig. 1.1).[3,4] Type 1 is diagnostic of Brugada syndrome and is characterized by a coved ST segment elevation ≥2 mm (0.2 mV) followed by a negative T wave. Type 2 has a saddleback appearance with a high take-off ST segment elevation of ≥2 mm followed by a trough displaying ≥1 mm ST elevation followed by either a positive or biphasic T wave. Type 3 has either a saddleback or coved appearance with an ST segment elevation of <1 mm. These three patterns may be observed sequentially in the same patient or following the introduction of specific drugs.

Placing the right precordial leads in a superior position (up to the 2nd intercostal spaces above normal) can increase the sensitivity of the ECG for detecting the Brugada phenotype in some patients, both in the presence or absence of a drug challenge (Fig. 1.2),[10,11] although this altered configuration may reduce the specificity of the diagnosis.

Prolongation of the QT interval is sometimes observed associated with the ST segment elevation.[12–14] The QT interval is prolonged more in the

Table 1.1 Diagnostic criteria for Brugada syndrome (from 1st consensus document). ST segment abnormalities in leads V_1–V_3.

	Type 1	Type 2	Type 3
J point	≥2 mm	≥2 mm	≥2 mm
T wave	negative	positive or biphasic	positive
ST–T configuration	coved type	saddleback	saddleback
ST segment (terminal portion)	gradually descending	elevated ≥1 mm	elevated <1 mm

1 mm = 0.1 mV.

The terminal portion of the ST segment refers to the latter half of the ST segment.

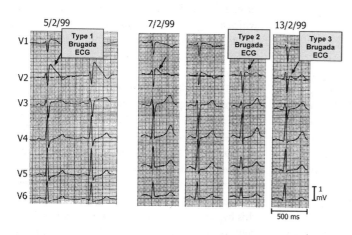

Figure 1.1 Three types of ST segment elevation generally observed in patients with the Brugada syndrome. Shown are precordial leads recorded from a patient diagnosed with the Brugada syndrome. Note the dynamic ECG changes occurring over a period of 2 days. The left panel shows a clear Type 1 ECG, which is diagnostic of the Brugada syndrome. A saddleback ST segment elevation (Type 2) is observed on 2–7–99. The ST segment is further normalized on 2–13–99 showing a Type 3 ECG. Modified from Ref. 4, with permission.

right versus left precordial leads, presumably due to a preferential prolongation of action potential duration (APD) in right ventricular (RV) epicardium secondary to accentuation of the action potential notch.[15] Depolarization abnormalities including prolongation of P wave duration, PR and QRS intervals are frequently observed, particularly in patients linked to *SCN5A* mutations.[16] PR prolongation likely reflects HV conduction delay.[12]

Recent reports indicate that up to 20% of Brugada syndrome patients develop supraventricular arrhythmias, including atrial fibrillation and Wolff–Parkinson–White syndrome.[17,18] It is as yet unknown whether atrial vulnerability is correlated with ventricular inducibility of arrhythmias or whether atrial arrhythmias may serve as triggering events for VT/VF, although the latter seems unlikely based on current knowledge. Slowed atrial conduction as well as atrial standstill have been reported in association with the syndrome.[19]

Observations from Japan suggest that in some cases arrhythmia initiation is bradycardia related.[20]

This may contribute to the higher incidence of sudden death at night in individuals with the syndrome and may account for the success of pacing in controlling the arrhythmia in isolated cases of the syndrome.[21] However, not all patients die at night and not all the cases are controlled with rapid ventricular pacing. South Asian patients who have the ECG pattern usually develop VT/VF during sleep at night.

VT/VF often terminates spontaneously in patients with the Brugada syndrome, as first reported by Bjerregaard *et al.*[22] This may explain why patients wake up at night after episodes of agonal respiration caused by the arrhythmia.

Sudden unexplained nocturnal death syndrome (SUNDS also known as SUDS), a disorder most prevalent in Southeast Asia, and Brugada syndrome have recently been shown to be phenotypically, genetically, and functionally the same disorder.[23] Sudden and unexpected death of young adults during sleep, known in the Philippines as *bangungut* ('to rise and moan in sleep'), was first described in the

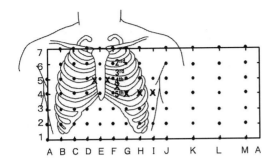

Upper Inter-costal Space

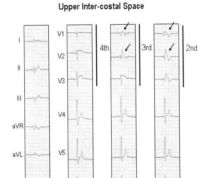

Figure 1.2 Shift of right precordial leads to 2nd and 3rd intercostal space unmasks a type 1 Brugada ECG. Top: Plot of 87 unipolar electrode sites (dots) and of 6 precordial electrocardiograms (ECG) (crosses). 87 lead points are arranged in a lattice-like pattern (13 × 7 matrix), except for four lead points on both midaxillary lines, and covered the entire thoracic surface. V_1 and V_2 leads of the ECG are located between D5 and E5, and between E5 and F5, respectively, whereas V_4, V_5, and V_6 are coincident with G4, H4 and I4, respectively. Bottom: Twelve lead electrocardiograms (ECG) in a patient with Brugada syndrome. Type 2 saddleback type segment elevation was observed in V_1 and V_2 of the standard 12 lead ECG (4th intercostal space), whereas typical Type 1 coved type ST segment elevation was apparent in V_1 and V_2 recorded from the 2nd and 3rd intercostal space (arrows).

Philippine medical literature in 1917. In Japan this syndrome, known as *pokkuri* ('sudden and unexpectedly ceased phenomena'), was reported as early as 1959.[24] In 1997, Nademanee *et al.*[25] reported that among 27 Thai men referred for aborted cases of what was known in Thailand as *Lai Tai* ('death during sleep'), as many as 16 had the ECG pattern of Brugada syndrome. In their review of the literature

in 1999, Alings and Wilde found that of the 163 patients who met the criteria for Brugada syndrome, 58% were of Asian origin.[12]

Relationship with structural heart disease

A subpopulation of arrhythmogenic right ventricular cardiomyopathy (ARVC) patients have been found to display an ST segment elevation and polymorphic VT characteristic of the Brugada syndrome.[26] In addition one case has been reported in which a patient with a Brugada phenotype required heart transplantation due to untreatable arrhythmias[27] and in whom severe fibrosis of the right ventricle was subsequently reported.

These facts notwithstanding, the vast majority of Brugada patients possess a structurally normal heart, consistent with the notion that this is a primary electrical heart disease.[28] It is not unreasonable to speculate that fibrosis and myocarditis, however mild, may occur and may exacerbate or indeed trigger events in patients with the Brugada syndrome, although definitive evidence in support of this hypothesis is lacking. It is noteworthy that recent studies suggest that some *SCN5A* defects may be capable of causing fibrosis in the conduction system and ventricular myocardium.[29]

ARVC and Brugada syndromes are distinct clinical entities both with respect to the clinical presentation and genetic predisposition (Table 1.2).[4] The only gene thus far linked to the Brugada syndrome is *SCN5A*, the gene that encodes for the α subunit of the cardiac sodium channel, whereas ARVC has been linked to ten different chromosomal loci and three putative genes independent to those responsible for the Brugada syndrome.[30] Only the ARVC5 locus has been mapped to a region overlapping with the second locus for Brugada syndrome, but neither gene has been identified as yet.[31,32] In Brugada syndrome, imaging techniques such as echocardiography, angiography, magnetic resonance imaging, and radionuclide scintigraphy show no evidence of overt structural heart disease, whereas ARVC patients characteristically display right ventricular morphological and functional changes (such as global dilatation, bulgings/aneurysms, and wall motion abnormalities). Ventricular arrhythmias in ARVC are most commonly monomorphic VT (LBBB

Table 1.2 Differential diagnosis between ARVC and Brugada syndrome.[123,142–145]

Clinical characteristics	ARVC	Brugada syndrome
Age	25–35	35–40
Sex (male/female)	M > F (3 : 1)	M > F (8 : 1)
Distribution	Worldwide (Italy)	Worldwide (Southeast Asia)
Inheritance	AD (AR)	AD
Chromosomes	1, 2, 3, 6, 10, 14 (17)	3
Gene	hRYR2, plakoglobin, desmoplakin	SCN5A
Symptoms	Palpitations, syncope, cardiac arrest	Syncope, cardiac arrest
Circumstances	Effort	Rest
Imaging	Normal	Morpho-functional RV (and LV) abnormalities
Pathology	Fibrofatty replacement	Normal
ECG repolarization	Inverted T waves in right precordial leads	High take-off ST segment V_1–V_3
ECG depolarization	Epsilon waves, QRS prolongation, late potentials	RBBB/LAD, late potentials
AV conduction	Normal	50% abnormal PR/HV intervals
Atrial arrhythmias	Late (secondary)	Early (primary 10–25%)
ECG changes	Fixed (mostly)	Variable
Ventricular arrhythmias	Monomorphic VT/VF	Polymorphic VT/VF
Mechanism of arrhythmias	Scar-related reentry	Phase 2 reentry
Drug effect class I	↓	↑
Drug effect class II	↓	↑
Drug effect class III	↓	–/↑
Drug effect class IV	–/↓	–
Beta-stimulation	↑	↓
Natural history	Sudden death, heart failure	Sudden death

Arrows denote changes in ST segment elevation (↑, increased; ↓, decreased; –/, small change, if any). Modified from Ref. 4, with permission.

type), often precipitated by catecholamines or exercise, accounting for sudden death of young competitive athletes. In contrast, ST segment elevation and arrhythmias in Brugada patients are enhanced by vagotonic agents or β-adrenergic blockers, and polymorphic VT most commonly occurs during rest or sleep. Unlike Brugada syndrome, the ECG abnormalities in ARVC are not dynamic, displaying a constant T wave inversion, epsilon waves, and, in the progressive stage, reduction of the R amplitude, which are largely unaffected by sodium channel blocker administration.

Electron beam computed tomography has uncovered wall motion abnormalities in a series of Brugada patients tested.[33] Although such contractile abnormalities are commonly considered pathognomonic of structural disease, recent studies[34,35] suggest that such contractile dysfunction can result from loss of the action potential dome in regions of right ventricular epicardium, and thus may be unrelated to any type of morphological defect. Loss of the dome leads to contractile dysfunction because calcium entry into the cells is greatly diminished and sarcoplasmic reticulum calcium stores are depleted. Signal-averaged ECG (SAECG) recordings have demonstrated late potentials in patients with the Brugada syndrome, especially in the anterior wall of the right ventricular outflow tract (RVOT),[36,37] and recordings from the epicardial surface of the anterior wall of the RVOT have revealed delayed potentials.[38] Although these type of potentials are commonly considered to be representative of delayed activation of the myocardium secondary to structural defects, recent studies suggest that in the case of the Brugada syndrome these late and delayed potentials may represent the delayed second upstroke of the epicardial action potential or local phase 2 reentry.[35]

Diagnostic criteria

ST segment elevation is associated with a wide variety of benign as well as malignant pathophysiologic conditions. A differential diagnosis is at times difficult, particularly when the degree of ST segment elevation is relatively small and the specificity of sodium channel blockers such as flecainide, ajmaline, procainamide, disopyramide, propafenone, and pilsicainide[7,14,39] to identify patients at risk is uncertain. The recommended dosage regimens are listed in Table 1.3. The test should monitored with a continuous ECG recording (speed 10 mm/s and interposed 50 mm/s) and should be terminated when (1) the diagnostic Type 1 Brugada ECG develops; (2) ST segment in Type 2 ECG increases by ≥2 mm; (3) premature ventricular beats or other arrhythmias develop; or (4) QRS widens to ≥130% of baseline. These sodium channel blockers should be used with particular caution in the presence of atrial and/or ventricular conduction disease (suspected cases of Lev–Lenègre disease or in the presence of wide QRS, wide P waves, or prolonged PR intervals). Mechanoelectrical dissociation has been encountered in isolated cases. Isoproterenol and sodium lactate may be effective antidotes.

Three types of repolarization patterns have been identified, as discussed above (Table 1.1 and Fig. 1.1). Brugada syndrome is definitively diagnosed when a Type 1 ST segment elevation is observed in more than one right precordial lead (V_1–V_3), in the presence or absence of sodium channel block, and in conjunction with one of the following: documented ventricular fibrillation, self-terminating polymorphic ventricular tachycardia, a family history of SCD (<45 years), coved type ECGs in family members, inducibility of VT with programmed electrical stimulation, syncope, or nocturnal agonal respiration. Importantly, confounding factor(s) that could account for the ECG abnormality should be carefully excluded (see Table 1.4). Striking ST segment elevation is sometimes observed for a brief period following DC cardioversion, although it is not known whether these patients are gene carriers for Brugada syndrome.[40] Another prominent confounding factor is the ST elevation encountered in well trained athletes (Fig. 1.3). Distinguishing features include the fact that in the athlete, the ST segment elevation is up-sloping rather than down-sloping and is largely unaffected by challenge with a sodium channel blocker. In addition, a variety of drugs have been reported to produce a Brugada-like ST

Table 1.4 ECG abnormalities that can lead to ST segment elevation in the right precordial leads.

Atypical right bundle branch block
Left ventricular hypertrophy
Early repolarization
Acute pericarditis
Acute myocardial ischemia or infarction
Pulmonary embolism
Prinzmetal's angina[94]
Dissecting aortic aneurysm[95]
Various central and autonomic nervous system abnormalities[96,97]
Duchenne muscular dystrophy[98]
Thiamine deficiency[99]
Hyperkalemia[95,100,101]
Hypercalcemia[102,103]
Arrhythmogenic right ventricular dysplasia/cardiomyopathy[26,104]
Hypothermia[105,106]
Mechanical compression of right ventricular outflow tract as with mediastinal tumor[107]
Hemopericardium[108]

Table 1.3 Drugs used to unmask the Brugada syndrome.

Drug	Concentration
Ajmaline	1 mg/kg/5 min, i.v.
Flecainide	2 mg/kg/10 min, i.v. (400 mg, p.o.)
Procainamide	10 mg/kg/10 min, i.v.
Pilsicainide	1 mg/kg, i.v./10 min

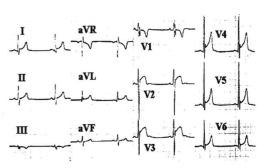

Figure 1.3 Twelve lead ECG of a well-trained athlete without the Brugada syndrome.

segment elevation (Table 1.5), although it is not as yet clear whether or to what extent a genetic predisposition may be involved.

The diagnosis of Brugada syndrome is also considered positive when a Type 2 (saddleback pattern) or Type 3 ST segment elevation is observed in more than one right precordial lead under baseline conditions and conversion to the diagnostic Type 1 pattern occurs after sodium channel blocker administration (ST segment elevation should be ≥2 mm). One or more of the clinical criteria described above should also be present.

Drug-induced conversion of Type 3 to Type 2 ST segment elevation is considered inconclusive for diagnosis of Brugada syndrome.

While most cases of Brugada syndrome display right precordial ST segment elevation, isolated cases of inferior lead[41] or left precordial lead[42] ST segment elevation have been reported in Brugada-like syndromes, in some cases associated with SCN5A mutations.

Risk stratification

Identification of patients at risk for sudden death is an important goal of investigators worldwide.[43,44] Brugada et al.[43] found that patients initially presenting with aborted sudden death are at the highest risk for a recurrence (69%), whereas those presenting with syncope and a spontaneously appearing Brugada ECG sign have a recurrence rate of 19%. An 8% occurrence of cardiac events was observed in initially asymptomatic patients. Among asymptomatic patients, those at highest risk displayed the Brugada sign spontaneously; those in whom ST segment elevation appeared only after provocation with sodium channel blockers appear to be at minimal or no risk for arrhythmic events. Brugada patients at highest risk are: (1) males with (2) inducible VT/VF and (3) a spontaneously elevated ST segment.

Recent studies have suggested that combined electrocardiographic markers may be helpful in risk stratification. Atarashi et al.[45] used the width of the S wave and the ST segment elevation magnitude, whereas Morita et al.[46] combined ST segment elevation and the presence of late potentials.

Brugada et al.[43] recently reported that among asymptomatic patients inducibility of VT during electrophysiologic study (EPS) may forecast risk.

Table 1.5 Drug-induced Brugada-like ECG patterns.

I Antiarrhythmic drugs
1. Na+ channel blockers — Class IC drugs (flecainide,[7,39,109–111] pilsicainide,[112,113] propafenone[114]); Class IA drugs (ajmaline,[7,115] procainamide,[7,8] disopyramide,[4,8] cibenzoline[116])
2. Ca2+ channel blockers — Verapamil
3. β blockers — Propranolol etc.

II Antianginal drugs
1. Ca2+ channel blockers — Nefedipine, diltiazem
2. Nitrate — Isosorbide dinitrate, nitroglycerine[117]
3. K+ channel openers — Nicorandil

III Psychotropic drugs
1. Tricyclic antidepressants — Amitriptyline,[118,119] nortriptyline,[68] desipramine,[66] clomipramine[67]
2. Tetracyclic antidepressants — Maprotiline[118]
3. Phenothiazine — Perphenazine,[118] cyamemazine[120]
4. Selective serotonin reuptake inhibitors — Fluoxetine[119]

IV Other drugs
1. Histaminic H1 receptor antagonists — Dimenhydrinate[121]
2. Cocaine intoxication[70,122]
3. Alcohol intoxication

Studies by Priori *et al.*,[44] Kanda *et al.*,[47] and Eckardt *et al.*,[18] however, failed to find an association between inducibility and recurrence of VT/VF among Brugada patients (both asymptomatic and symptomatic). These discrepancies may be due to differences in patient characteristics and the use of multiple testing centers with non-standardized or non-comparable stimulation protocols.[18] Additional studies are needed to further define risk stratification strategies for asymptomatic patients.

A recent study by Brugada *et al.*[48] reported on 547 individuals diagnosed with the Brugada syndrome and no previous cardiac arrest. In 124 patients the abnormal electrocardiogram was identified after one or multiple episodes of syncope and in 423 individuals during routine electrocardiographic screening or during study because they were family members of patients with the syndrome. Structural disease was ruled out in all patients. This study, evaluating the clinical outcome of the largest population of Brugada patients thus far reported, concluded the following.

1 Patients have a high risk for sudden arrhythmic death, even in the absence of a history of prior cardiac arrest: 8.2% experienced sudden death or at least one documented episode of ventricular fibrillation during a mean follow up of 24 ± 33 months. A spontaneously abnormal Type I ECG carried a 7.7-fold higher risk of developing an arrhythmic event during a lifetime as compared to individuals in whom the electrocardiogram diagnostic of Brugada syndrome was evident only after sodium channel blocker challenge.

2 Male gender is another risk factor for sudden death, because males had a 5.5-fold higher risk of sudden death as compared to females.

3 Programmed electrical stimulation resulting in inducibility of a sustained ventricular arrhythmia is the strongest marker of risk, associated with an 8-fold higher risk of (aborted) sudden death than non-inducible patients.

4 Familial forms of the disease are not associated with a worse prognosis than sporadic cases, because a positive family history of Brugada syndrome did not predict outcome.

They found a 27.2% probability of an event by logistic regression analysis in a patient with a spontaneously abnormal ECG, a previous history of syncope, and inducible sustained ventricular arrhythmias. Thus, inducibility of ventricular arrhythmias and a previous history of syncope are suggested to be markers of a poor prognosis in Brugada syndrome. Symptomatic patients require protective treatment even when they are not inducible. Asymptomatic patients can be reassured if they are non-inducible.

Genetic factors underlying the Brugada syndrome

Inheritance of the Brugada syndrome is via an autosomal dominant mode of transmission. The first and only gene to be linked to the Brugada syndrome is *SCN5A*, the gene encoding for the α subunit of the cardiac sodium channel gene.[49] Figure 1.4 shows a schematic illustration of *SCN5A*, highlighting the various mutations thus far associated with the Brugada syndrome. Mutations in *SCN5A* are also responsible for the LQT3 form of the long QT syndrome and cardiac conduction disease. A number of mutations have been reported to cause overlapping syndromes.

Approximately 60 mutations in *SCN5A* have been linked to the syndrome in recent years (see Refs 44 and 50–52 for references—also see http://pc4.fsm.it:81/cardmoc/SCN5A_bruada_mut.htm). About 24 of the these mutations have been studied in expression systems and shown to result in loss of function due to: (1) failure of the sodium channel to express; (2) a shift in the voltage- and time-dependence of I_{Na} activation, inactivation, or reactivation; (3) entry of the sodium channel into an intermediate state of inactivation from which it recovers more slowly; or (4) accelerated inactivation of the sodium channel (Table 1.6). The premature inactivation of the sodium channel is sometimes observed at physiologic temperatures, but not at room temperature.[53] Because this characteristic of the mutant channel was exaggerated at temperatures above the physiologic range, it was suggested that the syndrome may be unmasked, and that patients with the Brugada syndrome may be at an increased risk during a febrile state.[53] A number of Brugada patients displaying fever-induced polymorphic VT have been identified since the publication of this report (see Ref. 9 for references).

Another locus on chromosome 3, close to but distinct from *SCN5A*, has recently been linked to the syndrome[31] in a large pedigree in which the syndrome is associated with progressive conduction disease, a low sensitivity to procainamide, and a relatively good prognosis.

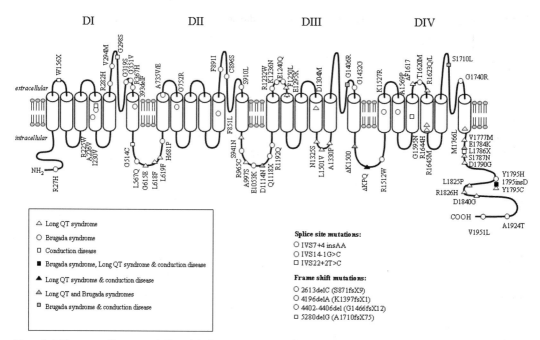

Figure 1.4 Diagrammatic representation of the human cardiac sodium channel, displaying locations of mutations associated with long QT syndrome type 3, Brugada syndrome, isolated cardiac conduction disease, and overlap syndromes. DI, domain I; DII, domain II; DIII, domain III; DIV, domain IV. From Ref. 143, with permission.

SCN5A mutations account for approximately 18–30% of Brugada syndrome cases. A higher incidence of *SCN5A* mutations has been reported in familial than in sporadic cases.[54] Of note, negative *SCN5A* results generally do not rule out causal gene mutations, since in general the promoter region, cryptic splicing mutations, or presence of gross rearrangements are not part of routine investigation.

Based on findings to date, knowledge of a specific mutation may not provide guidance in formulating a diagnosis or determining a prognosis. Mutations have been reported throughout the *SCN5A* gene, and it is not as yet clear which of these if any are associated with a greater risk of arrhythmic events or sudden death. Genetic testing is recommended for support of the clinical diagnosis, for early detection of relatives at potential risk and particularly for the purpose of advancing research and consequently our understanding of genotype–phenotype relations.

Cellular and ionic mechanisms

Phase 2 reentry and other characteristics of strong sodium channel blockade, which give rise to a Bru-gada-like syndrome, were described in the early 1990s and evolved in parallel with the clinical syndrome.[2,55–57] Studies conducted since the mid-1990s suggest that rebalancing of the currents active at the end of phase 1, leading to an accentuation of the action potential notch in right ventricular epicardium, is responsible for the accentuated J wave or ST segment elevation associated with the Brugada syndrome (see Ref. 50 for references). In larger mammals, the presence of a transient outward current (I_{to})-mediated spike and dome morphology, or notch, in ventricular epicardium, but not endocardium, creates a transmural voltage gradient responsible for the inscription of the electrocardiographic J wave (Fig. 1.5A).[58,59] The ST segment is isoelectric due to the absence of transmural voltage gradients at the level of the action potential plateau. Accentuation of the right ventricular action potential notch under pathophysiologic conditions leads to exaggeration of transmural voltage gradients and thus to accentuation of the J wave or to J point elevation. If the epicardial action potential continues to repolarize before that of endocardium, the T wave will remain positive, giving rise to a saddleback

Table 1.6 Biophysical changes of *SCN5A* mutations in Brugada syndrome.

Mutation	Localization	Reference	τfast current decay	Intermediate inact	Persistent current	Current density	V1/2 inact, mV −shift	V1/2 inact, mV +shift	V1/2 act, mV −shift	V1/2 act, mV +shift
G351V	DIS5S6	123	↑	—	—	↓	=		=	
R367H	DIS5S6	23	—	—	—	0	—		—	
L567Q	DIDII	124	↓	—	—	=	−11.3			6.9
H681P	DIIDIII	125	—	—	—	—	−17.3		−9.5	
A735V	DIIS1	23	=	—	—	=	=			6.7
G752R	DIIS2	126	—	—	—	↓		12.0		30
R1192Q	DIIDIII	23	↓	—	—	—		3.9	=	
R1232W	DIIIS1S2	127	—	—	—	=	−5.7		=	
R1232W+	DIIIS1S2+	127	—	—	—	0	—		—	
T1620M+β	DIVS3S4	128	—	—	—	↓		6.3	=	
R1232W+		128	—	—	—	=		6.5	=	
T1620M−β		49	—	—	=	—		8.8	=	
K1397R+1X	DIIIS5S6	49	—	—	—	0	—		—	
G1406R	DIIIS5S6	129	—	—	—	0	—		—	
R1432G	DIIIS5S6	130	—	—	—	0	—		—	
in oocytes		131	—	—	—	=	—		—	
in TSA cells		131	—	—	—	0	—		—	
R1512W	DIIIDIV	130	↑	—	=	=	=		=	
	132	=	—	—	—	−3.8		−5.1		
T1620M	DIVS3S4	127	—	—	—	—	−8.5		−2.5	
	133	=	=	=	—		13.1		6.8	
in oocytes		134	=	—	—	—		10.4	—	
in TSA cells		134	—	—	—	—	=		=	
T1620M at 22°C		53	=	—	—	—	=		=	
T1620M at 32°C		53	↓	—	—	—	=			10.7
T1620M at 22°C		135	=	↑	—	—	—		—	
T1620M at 32°C		135	=	↑	—	—	=		=	
T1620M+β		136	=	—	=	—		10.5	=	
T1620M−β		136	=	—	=	—		4.8	=	
S1710L	DIVS5S6	133	↓	↑	=	—	−21.7			18.7
	137	↓	—	—	—	−24.3			17.7	
1795insD	C terminus	13	=	—	=	↓	−7.3			8.1
	138	=	↑	↑	—	−9.7		=		
	139	—	↑	—	—	—		—		
	140	—	—	↑	↓	−19.2			9.1	
Y1795H	C terminus	141	↓	↑	↑	↓	−10.5		=	
A1924T	C terminus	142	↓	↓	—	—	—		—	
	132	↑	—	—	—	=		−9.0		

τfast current decay: time constant of fast component of sodium current decay (fast inactivation); inact: inactivation; V1/2 inact: voltage at which 50% of sodium channels are inactivated; V1/2 act: voltage at which 50% of sodium channels are activated; ↓: reduction; ↑: increase; +shift: shift to positive voltage; −shift: shift to negative voltage; =: unchanged; -: not reported.

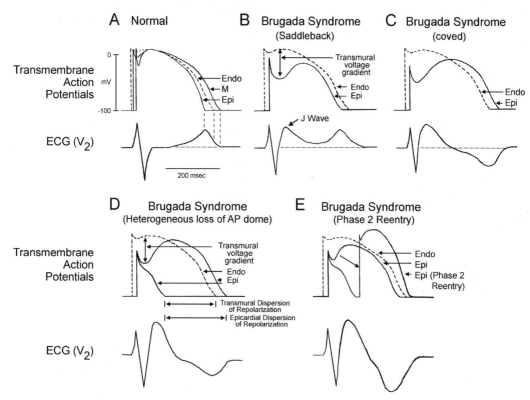

Figure 1.5 Schematic representation of right ventricular epicardial action potential changes proposed to underlie the electrocardiographic manifestation of the Brugada syndrome. Modified from Ref. 59, with permission.

configuration of the ST segment elevation (Fig. 1.5B). Further accentuation of the notch may be accompanied by a prolongation of the epicardial action potential such that the direction of repolarization across the right ventricular wall and transmural voltage gradients are reversed, leading to the development of a coved-type ST segment elevation and inversion of the T wave, typically observed in the ECG of Brugada patients (Fig. 1.5C). A delay in epicardial activation may also contribute to inversion of the T wave. The down-sloping ST segment elevation, or accentuated J wave, observed in the experimental wedge models often appears as an R', suggesting that the appearance of a right bundle branch block (RBBB) morphology in Brugada patients may be due at least in part to early repolarization of right ventricular (RV) epicardium, rather to impulse conduction block in the right bundle. Rigorous application of RBBB criteria reveals that a large majority of RBBB-like morphologies encountered in cases of Brugada syndrome do not fit the cri-

teria for RBBB.[60] Of note, attempts by Miyazaki and coworkers to record delayed activation of the RV in Brugada patients met with failure.[8]

Despite the appearance of a typical Brugada sign, the electrophysiological changes shown in Fig. 1.5C do not give rise to an arrhythmogenic substrate. The arrhythmogenic substrate is thought to develop with a further shift in the balance of current leading to loss of the action potential dome at some epicardial sites but not others (Fig. 1.5D). Loss of the action potential dome in epicardium but not endocardium results in the development of a marked transmural dispersion of repolarization and refractoriness, responsible for the development of a vulnerable window, which can be captured by a premature impulse or extrasystole to trigger a reentrant arrhythmia. Loss of the action potential dome in epicardium is usually heterogeneous, leading to the development of epicardial dispersion of repolarization. Conduction of the action potential dome from sites at which it is maintained to sites at which it is lost causes local re-excitation via phase 2 reentry (Fig. 1.5E), leading to the development of a very closely coupled extrasystole, which captures the vulnerable window across the wall, thus triggering a circus movement reentry in the form of VT/VF.[61,62] The phase 2 reentrant beat fuses with the negative T wave of the basic response. Because the extrasystole originates in epicardium, the QRS complex is largely comprised of a negative Q wave, which sums with the T wave to accentuate the negative deflection of the inverted T wave, giving the ECG a symmetrical appearance, often observed in the clinic preceding the onset of polymorphic VT. Support for these hypotheses derives from experiments involving the arterially perfused right ventricular wedge prepara-

tion[62] and from recent studies in which MAP electrodes where positioned on the epicardial and endocardial surfaces of the RVOT in patients with the Brugada syndrome.[2,63]

The ability of local pressure to give rise to an ST segment elevation has been demonstrated experimentally in the arterially perfused right ventricular wedge preparation.[64] Focal pressure was shown to cause loss of the action potential dome at some right epicardial sites but not others and to give rise to closely coupled phase 2 re-entrant extrasystoles and VT (Fig. 1.6).

An interesting aspect of the Brugada syndrome is that despite equal genetic transmission of the disease, the clinical phenotype is 8 to 10 times more

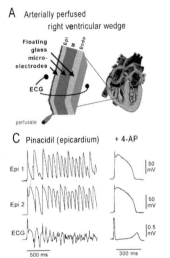
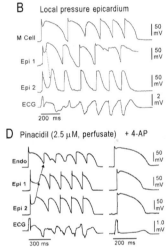
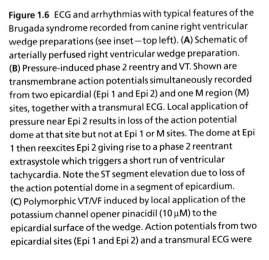

Figure 1.6 ECG and arrhythmias with typical features of the Brugada syndrome recorded from canine right ventricular wedge preparations (see inset—top left). (**A**) Schematic of arterially perfused right ventricular wedge preparation. (**B**) Pressure-induced phase 2 reentry and VT. Shown are transmembrane action potentials simultaneously recorded from two epicardial (Epi 1 and Epi 2) and one M region (M) sites, together with a transmural ECG. Local application of pressure near Epi 2 results in loss of the action potential dome at that site but not at Epi 1 or M sites. The dome at Epi 1 then reexcites Epi 2 giving rise to a phase 2 reentrant extrasystole which triggers a short run of ventricular tachycardia. Note the ST segment elevation due to loss of the action potential dome in a segment of epicardium. (**C**) Polymorphic VT/VF induced by local application of the potassium channel opener pinacidil (10 µM) to the epicardial surface of the wedge. Action potentials from two epicardial sites (Epi 1 and Epi 2) and a transmural ECG were

simultaneously recorded. Loss of the dome at Epi 1 but not Epi 2 creates a marked dispersion of repolarization, giving rise to a phase 2 reentrant extrasystole. The extrasystolic beat then triggers a long episode of ventricular fibrillation (22 s). Right panel: Addition of 4-aminopyridine (4-AP, 2 mM), a specific I_{to} blocker, to the perfusate restored the action potential dome at Epi 1, thus reducing dispersion of repolarization and suppressing all arrhythmic activity. BCL = 2000 ms. (**D**) Phase 2 reentry gives rise to VT following addition of pinacidil (2.5 µM) to the coronary perfusate. Transmembrane action potentials form 2 epicardial sites (Epi 1 and Epi 2) and one endocardial site (Endo) as well as a transmural ECG were simultaneously recorded. Right panel: 4-AP (1 mM) markedly reduces the magnitude of the action potential notch in epicardium, thus restoring the action potential dome throughout the preparation and abolishing all arrhythmic activity. (**D**) is from Ref. 62, with permission.

prevalent in males than in females. The basis for this sex-related distinction was recently shown to be due to a more prominent transient outward current (I_{to})-mediated action potential notch in the right ventricular (RV) epicardium of males versus females.[65] The more prominent I_{to} causes the end of phase 1 of the RV epicardial action potential to repolarize to more negative potentials in tissue and arterially perfused wedge preparations from males, facilitating loss of the action potential dome and the development of phase 2 reentry and polymorphic VT (Figs 1.7 and 1.8).

A rebalancing of currents active at the end of phase 1 underlies the unmasking of the syndrome in response to drugs. Vagotonic agents, I_{K-ATP} activators, and hypokalemia achieve this by augmenting outward currents, whereas sodium channel blockers, β blockers, cocaine, antidepressants, and antihistamines like terfenadine are thought to accomplish this by reducing inward currents.

Figure 1.9 summarizes the proposed cellular mechanism for the Brugada syndrome. The available data support the hypothesis that the Brugada syndrome results from amplification of heterogeneities intrinsic to the early phases of the action potential among the different transmural cell types. The amplification is secondary to a rebalancing of currents active during phase 1, including a decrease in I_{Na} or I_{Ca} or augmentation of any one of a number of outward currents. ST segment elevation similar to that observed in patients with the Brugada syn-

drome occurs as a consequence of the accentuation of the action potential notch, eventually leading to loss of the action potential dome in right ventricular epicardium, where I_{to} is most prominent. Loss of the dome gives rise to both transmural as well as epicardial dispersion of repolarization. The transmural dispersion is responsible for the development of ST segment elevation and the creation of a vulnerable window across the ventricular wall, whereas the epicardial dispersion gives rise to phase 2 reentry which provides the extrasystole that captures the vulnerable window, thus precipitating VT/VF. The VT generated is usually polymorphic, resembling a very rapid form of *torsade de pointes*.

Precipitating and modulating factors

ST segment elevation in the Brugada syndrome can be very dynamic. The Brugada ECG is often concealed, but may be unmasked or modulated by sodium channel blockers, a febrile state, vagotonic agents, α adrenergic agonists, β-adrenergic blockers, tricyclic or tetracyclic antidepressants, first generation antihistaminics (dimenhydrinate), a combination of glucose and insulin, hyperkalemia, hypokalemia, hypercalcemia, and by alcohol and cocaine toxicity (Fig. 1.10).[6–8,66–72] These agents may also induce acquired forms of the Brugada syndrome (Table 1.5). Until a definitive list of drugs to avoid in the Brugada syndrome is formulated, the

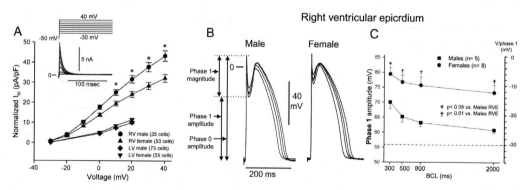

Figure 1.7 Sex-based and interventricular differences in I_{to}. **(A)** Mean I-V relationship for I_{to} recorded from RV epicardial cells isolated from hearts of male and female dogs. Inset, Representative I_{to} current traces and voltage protocol. I_{to} density was significantly greater in male versus female RV epicardial cells. No sex differences were observed in LV.

(B) Transmembrane action potentials recorded from isolated canine RV epicardial male and female tissue slices. BCLs 300, 500, 800, and 2000 ms. **(C)** Rate dependence of phase 1 amplitude and voltage at end of phase 1 (V/phase 1, mV) in males (solid squares) versus females (solid circles). Modified from Ref. 65, with permission.

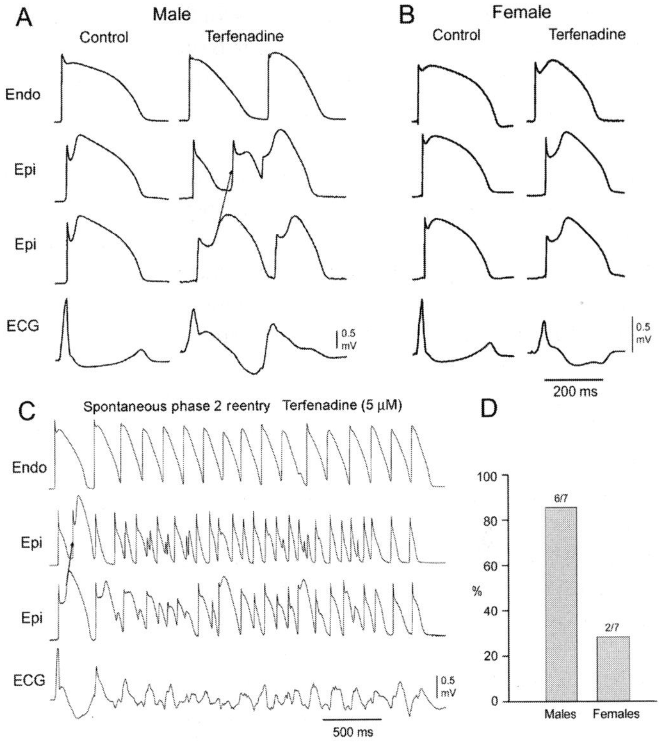

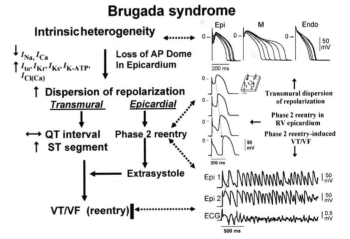

Figure 1.8 Terfenadine induces Brugada phenotype more readily in male than female RV wedge preparations. Each panel shows action potentials recorded from two epicardial sites and one endocardial site, together with a transmural ECG. Control recordings were obtained at a BCL of 2000 ms, whereas terfenadine data were recorded at a BCL of 800 ms after a brief period of pacing at a BCL of 400 ms. **(A)** Terfenadine (5 μM) – induced, heterogeneous loss of action potential dome, ST segment elevation, and phase 2 reentry (arrow) in a male RV wedge preparation. **(B)** Terfenadine fails to induce Brugada phenotype in a female RV wedge preparation. **(C)** Polymorphic VT triggered by spontaneous phase 2 reentry in a male preparation. **(D)** Incidence of phase 2 reentry in male (6 of 7) versus female (2 of 7) RV wedge preparations when perfused with 5 μM terfenadine for up to 2 hours. Modified from Ref. 65, with permission.

Figure 1.9 Proposed mechanism for the Brugada syndrome. A shift in the balance of currents serves to amplify existing heterogeneities by causing loss of the action potential dome at some epicardial sites, but not endocardial sites. A vulnerable window develops as a result of the dispersion of repolarization and refractoriness within epicardium as well as across the wall. Epicardial dispersion leads to the development of phase 2 reentry, which provides the extrasystole that captures the vulnerable window and initiates VT/VF via a circus movement re-entry mechanism. Modified from Ref. 144, with permission.

list of agents in Table 1.5 may provide some guidance.

Acute ischemia or myocardial infarction due to vasospasm involving the RVOT mimics ST segment elevation similar to that in Brugada syndrome. This effect is secondary to the depression of I_{Ca} and the activation of $I_{K\text{-}ATP}$ during ischemia, and suggests that patients with congenital and possibly acquired forms of Brugada syndrome may be at a higher risk for ischemia-related sudden cardiac death.[73]

VF and sudden death in the Brugada syndrome usually occur at rest and at night. Circadian variation of sympatho-vagal balance, hormones, and other metabolic factors are likely to contribute this

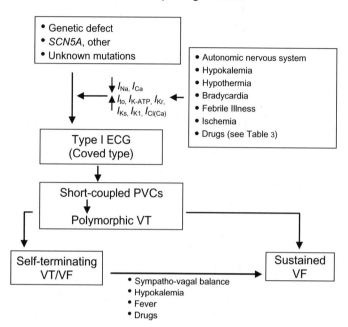

Pathophysiologic Mechanism of Brugada Syndrome: Predisposing Factors

Figure 1.10 Factors predisposing to the electrocardiographic and arrhythmic manifestations of the Brugada syndrome. Modified from Ref. 145, with permission.

circadian pattern. Bradycardia, due to altered sympatho-vagal balance or other factors, may contribute to arrhythmia initiation.[20,21,74] Abnormal ^{123}I-MIBG uptake was found in 8 (17%) of the 17 Brugada syndrome patients but none in the control group demonstrated by Wichter *et al.*[75] There was segmental reduction of ^{123}I-MIBG in the inferior and the septal left ventricular wall indicating presynaptic sympathetic dysfunction. Of note, imaging of the right ventricle, particularly the RVOT, is difficult with this technique, so that insufficient information is available concerning sympathetic function in the regions known to harbor the arrhythmogenic substrate. Moreover, it remains unclear what role the reduced uptake function plays in the arrhythmogenesis of the Brugada syndrome. If the RVOT is similarly affected, this defect may indeed alter the sympatho-vagal balance in favor of the development of an arrhythmogenic substrate.[62,76]

Hypokalemia has been implicated as a contributing cause for the high prevalence of SUDS in the Northeastern region of Thailand, where potassium deficiency is endemic.[72,77] Serum potassium in the Northeastern population is significantly lower than that of the population in Bangkok, which lies in the central part of Thailand where potassium is abundant in the food. A recent case report highlights the ability of hypokalemia to induce VF in a 60-year-old man who had asymptomatic Brugada syndrome, without a family history of sudden cardiac death.[72] This patient was initially treated for asthma by steroids, which lowered serum potassium from 3.8 mmol/L on admission to 3.4 and 2.9 mmol/L on the 7th day and 8th day of admission, respectively. Both were associated with unconsciousness. VF was documented during the last episode, which reverted spontaneously to sinus rhythm.

The Thai Ministry of Public Health Report (1990) found an association between a large meal of glutinous rice ('sticky rice') or carbohydrates ingested on the night of death in SUNDS patients.[77] Consistent with this observation, a recent study by Nogami *et al.* found that glucose and insulin could unmask the Brugada ECG.[71]

Premature inactivation of the sodium channel in *SCN5A* mutations associated with the Brugada syndrome has been shown to be accentuated at higher temperatures[53] suggesting that a febrile state may unmask the Brugada syndrome. Indeed, several case reports have emerged recently demonstrating that febrile illness could reveal the Brugada ECG and precipitate VF.[9,78–82] Anecdotal data point to hot baths as a possible precipitating factor. Of note, the Northeastern part of Thailand, where the Brugada syndrome is most prevalent, is known for its very hot climate. A study is underway to assess whether this extreme climate influences the prognosis of the disease.

Therapy of congenital Brugada syndrome

Despite impressive strides in the identification and characterization of the Brugada syndrome since the mid-1900s, progress relative to therapy has been less noteworthy. The various device and pharmacologic therapies tested clinically or suggested based on experimental evidence are listed in Table 1.7. Currently, an implantable cardioverter defibrillator (ICD) is the only proven effective treatment for the disease.[83,84] In a multicenter trial of 690 patients with Brugada syndrome, in which 258 individuals received an ICD, efficacy of the device in reverting VF and preventing sudden cardiac death was 100%, appropriate shocks were delivered in 14%, 20%, 29%, 38%, and 52% of cases at 1, 2, 3, 4, and 5 years of follow-up, respectively (Fig. 1.11). In the case

of initially asymptomatic patients, appropriate ICD discharge was delivered 4%, 6%, 9%, 17%, and 37% at 1, 2, 3, 4, and 5 years of follow-up, respectively.

Current recommendations for ICD implantation are summarized as follows.

1 Symptomatic patients displaying the Type 1 Brugada ECG (either spontaneously or after sodium channel blockade) who present with aborted sudden death should receive an ICD without additional need for electrophysiologic study (EPS). Similar patients presenting with related symptoms such as syncope, seizure or noctural agonal respiration should also undergo ICD implantation after noncardiac causes of these symptoms have been carefully ruled out. EPS is recommended in symptomatic patients only for the assessment of supraventricular arrhythmia.

2 Asymptomatic patients displaying a Type 1 Brugada ECG (spontaneously or after sodium channel block) should undergo EPS if there is a family history of sudden cardiac death suspected to be due to Brugada syndrome. EPS may be justified when the family history is negative for sudden cardiac death if the Type 1 ECG occurs spontaneously. If inducible for ventricular arrhythmia, the patient should receive an ICD. Asymptomatic patients who have no family history and who develop a Type I ECG only

Table 1.7 Device and pharmacologic considerations for therapy in the Brugada syndrome.

Devices
✓ ICD—only established effective therapy
? Pacemaker
? Ablation or cryosurgery

Pharmacologic
✗ Amiodarone—does not protect[86]
✗ β Blockers—do not protect[86]
✓ β Adrenergic agonists—Isoproterenol[8,10]
✓ Phosphodiesterase inhibitors—cilostazol[93]
✗ Class IC antiarrhythmics—flecainide, propafenone—contraindicated
Class IA antiarrhythmics
✗ Procainamide, disopyramide—contraindicated
✓ Quinidine[62,88,89,92]
? Tedisamil
✓ I_{to} blockers—cardioselective and ion channel specific

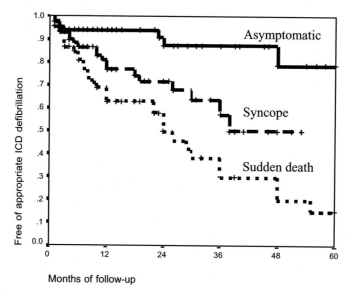

Cumulative ventricular events

	12 months	24 months	36 months	48 months	60 months
Asymptomatic	4%	6%	9%	17%	37%
Syncope	18%	23%	30%	36%	51%
Resuscitated SAD	45%	56%	76%	84%	88%

Figure 1.11 Kaplan–Meier curve of effectiveness of the ICD in 258 patients with electrocardiographic pattern of Brugada syndrome according to symptoms. Modified from Ref. 48, with permission. ICD, implantable cardioverter defibrillator; SAD, sudden arrhythmic death.

after sodium channel blockade should be closely followed-up.

As additional data become available, these recommendations will no doubt require further refinement.

ICD therapy is not an adequate solution for infants and young children or for patients residing in regions of the world where an ICD is unaffordable. Although arrhythmias and sudden cardiac death generally occur during sleep or at rest and have been associated with slow heart rates, a potential therapeutic role for cardiac pacing is largely unexplored. Data relative to a cryosurgical approach or the use of ablation therapy are limited to date. A recent report by Haissaguerre and coworkers[85] indicates that focal radiofrequency ablation may be a potentially valuable tool in controlling arrhythmogenesis by focal ablation of the ventricular premature beats that trigger VT/VF in the Brugada syndrome.

A pharmacologic approach to therapy has been tailored to a rebalancing of currents active during the early phases of the epicardial action potential in the right ventricle so as to reduce the magnitude of the action potential notch and/or restore the action potential dome (Table 1.7). Amiodarone and β blockers have been shown to be ineffective.[86] Class IC antiarrhythmic drugs (such as flecainide and propafenone) and class IA agents (such as procainamide and disopyramide) are contraindicated for reasons previously discussed. Other class IA agents, such as quinidine and tedisamil, however, may exert a therapeutic action because of their I_{to}-blocking properties. Because the presence of a prominent transient outward current, I_{to}, in the right ventricle is at the heart of the mechanism underlying the Brugada syndrome, any agent that inhibits this current may be protective, as a reduced I_{to} protects females from developing the electrocardiographic and arrhythmic manifestations of the Brugada syndrome. Unfortunately, cardioselective

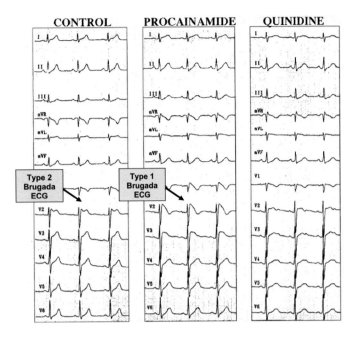

Figure 1.12 Twelve-lead electrocardiogram (ECG) tracings in an asymptomatic 26-year-old man with the Brugada syndrome. Left: Baseline: Type 2 ECG (not diagnostic) displaying a 'saddleback-type' ST segment elevation in V_2. Center: After intravenous administration of 750 mg procainamide, the Type 2 ECG is converted to the diagnostic Type 1 ECG consisting of a 'coved-type' ST segment elevation. Right: A few days after oral administration of quinidine bisulfate (1500 mg/day, serum quinidine level 2.6 mg/L), ST segment elevation is attenuated displaying a nonspecific (neither Type 1–3 Brugada ECG) abnormal pattern in the right precordial leads. VF could be induced during control and procainamide infusion, but not after quinidine. Reproduced from Ref. 88, with permission.

and I_{to}-specific blockers are currently not available. The only agent on the market in the United States with significant I_{to}-blocking properties is quinidine. It is for this reason that it was recommended for treatment of the Brugada syndrome.[62,87] Studies have shown quinidine to be effective in restoring the epicardial action potential dome, thus normalizing the ST segment and preventing phase 2 reentry and polymorphic VT in experimental models of the Brugada syndrome.[62] Clinical evidence of the effectiveness of quinidine in normalizing ST segment elevation in patients with the Brugada syndrome has been reported (Fig. 1.12),[88,89] although clinical trials designed to assess the efficacy of this agent are not available. Agents that boost the L-type calcium current, such as isoproterenol, may be useful as well.[50,62] Both types of agents (I_{to} blocker and agents that augment I_{Ca}) have been shown to be effective in normalizing ST segment elevation in patients with the Brugada syndrome and in controlling 'electrical storms', particularly in children.[10,88–91] A study by Belhassen and coworkers is the only one available demonstrating long-term efficacy of quinidine in the prevention of sudden cardiac death.[88,92]

The phosphodiesterase III inhibitor, cilostazol,[93] is the most recent addition to the pharmacologic armamentarium. Cilostazol normalizes the ST seg-ment most likely by augmenting calcium current (I_{Ca}) as well as by reducing I_{to} secondary to an increase in heart rate. Finally, an experimental antiarrhythmic agent, tedisamil, with potent actions to block I_{to}, among other outward currents, has been suggested as a therapeutic candidate.[50] Tedisamil may be more potent than quinidine because it lacks the relatively strong inward current blocking actions of quinidine. The development of a cardioselective and I_{to}-specific blocker is important for the future to complement the limited therapeutic armamentarium currently available to combat this disease. Appropriate clinical trials are needed to establish the effectiveness of all of the above pharmacologic agents as well as the possible role of pacemakers. Further studies evaluating the effectiveness of ablation and/or cryosurgical approaches to therapy are needed as well.

Supported by grants HL47678 and HL066169 from NHLBI, American Heart Association, and NYS and Florida Grand Lodges.

References

1 Brugada P, Brugada J. Right bundle branch block, persistent ST segment elevation and sudden cardiac death: a distinct clinical and electrocardiographic

syndrome: a multicenter report. *J. Am. Coll. Cardiol.* 1992; **20**: 1391–1396.

2 Antzelevitch C, Brugada P, Brugada J *et al.* Brugada syndrome: a decade of progress. *Circ. Res.* 2002; **91**: 1114–1118.

3 Wilde AA, Antzelevitch C, Borggrefe M *et al.* Proposed diagnostic criteria for the Brugada syndrome. *Eur. Heart J.* 2002; **23**: 1648–1654.

4 Wilde AA, Antzelevitch C, Borggrefe M *et al.* Proposed diagnostic criteria for the Brugada syndrome: consensus report. *Circulation* 2002; **106**: 2514–2519.

5 Brugada P, Brugada R, Antzelevitch C *et al.* The Brugada syndrome, in Gussak I, Antzelevitch C, eds.: *Cardiac Repolarization. Bridging Basic and Clinical Sciences.* Totowa, NJ, Humana Press, 2003: 427–446.

6 Brugada P, Brugada J, Brugada R. Arrhythmia induction by antiarrhythmic drugs. *Pacing Clin. Electrophysiol.* 2000; **23**: 291–292.

7 Brugada R, Brugada J, Antzelevitch C *et al.* Sodium channel blockers identify risk for sudden death in patients with ST-segment elevation and right bundle branch block but structurally normal hearts. *Circulation* 2000; **101**: 510–115.

8 Miyazaki T, Mitamura H, Miyoshi S *et al.* Autonomic and antiarrhythmic drug modulation of ST segment elevation in patients with Brugada syndrome. *J. Am. Coll. Cardiol.* 1996; **27**: 1061–1070.

9 Antzelevitch C, Brugada R. Fever and the Brugada syndrome. *Pacing Clin. Electrophysiol.* 2002; **25**: 1637–1639.

10 Shimizu W, Matsuo K, Takagi M *et al.* Body surface distribution and response to drugs of ST segment elevation in Brugada syndrome: clinical implication of eighty-seven-lead body surface potential mapping and its application to twelve-lead electrocardiograms. *J. Cardiovasc. Electrophysiol.* 2000; **11**: 396–404.

11 Sangwatanaroj S, Prechawat S, Sunsaneewitayakul B *et al.* New electrocardiographic leads and the procainamide test for the detection of the Brugada sign in sudden unexplained death syndrome survivors and their relatives. *Eur. Heart J.* 2001; **22**: 2290–2296.

12 Alings M, Wilde A. 'Brugada' syndrome: clinical data and suggested pathophysiological mechanism [see comments]. *Circulation* 1999; **99**: 666–673.

13 Bezzina C, Veldkamp MW, van Den Berg MP *et al.* A single Na(+) channel mutation causing both long-QT and Brugada syndromes. *Circ. Res.* 1999; **85**: 1206–1213.

14 Priori SG, Napolitano C, Gasparini M *et al.* Clinical and genetic heterogeneity of right bundle branch block and ST-segment elevation syndrome: a prospective evaluation of 52 families [In Process Citation]. *Circulation* 2000; **102**: 2509–2515.

15 Pitzalis MV, Anaclerio M, Iacoviello M *et al.* QT-interval prolongation in right precordial leads: an additional electrocardiographic hallmark of Brugada syndrome. *J. Am. Coll. Cardiol.* 2003; **42**: 1632–1637.

16 Smits JP, Eckardt L, Probst V *et al.* Genotype–phenotype relationship in Brugada syndrome: electrocardiographic features differentiate *SCN5A*-related patients from non-*SCN5A*-related patients. *J. Am. Coll. Cardiol.* 2002; **40**: 350–356.

17 Morita H, Kusano-Fukushima K, Nagase S *et al.* Atrial fibrillation and atrial vulnerability in patients with Brugada syndrome. *J. Am. Coll. Cardiol.* 2002; **40**: 1437.

18 Eckardt L, Kirchhof P, Johna R *et al.* Wolff–Parkinson–White syndrome associated with Brugada syndrome. *Pacing Clin. Electrophysiol.* 2001; **24**: 1423–1424.

19 Takehara N, Makita N, Kawabe J *et al.* A cardiac sodium channel mutation identified in Brugada syndrome associated with atrial standstill. *J Intern. Med* 2004; **255**: 137–142.

20 Kasanuki H, Ohnishi S, Ohtuka M *et al.* Idiopathic ventricular fibrillation induced with vagal activity in patients without obvious heart disease. *Circulation* 1997; **95**: 2277–2285.

21 Proclemer A, Facchin D, Feruglio GA *et al.* Recurrent ventricular fibrillation, right bundle-branch block and persistent ST segment elevation in V1-V3: a new arrhythmia syndrome? A clinical case report (see comments). *G. Ital. Cardiol.* 1993; **23**: 1211–1218.

22 Bjerregaard P, Gussak I, Kotar Sl *et al.* Recurrent syncope in a patient with prominent J-wave. *Am. Heart J.* 1994; **127**: 1426–1430.

23 Vatta M, Dumaine R, Varghese G *et al.* Genetic and biophysical basis of sudden unexplained nocturnal death syndrome (SUNDS), a disease allelic to Brugada syndrome. *Hum. Mol. Genet.* 2002; **11**: 337–345.

24 Sugai MA. Pathological study on sudden and unexpected death, especially on the cardiac death autopsied by medical examiners in Tokyo. *Acta Pathol. Jpn* 1959; **9** (suppl): 723–752.

25 Nademanee K, Veerakul G, Nimmannit S *et al.* Arrhythmogenic marker for the sudden unexplained death syndrome in Thai men. *Circulation* 1997; **96**: 2595–2600.

26 Corrado D, Basso C, Buja G *et al.* Right bundle branch block, right precordial ST-segment elevation, and sudden death in young people. *Circulation* 2001; **103**: 710–717.

27 Ayerza MR, de Zutter M, Goethals M *et al.* Heart transplantation as last resort against Brugada syndrome. *J. Cardiovasc. Electrophysiol.* 2002; **13**: 943–944.

28 Remme CA, Wever EFD, Wilde AAM *et al.* Diagnosis and long-term follow-up of Brugada syndrome in patients with idiopathic ventricular fibrillation. *Eur. Heart J.* 2001; **22**: 400–409.

29 Bezzina CR, Rook MB, Groenewegen WA *et al.* Compound heterozygosity for mutations (W156X and

R225W) in *SCN5A* associated with severe cardiac conduction disturbances and degenerative changes in the conduction system. *Circ. Res.* 2003; **92**: 159–168.

30 Antzelevitch C. Molecular genetics of arrhythmias and cardiovascular conditions associated with arrhythmias. Invited Review – NASPE 25th Anniversary. *J. Cardiovasc. Electrophysiol.* 2003; **14**: 1259–1272.

31 Weiss R, Barmada MM, Nguyen T *et al.* Clinical and molecular heterogeneity in the Brugada syndrome. A novel gene locus on chromosome 3. *Circulation* 2002; **105**: 707–713.

32 Ahmed F, Li D, Karibe A *et al.* Localization of a gene responsible for arrhythmogenic right ventricular dysplasia to chromosome 3p23. *Circulation* 1998; **98**: 2791–2795.

33 Takagi M, Aihara N, Kuribayashi S *et al.* Localized right ventricular morphological abnormalities detected by electron-beam computed tomography represent arrhythmogenic substrates in patients with the Brugada syndrome. *Eur. Heart J.* 2001; **22**: 1032–1041.

34 Antzelevitch C. Brugada syndrome: historical perspectives and observations. *Eur. Heart J.* 2002; **23**: 676–678.

35 Antzelevitch C. Late potentials and the Brugada syndrome. *J. Am. Coll. Cardiol.* 2002; **39**: 1996–1999.

36 Futterman LG, Lemberg L. Brugada. *Am. J. Crit. Care* 2001; **10**: 360–364.

37 Fujiki A, Usui M, Nagasawa H *et al.* ST segment elevation in the right precordial leads induced with class IC antiarrhythmic drugs: insight into the mechanism of Brugada syndrome [see comments]. *J. Cardiovasc. Electrophysiol.* 1999; **10**: 214–218.

38 Nagase S, Kusano KF, Morita H *et al.* Epicardial electrogram at the right ventricular outflow tract in patients with Brugada syndrome – using epicardial lead. *J. Am. Coll. Cardiol.* 2002; **39**: 1992–1995.

39 Shimizu W, Antzelevitch C, Suyama K *et al.* Effect of sodium channel blockers on ST segment, QRS duration, and corrected QT interval in patients with Brugada syndrome. *J. Cardiovasc. Electrophysiol.* 2000; **11**: 1320–1329.

40 Gurevitz O, Glikson M. Cardiac resynchronization therapy: a new frontier in the management of heart failure. *Isr. Med. Assoc. J.* 2003; **5**: 571–575.

41 Kalla H, Yan GX, Marinchak R. Ventricular fibrillation in a patient with prominent J (Osborn) waves and ST segment elevation in the inferior electrocardiographic leads: a Brugada syndrome variant? *J. Cardiovasc. Electrophysiol.* 2000; **11**: 95–98.

42 Horigome H, Shigeta O, Kuga K *et al.* Ventricular fibrillation during anesthesia in association with J waves in the left precordial leads in a child with coarctation of the aorta. *J. Electrocardiol.* 2003; **36**: 339–343.

43 Brugada J, Brugada R, Antzelevitch C *et al.* Long-term follow-up of individuals with the electrocardiographic pattern of right bundle-branch block and ST-segment elevation in precordial leads V(1) to V(3). *Circulation* 2002; **105**: 73–78.

44 Priori SG, Napolitano C, Gasparini M *et al.* Natural history of Brugada syndrome: insights for risk stratification and management. *Circulation* 2002; **105**: 1342–1347.

45 Atarashi H, Ogawa S, For the idiopathic ventricular fibrillation investigators: new ECG criteria for high-risk Brugada syndrome. *Circ. J.* 2003; **67**: 8–10.

46 Morita H, Takenaka-Morita S, Fukushima-Kusano K *et al.* Risk stratification for asymptomatic patients with Brugada syndrome. *Circ. J.* 2003; **67**: 312–316.

47 Kanda M, Shimizu W, Matsuo K *et al.* Electrophysiologic characteristics and implications of induced ventricular fibrillation in symptomatic patients with Brugada syndrome. *J. Am. Coll. Cardiol.* 2002; **39**: 1799–1805.

48 Brugada J, Brugada R, Brugada P. Determinants of sudden cardiac death in individuals with the electrocardiographic pattern of Brugada syndrome and no previous cardiac arrest. *Circulation* 2003; **108**: 3092–3096.

49 Chen Q, Kirsch GE, Zhang D *et al.* Genetic basis and molecular mechanisms for idiopathic ventricular fibrillation. *Nature* 1998; **392**: 293–296.

50 Antzelevitch C. The Brugada syndrome: ionic basis and arrhythmia mechanisms. *J. Cardiovasc. Electrophysiol.* 2001; **12**: 268–272.

51 Balser JR. The cardiac sodium channel: gating function and molecular pharmacology. *J. Mol. Cell. Cardiol.* 2001; **33**: 599–613.

52 Tan HL, Bezzina CR, Smits JP *et al.* Genetic control of sodium channel function. *Cardiovasc. Res.* 2003; **57**: 961–973.

53 Dumaine R, Towbin JA, Brugada P *et al.* Ionic mechanisms responsible for the electrocardiographic phenotype of the Brugada syndrome are temperature dependent. *Circ. Res.* 1999; **85**: 803–809.

54 Schulze-Bahr E, Eckardt L, Breithardt G *et al.* Sodium channel gene (*SCN5A*) mutations in 44 index patients with Brugada syndrome: different incidences in familial and sporadic disease. *Human Mut. online.* 2003.

55 Antzelevitch C, Sicouri S, Litovsky SH *et al.* Heterogeneity within the ventricular wall: electrophysiology and pharmacology of epicardial, endocardial and M cells. *Circ. Res.* 1991; **69**: 1427–1449.

56 Krishnan SC, Antzelevitch C. Sodium channel blockade produces opposite electrophysiologic effects in canine ventricular epicardium and endocardium. *Circ. Res.* 1991; **69**: 277–291.

57 Krishnan SC, Antzelevitch C. Flecainide-induced arrhythmia in canine ventricular epicardium: Phase 2 Reentry? *Circulation* 1993; **87**: 562–572.

58 Yan GX, Antzelevitch C. Cellular basis for the electrocardiographic J wave. *Circulation* 1996; **93**: 372–379.

59 Antzelevitch C. The Brugada syndrome: ionic basis and arrhythmia mechanisms. *J. Cardiovasc. Electrophysiol.* 2001; **12**: 268–272.

60 Gussak I, Antzelevitch C, Bjerregaard P et al. The Brugada syndrome: clinical, electrophysiological and genetic aspects. *J. Am. Coll. Cardiol.* 1999; **33**: 5–15.

61 Lukas A, Antzelevitch C. Phase 2 reentry as a mechanism of initiation of circus movement reentry in canine epicardium exposed to simulated ischemia. The antiarrhythmic effects of 4-aminopyridine. *Cardiovasc. Res.* 1996; **32**: 593–603.

62 Yan GX, Antzelevitch C. Cellular basis for the Brugada syndrome and other mechanisms of arrhythmogenesis associated with ST segment elevation. *Circulation* 1999; **100**: 1660–1666.

63 Kurita T, Shimizu W, Inagaki M et al. The electrophysiologic mechanism of ST-segment elevation in Brugada syndrome. *J. Am. Coll. Cardiol.* 2002; **40**: 330–334.

64 Antzelevitch C, Dumaine R. Electrical heterogeneity in the heart: physiological, pharmacological and clinical implications. In Page E, Fozzard HA, Solaro RJ, eds. *Handbook of Physiology. The Heart.* New York: Oxford University Press, 2001: 654–692.

65 Di Diego JM, Cordeiro JM, Goodrow RJ et al. Ionic and cellular basis for the predominance of the Brugada syndrome phenotype in males. *Circulation* 2002; **106**: 2004–2011.

66 Babaliaros VC, Hurst JW. Tricyclic antidepressants and the Brugada syndrome: an example of Brugada waves appearing after the administration of desipramine. *Clin. Cardiol.* 2002; **25**: 395–398.

67 Goldgran-Toledano D, Sideris G, Kevorkian JP. Overdose of cyclic antidepressants and the Brugada syndrome. *N. Engl. J. Med.* 2002; **346**: 1591–1592.

68 Tada H, Sticherling C, Oral H et al. Brugada syndrome mimicked by tricyclic antidepressant overdose. *J. Cardiovasc. Electrophysiol.* 2001; **12**: 275.

69 Pastor A, Nunez A, Cantale C et al. Asymptomatic Brugada syndrome case unmasked during dimenhydrinate infusion. *J. Cardiovasc. Electrophysiol.* 2001; **12**: 1192–1194.

70 Ortega-Carnicer J, Bertos-Polo J, Gutierrez-Tirado C. Aborted sudden death, transient Brugada pattern, and wide QRS dysrrhythmias after massive cocaine ingestion. *J. Electrocardiol.* 2001; **34**: 345–349.

71 Nogami A, Nakao M, Kubota S et al. Enhancement of J-ST-segment elevation by the glucose and insulin test in Brugada syndrome. *Pacing Clin. Electrophysiol.* 2003; **26**: 332–337.

72 Araki T, Konno T, Itoh H et al. Brugada syndrome with ventricular tachycardia and fibrillation related to hypokalemia. *Circ. J.* 2003; **67**: 93–95.

73 Noda T, Shimizu W, Taguchi A et al. ST-segment elevation and ventricular fibrillation without coronary spasm by intracoronary injection of acetylcholine and/or ergonovine maleate in patients with Brugada syndrome. *J. Am. Coll. Cardiol.* 2002; **40**: 1841–1847.

74 Mizumaki K, Fujiki A, Tsuneda T et al. Vagal activity modulates spontaneous augmentation of ST elevation in daily life of patients with Brugada syndrome. *J. Cardiovasc. Electrophysiol.* 2004; **15**: 667–673.

75 Wichter T, Matheja P, Eckardt L et al. Cardiac autonomic dysfunction in Brugada syndrome. *Circulation* 2002; **105**: 702–706.

76 Litovsky SH, Antzelevitch C. Differences in the electrophysiological response of canine ventricular subendocardium and subepicardium to acetylcholine and isoproterenol. A direct effect of acetylcholine in ventricular myocardium. *Circ. Res.* 1990; **67**: 615–627.

77 Nimmannit S, Malasit P, Chaovakul V et al. Pathogenesis of sudden unexplained nocturnal death (lai tai) and endemic distal renal tubular acidosis. *Lancet* 1991; **338**: 930–932.

78 Gonzalez Rebollo G, Madrid H, Carcia A et al. Reccurrent ventricular fibrillation during a febrile illness in a patient with the Brugada syndrome. *Rev. Esp. Cardiol.* 2000; **53**: 755–757.

79 Madle A, Kratochvil Z, Polivkova A. [The Brugada syndrome]. *Vnitr. Lek.* 2002; **48**: 255–258.

80 Saura D, Garcia-Alberola A, Carrillo P et al. Brugada-like electrocardiographic pattern induced by fever. *Pacing Clin. Electrophysiol.* 2002; **25**: 856–859.

81 Porres JM, Brugada J, Urbistondo V et al. Fever unmasking the Brugada syndrome. *Pacing Clin. Electrophysiol.* 2002; **25**: 1646–1648.

82 Kum L, Fung JWH, Chan WWL et al. Brugada syndrome unmasked by febrile illness. *Pacing Clin. Electrophysiol.* 2002; **25**: 1660–1661.

83 Brugada J, Brugada R, Brugada P. Pharmacological and device approach to therapy of inherited cardiac diseases associated with cardiac arrhythmias and sudden death. *J. Electrocardiol.* 2000; **33** Suppl: 41–47.

84 Brugada P, Brugada R, Brugada J et al. Use of the prophylactic implantable cardioverter defibrillator for patients with normal hearts. *Am. J. Cardiol.* 1999; **83**: 98D–100D.

85 Haissaguerre M, Extramiana F, Hocini M et al. Mapping and ablation of ventricular fibrillation associated with long-QT and Brugada syndromes. *Circulation* 2003; **108**: 925–928.

86 Brugada J, Brugada R, Brugada P. Right bundle-branch block and ST-segment elevation in leads V_1 through V_3. A marker for sudden death in patients without demonstrable structural heart disease. *Circulation* 1998; **97**: 457–460.

87 Antzelevitch C, Brugada P, Brugada J et al. The Brugada Syndrome. Armonk, NY: Futura Publishing Company, Inc., 1999: 1–99.

88 Belhassen B, Viskin S, Antzelevitch C. The Brugada syndrome: is ICD the only therapeutic option? Pacing Clin. Electrophysiol. 2002; 25: 1634–1640.

89 Alings M, Dekker L, Sadee A et al. Quinidine induced electrocardiographic normalization in two patients with Brugada syndrome. Pacing Clin. Electrophysiol. 2001; 24: 1420–1422.

90 Suzuki H, Torigoe K, Numata O et al. Infant case with a malignant form of Brugada syndrome. J. Cardiovasc. Electrophysiol. 2000; 11: 1277–1280.

91 Tanaka H, Kinoshita O, Uchikawa S et al. Successful prevention of recurrent ventricular fibrillation by intravenous isoproterenol in a patient with Brugada syndrome. Pacing Clin. Electrophysiol. 2001; 24: 1293–1294.

92 Belhassen B, Viskin S, Fish R et al. Effects of electrophysiologic-guided therapy with Class IA antiarrhythmic drugs on the long-term outcome of patients with idiopathic ventricular fibrillation with or without the Brugada syndrome [see comments]. J. Cardiovasc. Electrophysiol. 1999; 10: 1301–1312.

93 Tsuchiya T, Ashikaga K, Honda T et al. Prevention of ventricular fibrillation by cilostazol, an oral phosphodiesterase inhibitor, in a patient with Brugada syndrome. J. Cardiovasc. Electrophysiol. 2002; 13: 698–701.

94 Wang K, Asinger RW, Marriott HJ. ST-segment elevation in conditions other than acute myocardial infarction. N. Engl. J. Med. 2003; 349: 2128–2135.

95 Myers GB. Other QRS-T patterns that may be mistaken for myocardial infarction. IV. Alterations in blood potassium; myocardial ischemia; subepicardial myocarditis; distortion associated with arrhythmias. Circulation 1950; 2: 75–93.

96 Abbott JA, Cheitlin MD. The nonspecific camel-hump sign. JAMA 1976; 235: 413–414.

97 Hersch C. Electrocardiographic changes in head injuries. Circulation 1961; 23: 853–860.

98 Perloff JK, Henze E, Schelbert HR. Alterations in regional myocardial metabolism, perfusion, and wall motion in Duchenne muscular dystrophy studied by radionuclide imaging. Circulation 1984; 69: 33–42.

99 Read DH, Harrington DD. Experimentally induced thiamine deficiency in beagle dogs: clinical observations. Am. J. Vet. Res. 1981; 42: 984–991.

100 Merrill JP, Levine HD, Somerville W et al. Clinical recognition and treatment of acute potassium intoxication. Ann. Intern. Med. 1950; 33: 797–830.

101 Ortega-Carnicer J, Benezet J, Ruiz-Lorenzo F et al. Transient Brugada-type electrocardiographic abnormalities in renal failure reversed by dialysis. Resuscitation 2002; 55: 215–219.

102 Douglas PS, Carmichael KA, Palevsky PM. Extreme hypercalcemia and electrocardiographic changes. Am. J. Cardiol. 1984; 54: 674–675.

103 Sridharan MR, Horan LG. Electrocardiographic J wave of hypercalcemia. Am. J. Cardiol. 1984; 54: 672–673.

104 Corrado D, Nava A, Buja G et al. Familial cardiomyopathy underlies syndrome of right bundle branch block, ST segment elevation and sudden death [see comments]. J. Am. Coll. Cardiol. 1996; 27: 443–448.

105 Osborn JJ. Experimental hypothermia: respiratory and blood pH changes in relation to cardiac function. Am. J. Physiol. 1953; 175: 389–398.

106 Noda T, Shimizu W, Tanaka K et al. Prominent J wave and ST segment elevation: serial electrocardiographic changes in accidental hypothermia. J. Cardiovasc. Electrophysiol. 2003; 14: 223.

107 Tarin N, Farre J, Rubio JM et al. Brugada-like electrocardiographic pattern in a patient with a mediastinal tumor. Pacing Clin. Electrophysiol. 1999; 22: 1264–1266.

108 Tomcsanyi J, Simor T, Papp L. Images in cardiology. Haemopericardium and Brugada-like ECG pattern in rheumatoid arthritis. Heart 2002; 87: 234.

109 Krishnan SC, Josephson ME. ST segment elevation induced by class IC antiarrhythmic agents: underlying electrophysiologic mechanisms and insights into drug-induced proarrhythmia. J. Cardiovasc. Electrophysiol. 1998; 9: 1167–1172.

110 Fujiki A, Usui M, Nagasawa H et al. ST segment elevation in the right precordial leads induced with class IC antiarrhythmic drugs: insight into the mechanism of Brugada syndrome [see comments]. J. Cardiovasc. Electrophysiol. 1999; 10: 214–218.

111 Gasparini M, Priori SG, Mantica M et al. Flecainide test in Brugada syndrome: a reproducible but risky tool. Pacing Clin. Electrophysiol. 2003; 26: 338–341.

112 Takenaka S, Emori T, Koyama S et al. Asymptomatic form of Brugada syndrome. Pacing Clin. Electrophysiol. 1999; 22: 1261–1263.

113 Shimizu W, Aiba T, Kurita T et al. Paradoxic abbreviation of repolarization in epicardium of the right ventricular outflow tract during augmentation of Brugada-type ST segment elevation. J. Cardiovasc. Electrophysiol. 2001; 12: 1418–1421.

114 Matana A, Goldner V, Stanic K et al. Unmasking effect of propafenone on the concealed form of the Brugada phenomenon. Pacing Clin. Electrophysiol. 2000; 23: 416–418.

115 Rolf S, Bruns HJ, Wichter T et al. The ajmaline challenge in Brugada syndrome: diagnostic impact, safety, and recommended protocol. Eur. Heart J. 2003; 24: 1104–1112.

116 Tada H, Nogami A, Shimizu W et al. ST segment and T wave alternans in a patient with Brugada syndrome. Pacing Clin. Electrophysiol. 2000; 23: 413–415.

117 Matsuo K, Shimizu W, Kurita T *et al.* Dynamic changes of 12-lead electrocardiograms in a patient with Brugada syndrome. *J. Cardiovasc. Electrophysiol.* 1998; **9**: 508–512.

118 Bolognesi R, Tsialtas D, Vasini P *et al.* Abnormal ventricular repolarization mimicking myocardial infarction after heterocyclic antidepressant overdose. *Am. J. Cardiol.* 1997; **79**: 242–245.

119 Rouleau F, Asfar P, Boulet S *et al.* Transient ST segment elevation in right precordial leads induced by psychotropic drugs: relationship to the Brugada syndrome. *J. Cardiovasc. Electrophysiol.* 2001; **12**: 61–65.

120 Antzelevitch C. The Brugada syndrome. *J. Cardiovasc. Electrophysiol.* 1998; **9**: 513–516.

121 Pastor A, Nunez A, Cantale C *et al.* Asymptomatic Brugada syndrome case unmasked during dimenhydrinate infusion. *J. Cardiovasc. Electrophysiol.* 2001; **12**: 1192–1194.

122 Littmann L, Monroe MH, Svenson RH. Brugada-type electrocardiographic pattern induced by cocaine. *Mayo Clin. Proc.* 2000; **75**: 845–849.

123 Vatta M, Dumaine R, Antzelevitch C *et al.* Novel mutations in domain I of *SCN5A* cause Brugada syndrome. *Mol. Genet. Metab.* 2002; **75**: 317–324.

124 Wan X, Chen S, Sadeghpour A *et al.* Accelerated inactivation in a mutant Na(+) channel associated with idiopathic ventricular fibrillation. *Am. J. Physiol. Heart Circ. Physiol.* 2001; **280**: H354–H360.

125 Mok NS, Priori SG, Napolitano C *et al.* A newly characterized *SCN5A* mutation underlying Brugada syndrome unmasked by hyperthermia. *J Cardiovasc. Electrophysiol.* 2003; **14**: 407–411

126 Potet F, Mabo P, Le Coq G *et al.* Novel brugada *SCN5A* mutation leading to ST segment elevation in the inferior or the right precordial leads. *J. Cardiovasc. Electrophysiol.* 2003; **14**: 200–203.

127 Baroudi G, Acharfi S, Larouche C *et al.* Expression and intracellular localization of an *SCN5A* double mutant R1232W/T1620M implicated in Brugada syndrome. *Circ. Res.* 2002; **90**: E11–E16.

128 Wan X, Wang Q, Kirsch GE. Functional suppression of sodium channels by beta(1)-subunits as a molecular mechanism of idiopathic ventricular fibrillation [In Process Citation]. *J. Mol. Cell. Cardiol.* 2000; **32**: 1873–1884.

129 Kyndt F, Probst V, Potet F *et al.* Novel *SCN5A* mutation leading either to isolated cardiac conduction defect or Brugada syndrome in a large French family. *Circulation* 2001; **104**: 3081–3086.

130 Deschenes I, Baroudi G, Berthet M *et al.* Electrophysiological characterization of *SCN5A* mutations causing long QT (E1784K) and Brugada (R1512W and R1432G) syndromes. *Cardiovasc. Res.* 2000; **46**: 55–65.

131 Baroudi G, Pouliot V, Denjoy I *et al.* Novel mechanism for Brugada syndrome: defective surface localization of an *SCN5A* mutant (R1432G). *Circ. Res.* 2001; **88**: E78–E83.

132 Rook MB, Alshinawi CB, Groenewegen WA *et al.* Human *SCN5A* gene mutations alter cardiac sodium channel kinetics and are associated with the Brugada syndrome. *Cardiovasc. Res.* 1999; **44**: 507–517.

133 Shirai N, Makita N, Sasaki K *et al.* A mutant cardiac sodium channel with multiple biophysical defects associated with overlapping clinical features of Brugada syndrome and cardiac conduction disease. *Cardiovasc. Res.* 2002; **53**: 348–354.

134 Baroudi G, Carbonneau E, Pouliot V *et al. SCN5A* mutation (T1620M) causing Brugada syndrome exhibits different phenotypes when expressed in *Xenopus* oocytes and mammalian cells. *FEBS Lett.* 2000; **467**: 12–16.

135 Wang DW, Makita N, Kitabatake A *et al.* Enhanced Na(+) channel intermediate inactivation in Brugada syndrome. *Circ. Res.* 2000; **87**: E37–E43.

136 Kiehn J, Karle C, Thomas D *et al.* HERG potassium channel activation is shifted by phorbol esters via protein kinase A-dependent pathways. *J Biol. Chem.* 1998; **273**: 25 285–25 291.

137 Akai J, Makita N, Sakurada H *et al.* A novel *SCN5A* mutation associated with idiopathic ventricular fibrillation without typical ECG findings of Brugada syndrome. *FEBS Lett.* 2000; **479**: 29–34.

138 Veldkamp MW, Viswanathan PC, Bezzina C *et al.* Two distinct congenital arrhythmias evoked by a multidysfunctional Na(+) channel. *Circ. Res.* 2000; **86**: E91–E97.

139 Viswanathan PC, Bezzina CR, George AL, Jr. *et al.* Gating-dependent mechanisms for flecainide action in *SCN5A*-linked arrhythmia syndromes. *Circulation* 2001; **104**: 1200–1205.

140 Baroudi G, Chahine M. Biophysical phenotypes of *SCN5A* mutations causing long QT and Brugada syndromes. *FEBS Lett.* 2000; **487**: 224–228.

141 Rivolta I, Abriel H, Tateyama M *et al.* Inherited Brugada and LQT-3 syndrome mutations of a single residue of the cardiac sodium channel confer distinct channel and clinical phenotypes. *J. Biol. Chem.* 2001; **276**: 30 623–30 630.

142 Tan HL, Kupershmidt S, Zhang R *et al.* A calcium sensor in the sodium channel modulates cardiac excitability. *Nature* 2002; **415**: 442–447.

143 Tan HL. Biophysical analysis of mutant sodium channels in Brugada syndrome. In: Antzelevitch C, Brugada P, eds. *The Brugada Syndrome.* Elmsford: Blackwell Publishing, 2004.

144 Antzelevitch C. The Brugada syndrome. Diagnostic criteria and cellular mechanisms. *Eur. Heart J.* 2001; **22**: 356–363.

145 Nademanee K, Veerakul G, Schwab M. Predisposing factors in the Brugada syndrome. In: Antzelevitch C, Brugada P, eds. *The Brugada Syndrome.* Elmsford, Blackwell Publishing, 2004.

CHAPTER 2

History of the Brugada syndrome

I. Gussak, MD, PhD, *P. Bjerregaard,* MD

Introduction

Death is the inevitable consequence of life, and the postponement of death until it occurs naturally at an advanced age after a life of vigor and good health is a primary goal of medicine. The sudden and unexpected death of a young, apparently healthy, person is the antithesis of this goal.

In 1986 a desperate father fled Poland under cover of darkness to seek help for his ailing son. The patient was a 3-year-old boy who had had multiple episodes of loss of consciousness, requiring resuscitation by his father on many occasions. The boy's sister had died suddenly and without apparent cause aged 2 years, following repeated episodes of aborted cardiac death. At the time of her death, she had undergone implantation of a ventricular pacemaker and was being treated with amiodarone. Electrocardiograms of the two siblings were very similar and clearly abnormal and 'bizarre'. The identification of two additional patients with similar findings by Dr Pedro Brugada resulted in the presentation of preliminary data at the annual meeting of the North American Society of Pacing and Electrophysiology (NASPE) in 1991.[1] The first paper, which described eight patients, was published in 1992.[2]

Since that time, an exponential increase in the number of similarly afflicted patients has been recognized worldwide. From relative obscurity, this new clinical entity—which the medical and scientific community has termed the Brugada syndrome—has rapidly gained recognition as a major cause of sudden cardiac death. The recent discovery of genetic abnormalities linked to this syndrome lends support to the probability of its being a primary electrical disease, laying a foundation for the development of strategies for prevention and effective treatments of this form of sudden death in patients with a structurally normal heart.

Historical milestones

The history of the Brugada syndrome is very short but very enlightening, since it involves a series of remarkably insightful discoveries that have revolutionized our understanding of the clinical, genetic, ionic, cellular, and molecular mechanisms that underlie life-threatening arrhythmias, culminating in the discovery of a new clinical syndrome, identification of patients at risk, and prevention of sudden cardiac death.

ECG phenomenon and terminology

To our knowledge, the first clinical report of the unusual electrocardiographic pattern consistent with the ECG signature of the Brugada syndrome was published in 1953 by Osher and Wolff.[3] They described right bundle branch block (RBBB) with persistent elevation of the ST segment and inversion of the T wave in the right precordial leads with minor variations in three healthy males. One year later, Edeiken identified persistent and apparent RS-T segment elevation without RBBB in another ten asymptomatic males.[4] Levine *et al.* observed ST segment elevation in the right chest leads with some degree of conduction block in the right ventricle in patients with severe hyperkalemia. The authors named such RS-T segment shift as 'dialyzable current of injury' and postulated that the 'wax-and-wane' pattern of this ECG abnormality was dependent on the level of plasma potassium, and not related to the conduction block in the right ventricle.[5] In 1960, Roesler observed unusually 'high takeoff of the R(R')S-T segment' in the right precordial leads in four patients with hump-shaped elevation of the ST segment. In each case, the repolarization abnormality was more prominent in the high right chest leads, and neither RBBB nor reciprocal changes in the opposite leads were present.[6] Similarly, Calo noted that 'the triad of secondary R wave,

RS-T segment elevation and T wave inversion in the right precordial leads' was more prominent at higher levels of the electrode position than in routine right precordial leads. He noted a benign course in one patient during a 14-year follow-up period. This author also questioned the primary role of RBBB in the genesis of the elevated ST segment elevation.[7] Variations in the degree of plateau elevation of the right precordial ST segment dependent upon displacement of the exploring chest electrodes in an asymptomatic individual were included in the textbook on ECG by Marriott.[8]

Apparently, this striking ECG phenomenon had been largely ignored until Martini et al.[9] and Aihara and coworkers[10] called attention to a possible link between this ventricular repolarization abnormality and sudden death in one and four of their patients, respectively. In 1991, Pedro and Josep Brugada described an additional four patients with sudden and aborted cardiac death, in whom they found 'right bundle branch block and persistent ST segment elevation in leads V_1–V_3'.[3] In 1992, based on eight clinical cases, they outlined a new 'distinct clinical and electrocardiographic syndrome'.[2]

The term 'Brugada syndrome' was introduced during a cardiology conference on sudden cardiac death organized by the brothers Brugada in July 1995, held in the Cardiovascular Center OLV Hospital in Aalst, Belgium. Use of the term 'Brugada syndrome' (known in Belgium also as 'Brugi-Brugi syndrome') was proposed in lieu of the original lengthy description of the syndrome. The first literature reference to the newly named Brugada syndrome was documented in 1996; Yan and Antzelevitch[11] highlighted the importance of the ST segment elevation and apparent RBBB described by Brugada and Brugada as the basis for a substrate capable of giving rise to malignant arrhythmias. Kobayashi et al.[12] and Miyazaki et al.[13] followed suit the same year.

At the same conference, Nademanee pointed out similarities in both the electrocardiographic and the clinical presentations between patients with Brugada syndrome and victims of sudden unexplained death syndrome (SUDS), a disorder most prevalent in Southeast Asia. Sudden and unexpected death of young adults during sleep, known in the Philippines as *bangungut* ('to rise and moan in sleep'), was first described in the Philippine medical literature in 1917. In 1997, Nademanee et al.[14] reported that a majority of Thai men referred for aborted cases of what was known in Thailand as *Lai Tai* ('death during sleep') displayed ECG patterns typical of Brugada syndrome. Alings and Wilde reviewed the literature in 1999, and reported that of 163 patients who met the criteria for Brugada syndrome, 58% were of Asian origin.[15]

The terms 'transient, latent and manifested' and 'symptomatic and asymptomatic' forms of the syndrome were also introduced by the Brugada brothers, who held the largest database of affected patients and members of the family at any given time.

Clinical, experimental, and genetic perspectives

Certain electrophysiologic similarities have been found between ECG markers of the Brugada syndrome, early repolarization syndrome, hypothermia, and arrhythmogenic right ventricular cardiomyopathy.[16] The hereditary nature of the syndrome, characterized by an autosomal dominant mode of transmission, was first described by Corrado et al.[17] Chen and coworkers were the first to link the syndrome to the α subunit of the cardiac sodium channel gene, SCN5A, in 1998.[18] The concept of Brugada syndrome as a primary electrical disease was introduced by Gussak et al. in 1999.[16]

Investigation of the cellular mechanisms believed to underlie the Brugada syndrome evolved on a parallel but separate track from that of the clinical syndrome. The concept of all-or-none repolarization of the ventricular epicardial action potential and of phase 2 reentry secondary to sodium channel block or ischemia were developed in the early 1990s.[19–21] ST segment elevation in the Brugada syndrome is thought to be due to a rebalancing of the currents active at the end of phase 1, leading to an accentuation of the action potential notch in the right ventricular epicardium (see Ref. 22 for references).

Despite substantial progress in the identification and characterization of the Brugada syndrome since the mid-1990s, relatively little progress has been made in the approach to therapy. Implantable cardioverter-defibrillator (ICD) placement is the only established effective treatment for the disease.[16,23,24] This, however, is not an adequate solution for infants and young children or for people residing in regions of the world where ICD is not an option.

Epilogue

In the span of 10 years, the Brugada syndrome has gained broad recognition worldwide. The syndrome occupies a prominent portion of the time devoted to cardiac arrhythmias at national and international meetings, and publications on the subject continue to appear at a brisk rate. More questions than answers still remain with regard to etiology, pathogenesis, arrhythmogenesis, epidemiology, prevention, and treatment of the Brugada syndrome. These and other ambiguities concerning diagnosis of the Brugada syndrome have prompted the establishment of a special Arrhythmia Working Group of the European Society of Cardiology that is actively supported by the Brugada, Sr. Foundation (http://www.brugada.crtia.be/).

References

1 Brugada P, Brugada J. A distinct clinical and electrocardiographic syndrome: right bundle-branch block, persistent ST segment elevation with normal QT interval and sudden cardiac death (abstr). *Pacing Clin. Electrophysiol.* 1991; **14**: 746.

2 Brugada P, Brugada J. Right bundle-branch block, persistent ST segment elevation and sudden cardiac death: a distinct clinical and electrocardiographic syndrome. A multicenter Report. *J. Am. Coll. Cardiol.* 1992; **20**: 1391–1396.

3 Osher HL, Wolff L. Electrocardiographic pattern simulating acute myocardial injury. *Am. J. Med. Sci.* 1953; **226**: 541–545.

4 Edeiken J. Elevation of RS-T segment, apparent or real in right precordial leads as probable normal variant. *Am. Heart J.* 1954; **48**: 331–339.

5 Levine HD, Wanzer SH, Merrill JP. Dialyzable currents of injury in potassium intoxication resembling acute myocardial infarction or pericarditis. *Circulation* 1956; **13**: 29–36.

6 Roesler H. An electrocardiographic study of high take-off of the R(R)-T segment in right precordial leads. Altered repolarization. *Am. J. Cardiol.* 1960; **6**: 920–928.

7 Calo AA. The triad secondary R wave, RS-T segment elevation and T waves inversion in right precordial leads: a normal electrocardiographic variant. *G. Ital. Cardiol.* 1975; **5**: 955–960.

8 Marriott HJL. *Practical Electrocardiography*, 7th edn. Baltimore: Williams and Williams, 1988.

9 Martini B, Nava A, Thiene G *et al.* Ventricular fibrillation without apparent heart disease. Description of six cases. *Am. Heart J.* 1989; **118**: 1203–1209.

10 Aihara N, Ohe T, Kamakura S *et al.* Clinical and electrophysiologic characteristics of idiopathic ventricular fibrillation. *Shinzo* 1990; **22** (Suppl. 2): 80–86.

11 Yan GX, Antzelevitch C. Cellular basis for the electrocardiographic J wave. *Circulation* 1996; **93**: 372–379.

12 Kobayashi T, Shintani U, Yamamoto T *et al.* Familial occurrence of electrocardiographic abnormalities of the Brugada-type [see comments]. *Intern. Med.* 1996; **35**: 637–640.

13 Miyazaki T, Mitamura H, Miyoshi S *et al.* Autonomic and antiarrhythmic drug modulation of ST segment elevation in patients with Brugada syndrome. *J. Am. Coll. Cardiol.* 1996; **27**: 1061–1070.

14 Nademanee K, Veerakul G, Nimmannit S *et al.* Arrhythmogenic marker for the sudden unexplained death syndrome in Thai men. *Circulation* 1997; **96**: 2595–2600.

15 Alings M, Wilde A. 'Brugada' syndrome: clinical data and suggested pathophysiological mechanism [see comments]. *Circulation* 1999; **99**: 666–673.

16 Gussak I, Antzelevitch C, Bjerregaard P, Towbin JA, Chaitman BR. The Brugada syndrome: clinical, electrophysiological and genetic aspects. *J. Am. Coll. Cardiol.* 1999; **33**: 5–15.

17 Corrado D, Nava A, Buja G *et al.* Familial cardiomyopathy underlies syndrome of right bundle branch block, ST segment elevation and sudden death. *J. Am. Coll. Cardiol.* 1996; **27**: 443–448.

18 Chen Q, Kirsch GE, Zhang D *et al.* Genetic basis and molecular mechanisms for idiopathic ventricular fibrillation. *Nature* 1998; **392**: 293–296.

19 Antzelevitch C, Sicouri S, Litovsky SH *et al.* Heterogeneity within the ventricular wall: electrophysiology and pharmacology of epicardial, endocardial and M cells. *Circ. Res.* 1991; **69**: 1427–1449.

20 Krishnan SC, Antzelevitch C. Sodium channel blockade produces opposite electrophysiologic effects in canine ventricular epicardium and endocardium. *Circ. Res.* 1991; **69**: 277–291.

21 Krishnan SC, Antzelevitch C. Flecainide-induced arrhythmia in canine ventricular epicardium: phase 2 reentry? *Circulation* 1993; **87**: 562–572.

22 Antzelevitch C. The Brugada syndrome: ionic basis and arrhythmia mechanisms. *J. Cardiovasc. Electrophysiol.* 2001; **12**: 268–272.

23 Brugada J, Brugada R, Brugada P. Pharmacological and device approach to therapy of inherited cardiac diseases associated with cardiac arrhythmias and sudden death. *J. Electrocardiol.* 2000; **33** (Suppl): 41–47.

24 Brugada P, Brugada R, Brugada J, Geelen P. Use of the prophylactic implantable cardioverter defibrillator for patients with normal hearts. *Am. J. Cardiol.* 1999; **83**: 98D–100D.

CHAPTER 3

Biophysical analysis of mutant sodium channels in Brugada syndrome

H. Tan, MD, PhD

Brugada syndrome and sodium channel mutations

The only gene with a proven causal involvement in Brugada syndrome found so far is *SCN5A*, the gene encoding the main (α) subunit of the human cardiac sodium (Na) channel.[1] Various *SCN5A* mutations have been recognized in up to 30% of Brugada syndrome patients.[2,3] Another gene locus was mapped in close proximity to the *SCN5A* locus on chromosome 3 (3p22–25), but the causal gene was not identified.[4] It is clear that there is clinical as well as genetic variability in Brugada syndrome. Identification and functional analysis of other genes may further enhance our understanding of the pathophysiologic basis of Brugada syndrome.

Linkage of Brugada syndrome to mutant Na channels fits well with the clinical observations that Na channel dysfunction may cause life-threatening arrhythmias by various electrophysiologic mechanisms. For instance, during ischemia, reduced Na current may evoke reentrant tachyarrhythmias by causing conduction slowing or block.[5] Similarly, excess mortality in the CAST study among patients on Na channel blocking drugs befell those patients who had active ischemia.[6] Conversely, in the drug-induced or *SCN5A*-related inherited long QT (LQTS3) syndromes, enhanced Na current may trigger after-depolarizations and *torsade de pointes* ventricular tachycardia (VT).[7]

Structure and function of the cardiac Na channel

The cardiac Na channel is a trans-sarcolemmal protein composed of the main pore-forming α-subunit and two subsidiary β-subunits (β$_1$ and β$_2$). Some studies report that β-subunits may exert modulating effects on the function of (mutant) α-subunits,[8] but a physiological role of α-subunits remains controversial.[9] The α-subunit contains four homologous domains, each composed of six membrane-spanning segments, linked by linker segments (Fig. 3.1). These domains are bracketed by an intracellular N terminus and C terminus. In general, in their three-dimensional configuration, the membrane-spanning segments combine to create an ion-conducting channel. Based on this general structure, the Na channel assumes different conformations during the cardiac cycle. Upon depolarization, it transits from a resting (closed) to an ion-conducting activated (open) state. This state is short-lived, as channel opening is coupled to and rapidly followed by inactivation.[10] The channels have to recover from this state and return to their resting state before they can reopen. There are several inactivation processes, linked to conformational changes in distinct channel regions, which have clinical relevance. Fast inactivation (time constant, τ: few ms) and intermediate inactivation (τ: 50–100 ms) are distinguished by their speed of development and recovery. The magnitude of their time constants indicate that both processes are relevant for the cardiac action potential. Closed-state inactivation (inactivation from closed states without prior activation) may also be clinically relevant.[11] The transitions between these conformational states are summarized by the term 'gating'. All gating processes have specific time and voltage dependence. In general, transitions into the activated and inactivated

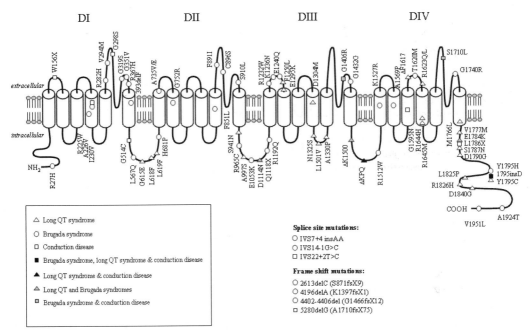

Figure 3.1 Diagrammatic representation of the human cardiac sodium channel displaying locations of mutations associated with long QT syndrome type 3, Brugada syndrome, isolated cardiac conduction disease, and overlap syndromes. DI, domain I; DII, domain II; DIII, domain III; DIV, domain IV.

states require depolarization (to less negative potentials), while recovery from inactivation requires hyperpolarization (to more negative potentials). The ion-conducting pore is lined by the linker segments (P loop) between transmembrane segments 5 and 6 in each domain. Some P loop residues confer ion selectivity.[12] Segment 4 in each domain contains positively charged residues, which impart sensitivity to the membrane voltage.[13] Outward S4 movement upon membrane depolarization opens the ion-conducting pore. Subsequent fast inactivation, coupled to this process,[10] involves a hinged lid process. The intracellular linker between domains III and IV acts as a lid, which docks at the inner vestibule of the pore to occlude it.[10,13,14] Intermediate inactivation involves residues within the outer pore and the C terminus.[15–17] The regions involved in closed-state inactivation await identification. This spatial organization of gating functions suggests that the effects of missense mutations or deletions are predictable from their position and alteration of charge or other biophysical properties. These predictions have been verified in some, but not all, mutations.

Similarly, mutations with equal gating changes may be clustered within the same segments, or be located apart. For instance, enhanced intermediate inactivation is observed in mutants in the C terminus,[18–20] but also remote from it.[21–23]

Biophysical analysis of mutant Na channels: the patch-clamp technique

After identification of the causative *SCN5A* defect using molecular genetics, and synthesis of the mutant gene using site-directed mutagenesis, the gating properties of the resulting mutant Na channel protein can be established using patch-clamp studies in heterologous expression systems. In general, cultured mammalian cells or oocytes of the frog *Xenopus laevis* are used. In mammalian cells (e.g., the human embryonic kidney cell line, HEK293, or its derivative, tsA201), cDNA of the mutant *SCN5A* gene is transfected by transiently exposing the cells to agents that render the plasma membrane permeable to cDNA. In oocytes, cRNA of the mutant

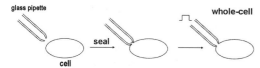

Figure 3.2 Patch-clamp technique. Left: glass pipette is positioned in close proximity to cell. Middle: using gentle suction, a high-resistance seal of several GΩ ('gigaseal') between pipette and cell is created. Right: this 'whole-cell' configuration is created by rupturing the membrane enclosed by the pipette through abrupt suction; the intracellular voltage is now controlled through the pipette.

SCN5A gene is injected by micro-injection. In both systems, the corresponding mutant Na channel protein is synthesized by the host cell, and its biophysical analysis is conducted after an incubation period (usually 24–72 hours after cDNA transfection/cRNA injection). These cell types are used, because they possess virtually no intrinsic Na or other sarcolemmal ion channels, and currents recorded during patch-clamp studies must therefore result from ion fluxes through the transfected Na channels.

Figure 3.2 summarizes the basic principles of the patch-clamp technique. In short, a glass micropipette with a polished tip, connected to an amplifier and recording system, is placed on a cell and gentle suction is applied to create an electrical seal between the cell and the pipette. This seal is in the magnitude of several GΩ ('gigaseal') and serves to minimize leak currents between cell and pipette, thereby reducing noise and ensuring that recorded currents result from nothing but ion fluxes through the mutant Na channels. Next, various configurations can be obtained. The whole-cell configuration is often used in studies of mutant Na channels in inherited arrhythmia syndromes. It is obtained by abrupt suction which results in rupture of the membrane enclosed by the pipette tip. As access to the intracellular milieu is gained, all Na channels within the sarcolemma can be controlled through the pipette and their gating properties analyzed. Pulses of varying durations and voltages (patch-clamp protocols) are imposed upon the cell to elicit Na currents and dissect various aspects of Na channel gating (see later). In addition to gating properties, current density (amplitude of macroscopic current per surface area) is measured. While the patch-

clamp technique is also being successfully used to study sarcolemmal ion channels in myocytes (isolated using enzymatic dissociation), this application in studies of Brugada syndrome is not feasible, given that cardiac biopsies from Brugada syndrome patients would be required to obtain myocytes, as animal models of Brugada syndrome are not yet available.

Reduced Na current

The overriding insight from patch-clamp studies of Brugada syndrome associated *SCN5A* mutations is that the mutant Na channels conduct less Na current. This may be caused by various mechanisms (see the next section).[1] The resulting reduction in net depolarizing force fits well with the postulated electrophysiologic mechanism of Brugada syndrome (see chapter 5), and the clinical observation that the characteristic ECG pattern can be evoked by Na channel blockers (see chapter 6). At the same time, it would be expected that Na channel reduction causes conduction slowing. Accordingly, *SCN5A* mutations that result in reduced Na current were also found in families with isolated cardiac conduction disease (i.e., in the absence of Brugada syndrome). Furthermore, Brugada syndrome patients with a proven *SCN5A* mutation have more conduction slowing than those without one.[2] Numerous other clinical observations support a key role of conduction slowing, particularly in the right ventricle, in Brugada syndrome.[24–29] Why mutant Na channels that conduct less Na current cause Brugada syndrome in some patients, while they result in isolated conduction disease in others, may have various reasons. It may be explained by differences in the extent of Na channel reduction, with Brugada syndrome patients having more severe Na current reduction than those with isolated conduction disease.[30] Alternatively, it may result from modulating factors, as Brugada syndrome and isolated conduction disease may coexist in the same family among family members who share the same *SCN5A* mutation (see below).[31]

The implications for arrhythmogenesis of reduced Na current were elegantly demonstrated in an experimental study on transgenic mice, in which one allele of *SCN5A* was knocked out.[32] Predictably, the resulting haplo-insufficiency caused a 50%

reduction in Na current density of ventricular myocytes isolated from these mice. *In vivo*, this resulted in slowed conduction, as witnessed by widening of the P wave and prolongation of the PR interval. Interestingly, the magnitude of slowing of these conduction parameters (26–37%) was in accordance with predictions from modeling studies in which Na current was reduced by 50%.[33] Studies in isolated perfused hearts of these mice also yielded indicators of slow conduction, most notably broadening of the ventricular complex and increased latency from the stimulus to the evoked electrogram. Furthermore, re-entrant ventricular tachycardias were induced by programmed electrical stimulation. Demonstration of a Brugada syndrome ECG was not provided, as this is virtually impossible in mice because their action potentials are very much shorter than those in humans, and ST segment elevation was not found, as an isoelectric ST segment is absent even in normal mice. Still, this study strongly supports some of the key elements in the proposed pathophysiologic basis of Brugada syndrome: conduction slowing and facilitation of reentrant ventricular tachyarrhythmias. Unexpectedly, there was also evidence of structural derangements. Mice in which both alleles of *SCN5A* were knocked out, exhibited gross derangements of ventricular structure (and died *in utero*). While gross structural abnormalities are not detected clinically by routine cardiologic examinations (as they are by definition absent from Brugada syndrome), microscopic derangements of the conduction system have also been reported in a family with widespread conduction disease due to compound heterozygosity for two *SCN5A* mutations (*W156X* and *R225W*).[34] These findings suggest that chronic disruptions in Na current may result in structural derangements. Further studies into these intriguing observations are awaited.

Biophysical mechanisms of Na current reduction

Several biophysical mechanisms have been shown to reduce Na current in *SCN5A* mutations. These mechanisms are here subdivided into those that involve reduced current density, and those that revolve around changes in gating (Table 3.1). In the first category, reduced Na current results from fewer functional Na channels or smaller currents being conducted by single Na channels. In the second category, the time- and/or voltage-dependent activation/inactivation properties are altered in such a way that this results in reduced Na current during the time/voltage range of the cardiac action potential. Table 3.2 summarizes the main biophysical alterations that result in reduced Na current of mutant Na channels in Brugada syndrome reported so far.[18,19,22,31,35–54] Table 3.3 shows those of mutant Na channels associated with isolated conduction disease.[21,30,31,34,37,55–58] Despite the general success of patch-clamp studies in reconciling the clinical observations with the biophysical changes, it has to be noted that a sizeable number of *SCN5A* mutations associated with Brugada syndrome have not been studied by patch-clamp analysis (Table 3.4).[59,60]

Reduction of current density
Truncation of Na channel protein

A premature stop codon may be created when the mutation causes a frameshift.[34] The resulting truncation of the Na channel protein culminates in reduced Na current. While intuition would predict that this reduction is more severe if the truncation is localized closer to the N terminus of the Na channel, clinical observations in patients with truncation causing *SCN5A* mutations so far show that this may not always be true. In particular, carriers of the *W156X* mutation, which truncates the protein in the linker segment between segments 1 and 2 of domain I (thereby leaving only 1 of 24 transmembrane segments intact), exhibit no conduction slowing.[34] In contrast, individuals carrying the 5280delG mutation, which results in truncation at codon 1786 in

Table 3.1 Biophysical mechanisms of Na current reduction.

Reduced current density
Truncation of Na channel protein
Mutation within the ion-conducting pore
Trafficking disorder

Changes in gating
Depolarizing shift in voltage-dependent activation
Hyperpolarizing shift in voltage-dependent inactivation
Enhanced closed-state inactivation
Accelerated fast inactivation
Enhanced intermediate inactivation

Table 3.2 Biophysical changes of *SCN5A* mutations in Brugada syndrome.

Mutation	Localization	Reference	τfast current decay	Intermediate inact	Persistent current	Current density	V½ inact, mV −shift	V½ inact, mV +shift	V½ act, mV −shift	V½ act, mV +shift
G351V	DIS5S6	123	↑	—	—	↓	=		=	
R367H	DIS5S6	23	—	—	—	0	—		—	
L567Q	DIDII	124	↓	—	—	=	−11.3			6.9
H681P	DIIDIII	125	—	—	—	—	−17.3		−9.5	
A735V	DIIS1	23	=	—	—	=	=			6.7
G752R	DIIS2	126	—	—	—	↓		12.0		30
R1192Q	DIIDIII	23	↓	—	—	—		3.9	=	
R1232W	DIIIS1S2	127	—	—	—	=	−5.7		=	
R1232W+	DIIIS1S2+	127	—	—	—	0	—		—	
T1620M+β	DIVS3S4	128	—	—	—	↓		6.3	=	
R1232W+		128	—	—	—	=		6.5	=	
T1620M-β		49	—	—	=	—		8.8	=	
K1397R+1X	DIIIS5S6	49	—	—	—	0	—		—	
G1406R	DIIIS5S6	129	—	—	—	0	—		—	
R1432G	DIIIS5S6	130	—	—	—	0	—		—	
in oocytes		131	—	—	—	=	—		=	
in TSA cells		131	—	—	—	0	—		—	
R1512W	DIIIDIV	130	↑	—	=	=	=		=	
		132	=	—	—	—	−3.8		−5.1	
T1620M	DIVS3S4	127	—	—	—	—	−8.5		−2.5	
		133	=	=	=	—		13.1		6.8
in oocytes		134	=	—	=	—		10.4	—	
in TSA cells		134	—	—	—	—	=		=	
T1620M at 22°C		53	=	—	—	—	=		=	
T1620M at 32°C		53	↓	—	—	—	=			10.7
T1620M at 22°C		135	=	↑	—	—	—		—	
T1620M at 32°C		135	=	↑	—	—	=		=	
T1620M+β		136	=	—	—	—		10.5	=	
T1620M-β		136	=	—	=	—		4.8	=	
S1710L	DIVS5S6	133	↓	↑	=	—	−21.7			18.7
		137	↓	—	—	—	−24.3			17.7
1795insD	C terminus	13	=	—	=	↓	−7.3			8.1
		138	=	↑	↑	—	−9.7		=	
		139	—	↑	—	—	—		—	
		140	—	—	↑	↓	−19.2			9.1
Y1795H	C terminus	141	↓	↑	↑	↓	−10.5		=	
A1924T	C terminus	142	↓	↓	—	—	—		—	
		132	↑	—	—	—	=		−9.0	

τfast current decay: time constant of fast component of sodium current decay (fast inactivation); inact: inactivation; V½ inact: voltage at which 50% of sodium channels are inactivated; V½ act: voltage at which 50% of sodium channels are activated; ↓: reduction; ↑: increase; + shift: shift to positive voltage; – shift: shift to negative voltage; =: unchanged; -: not reported.

Table 3.3 Biophysical changes of *SCN5A* mutations in isolated cardiac conduction disease.

Mutation	Localization	Reference	τ_{fast} current decay	Intermediate inact	Persistent current	Current density	$V_{1/2}$ inact, mV – shift	$V_{1/2}$ inact, mV + shift	$V_{1/2}$ act, mV – shift	$V_{1/2}$ act, mV + shift
W156X	DIS1S2	34	—	—	—	0	—		—	
R225W-β	DISIV	34	—	=	—	↓	=		=	
R225W+β		34	—	—	—	↓		11.1		14.0
G298S	DIS5S6	21	↑	↑	=	↓	7.4		=	
G514C	DI-DII	30	↓	—	—	=	6.9		10.1	
IV 22DS+2	DIIIS4S5	55-56	—	—	—	0	—		—	
G1406R	DIIIS5S6	31	—	—	—	0	—		—	
D1595N	DIVS3	57	↑	↑	=	↓	4.2		=	
S1710L	DIVS5S6	46	↓	↑	=	—	-21.7			18.7
L1786X (5280delG)	C terminus	58	—	—	—	0	—		—	

τ_{fast} current decay: time constant of fast component of sodium current decay (fast inactivation); inact: inactivation; $V_{1/2}$ inact: voltage at which 50% of sodium channels are inactivated; $V_{1/2}$ act: voltage at which 50% of sodium channels are activated; ↓: reduction; ↑: increase; + shift: shift to positive voltage; – shift: shift to negative voltage; =: unchanged; -: not reported.

the C terminal tail, thereby leaving all transmembrane segments intact, have distinct conduction slowing.[58] It has been proposed that this is based on the position of the stop codon within the transcript, with earlier stop codons resulting in decreased levels of transcript and, consequently, a milder phenotype.[34]

Mutations within the ion-conducting pore

Mutations may be located within the ion-conducting pore of the Na channel. It is comfortably envisaged that the resulting conformational changes within the pore may impede Na ion flow and reduce or abolish Na current.

Trafficking disorders

The mutant Na channels may not be expressed in the sarcolemma, because they are retained within the endoplasmic reticulum (ER). Figure 3.3 illustrates this.[40] While wild-type Na channels, coupled to a fluorescent marker, are expressed at the sarcolemma (panel A), the mutant *R1432G*, identified in a Brugada syndrome family, was trapped in the cytosol (panel B). Utilizing the ER-targeted marker calnexin, it was established that the mutant was retained within the ER (panel C).

The ER is the first compartment for the synthesis and processing of membrane proteins. When errors

in polypeptide folding occur, quality control mechanisms within the ER ensure that the misfolded polypeptides are recognized and degraded. Various strategies to correct diseases of protein folding are under investigation.[61,62] Trafficking-deficient mutants have been 'rescued' by lowering the incubation temperature or using 'chemical chaperones', e.g., glycerol and dimethyl sulfoxide.[63,64] These strategies may stabilize conformations, thereby saving them from degradation by the ER. The former is only applicable *in vitro* while 'chemical chaperones' are not clinically applicable since concentrations that would be needed to attain the desired effect are too high to be achieved *in vivo* and are unsafe. A more promising approach was demonstrated recently: substrates and blockers that bind to the mutant protein, and stabilize them.[65–68] The selectivity that can be achieved using such 'pharmacological chaperones' (ligand-mediated) makes it more likely that such a strategy could ultimately become clinically relevant. The feasibility of this approach was demonstrated for mutant HERG potassium channels that were rescued by the HERG blockers E-4031, astemizole, and cisapride. Importantly, rescue may be accomplished without inducing channel block.[69] Similarly, trafficking-deficient Na channels were rescued by the Na channel blocker mexiletine, as illustrated in Fig. 3.4.[70] Panel A shows wild-type Na current. Cells into

Table 3.4 *SCN5A* mutations in Brugada syndrome without biophysical analysis.

Mutation	Localization	Reference
R27H	N terminus	59
K126E	N terminus	35
A226V	DIS4	59
I230V	DIS4	59
IVS7DS + 4	DIS5-S6	59
R282H	DIS5-S6	59
V294M	DIS5-S6	59
G319S	DIS5-S6	60
F393del	DIS6	59
H681P	DIDII	59
A735E	DIIS2	60
IVS14–1G > C	DIIS2	60
F851L	DIIS5	59
S871fs + 9X	DIIS5S6	59
F892I	DIIS5S6	59
C896S	DIIS5S6	59
S910L	DIIS5S6	59
R965C	DIIDIII	60
E1053K	DIIDIII	60
D1114N	DIIDIII	60
Q1118X	DIIDIII	59
K1236N	DIIIS1S2	59
E1240Q	DIIIS2	59
F1293S	DIIIS3S4	59
V1398X	DIIIS5-S6	42
G1466fs + 12X	DIIIS6	59
K1500del	DIIIDIV	59
G1740R	DIVS5-S6	59
E1784K	C terminus	59
V1951L	C terminus	59

which the mutant *M1766L* (associated with LQTS3) was transfected exhibit strongly reduced Na current (panel B). However, incubation with mexiletine increased these currents (panel D). In contrast, mexiletine did not increase Na currents in wild-type Na channels (panel C). While it is clear that rescuing *SCN5A* mutants and enhancing Na current is a highly attractive novel concept with potentially far-reaching therapeutic implications, several theoretical and practical issues need to be resolved prior to its clinical application.[71]

Changes in gating
Voltage-dependent activation

Figure 3.5 demonstrates how voltage-dependent activation can be assessed.[30] The patch-clamp protocol shown in the inset consisted of sequential (superimposed in this schematic representation) depolarizing steps of 20 ms duration from −80 mV to 0 mV from a resting membrane potential (holding potential) of −140 mV. These depolarizing steps elicit Na current. The voltage dependence of this activation process is generally expressed as $V_{1/2}$, i.e., the voltage at which half-maximal activation is attained. In this instance, the mutant Na channel (*G514C*) was identified in a family afflicted with isolated conduction disease. This mutant exhibited a shift of voltage-dependent activation to depolarized voltages when compared to wild-type Na channels (wild-type $V_{1/2} = -48.6$ mV, mutant $V_{1/2} = -38.5$ mV). Such a shift implies that any given depolarization from the resting membrane potential causes less

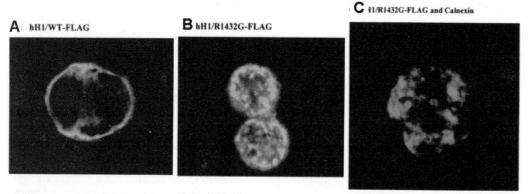

Figure 3.3 Trafficking disorder of mutant (*R1432G*) Na channel. Immunostaining of cultured cells (tsA201) expressing human cardiac Na channel protein (hH1). (**A**) Wild-type (WT) Na channels are expressed in the cell membrane. (**B**) *R1432G* Na channels are not expressed at the cell surface, as they are retained within the cytosol. (**C**) Anti-calnexin staining indicates that *R1432G* Na channels are localized within ER vesicles. Adapted from Ref. 44.

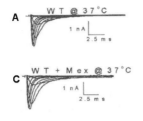

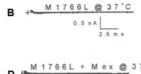

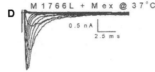

Figure 3.4 Pharmacological 'rescue' of mutant (*M1766L*) Na channel. Whole-cell current tracings from HEK293 cells expressing Na channels (these superimposed current tracings were elicited by depolarizing pulses to varying voltages). (**A**) Wild-type (WT) Na current. (**B**) M1766L Na channels conduct strongly reduced Na current. (**C**) Incubation with mexiletine (Mex) did not change density of wild-type Na current. (**D**) Incubation with mexiletine increased *M1766L* Na current. Adapted from Ref. 70.

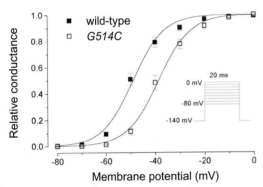

Figure 3.5 Depolarizing shift in voltage-dependent activation of mutant (*G514C*) Na channel. Voltage-dependent activation is assessed by depolarizing steps ranging from −80 mV to 0 mV from a holding potential of −140 mV, as indicated in the inset. In comparison with wild-type Na channels, G514C Na channels resist activation as indicated by a shift in the voltage of half-maximal activation ($V_{1/2}$) from −48.6 mV to −38.5 mV. This shift implies that any given depolarization results in less *G514C* Na current than wild-type Na current. Adapted from Ref. 30.

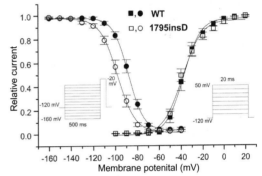

Figure 3.6 Hyperpolarizing shift in voltage-dependent inactivation of mutant (1795insD) Na channel (left part). Voltage-dependent inactivation is assessed by depolarizing steps from −160 mV to −40 mV, which precede the test pulse (−20 mV), as indicated in the left inset. $V_{1/2}$ of inactivation is shifted from −88.5 mV (wild-type, WT) to −98.2 mV (1795insD). This shift implies that 1795insD Na channels are more readily inactivated than wild-type channels, and that more 1795insD channels are inactivated at a given resting membrane potential. Adapted from Ref. 18.

Na channel activation. This results in reduced net Na current and is compatible with the clinical phenotype.

Voltage-dependent inactivation

Figure 3.6 (left part) demonstrates voltage-dependent inactivation of the mutant 1795insD, which was identified in a family afflicted with Brugada syndrome, conduction disturbances, sinus bradycardia, and LQTS3.[18] Superimposed in this figure is voltage-dependent activation (right part). As indicated in the left inset, prepulses of 500 ms duration ranging from −160 mV to −40 mV cause voltage-dependent Na channel inactivation. The magnitude of the residual Na current (i.e., the remaining proportion of Na channels that have escaped voltage-dependent inactivation) is assessed by the subsequent test pulse (20 ms, −20 mV). Voltage dependence is expressed as $V_{1/2}$, as in voltage-dependent activation. The mutant exhibited a hyperpolarizing shift of voltage-dependent inactivation (wild-type $V_{1/2}$ −88.5 mV, mutant $V_{1/2}$ −98.2 mV). This implies that the mutant inactivates more readily. In particular, at the resting membrane potential, more mutant Na channels are inactivated, and less are available for activation, resulting in smaller Na current.

Closed-state inactivation

Comparison of voltage-dependent inactivation (Fig. 3.6, left part) and voltage-dependent activation (Fig. 3.6, right part) reveals that inactivation occurs at voltages where Na channels have not opened.[18] For instance, although inactivation of wild-type Na channels starts at −110 mV, these channels are not activated until depolarized to −60 mV (or more positive potentials). In effect, this implies that some Na channels transit directly from their closed state to an inactivated state. While this closed-state inactivation process is present in wild-type Na channels, it may be more prominent in mutant Na channels. A more detailed characterization of closed-state inactivation may be obtained by patch-clamp protocols as shown in the inset of Fig. 3.7.[19] Depolarizing prepulses of varying duration (1–500 ms) that do not activate Na channels (−90 mV and −100 mV) cause inactivation of closed channels, as evidenced by the reduction in the number of Na channels that can be activated by the subsequent depolarizing test pulse (100 ms, −20 mV). At both depolarizing prepulses, closed-state inactivation is more severe in the 1795insD mutant than in wild-type. Studies of some

mutant Na channels have indicated that this inactivation process may underlie the enhanced sensitivity to tonic block (block at slow heart rates) of these mutants as imposed by class I antiarrhythmic drugs. The clinical correlate is the observation that these drugs may elicit Brugada-type ST elevations even in patients who carry LQTS3-associated *SCN5A* mutations.[72] These mutant Na channels not only exhibit noninactivating Na current to account for QT prolongation (see below), but also enhanced closed-state inactivation.[73] It is clear that delineation of the structural domains that underlie this gating process may aid in designing drugs that combine greater antiarrhythmic efficacy with smaller proarrhythmic potential. As such, analysis of mutant Na channels is a powerful tool to develop novel strategies that are applicable to antiarrhythmic drug design and management of common acquired disease.

Fast inactivation

Figure 3.8 A demonstrates two typical superimposed Na channel currents of a wild-type Na channel and a mutant responsible for isolated conduction disease (*G514C*).[30] The rapid decay of both currents is caused by the transition into the fast inactivated state. The faster decay of the mutant Na channel is expressed as a shorter time constant of this process (panel B) and results in a smaller area under the curve of the current transient, thereby reflecting reduced Na current. Conversely, disruptions of this process that lead to noninactivating Na current are a virtually universal finding in mutant Na channels that are responsible for the enhanced Na current during the action potential plateau that underlies action potential prolongation in LQTS3.[2,7]

Intermediate inactivation

Intermediate inactivation is an inactivation process with a slow onset and recovery (both have τ 50–100 ms). Given the slow recovery from intermediate inactivation, this gating process may determine Na channel availability at short diastolic intervals, i.e., at fast heart rates. In addition, intermediate inactivation has been implied in use-dependent Na channel block by class I antiarrhythmic agents.[17] To further illustrate its potential role in common disease, there is evidence that intermediate inactivation may be increased in the ischemic border zone in a chronic infarction model, thereby enhancing the likelihood of

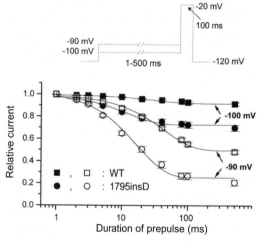

Figure 3.7 Enhanced closed-state inactivation of mutant (1795insD) Na channel. Closed-state inactivation is assessed by depolarizing steps to −100 and −90 mV of variable duration, which precede the test pulse (−20 mV), as indicated in the inset. In comparison with wild-type (WT) Na channels, 1795insD Na channels exhibit enhanced inactivation following the depolarizing prepulses, as indicated by the smaller Na currents that can be elicited by the test pulse. Adapted from Ref. 19.

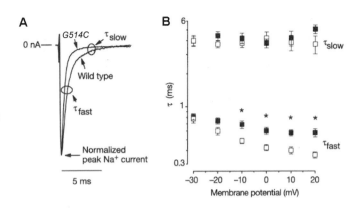

Figure 3.8 Faster current decay (fast inactivation) of mutant (*G514C*) Na channel. **(A)** superimposed Na current transients from wild-type Na channels and *G514C* Na channels. Current decay is fitted by a two-exponential function characterized by τ_{fast} and τ_{slow}. **(B)** Current decay is faster in *G514C* channels, as indicated by shorter τ_{fast}. * $p < 0.05$ versus wild-type. Adapted from Ref. 30.

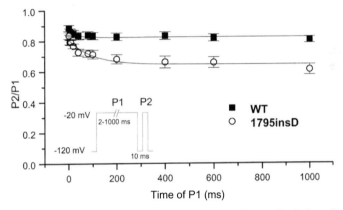

Figure 3.9 Enhanced intermediate inactivation of mutant (1795insD) Na channel. Intermediate inactivation is assessed by depolarizing steps to –20 mV of variable duration, followed by a brief (10 ms) hyperpolarizing (–120 mV) pulse (which causes recovery fro fast inactivation, but is too short to cause recovery from intermediate inactivation), and a final test pulse (–20 mV), as indicated in the inset. In comparison with wild-type (WT) Na channels, 1795insD Na channels exhibit enhanced intermediate inactivation, as indicated by the smaller Na currents that can be elicited by the test pulse. Adapted from Ref. 18.

reentrant arrhythmias.[74] To study intermediate inactivation, a distinction from fast inactivation must be made. In the patch-clamp protocol shown in the inset of Fig. 3.9, the cell is depolarized from its resting membrane potential to –20 mV for a varying duration (2–1000 ms).[18] During this depolarizing pulse, Na channels will activate and subsequently inactivate by passing into the fast inactivated and intermediate inactivated states; the number of channels that enter the intermediate inactivated state will increase as the duration of the depolarizing step lengthens. The subsequent hyperpolarizing pulse (10 ms, –120 mV) will recover the Na channels from their fast inactivated state, but is too short to result in recovery from intermediate inactivation. Consequently, the final depolarizing test pulse (10 ms, –20

mV) will activate only those Na channels that have recovered from fast inactivation, but not those that remain in the intermediate inactivated state. The mutant Na channel (1795insD), which is associated with Brugada syndrome, conduction disturbances, sinus bradycardia, and LQTS3, exhibits enhanced intermediate inactivation compared with wild-type Na channels. As theory would predict, this results in reduced Na current at fast heart rates. This is evidenced clinically by more severe right precordial ST elevation during exercise (Fig. 3.10). Equally, conduction slowing was more prominent at fast heart rates. Interestingly, patch-clamp studies also provided a satisfactory explanation for the LQTS3 features found in this family: noninactivating Na current; this gating defect was also found to be re-

1795insD

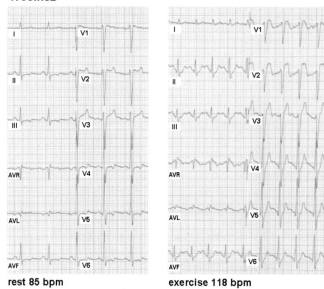

rest 85 bpm   exercise 118 bpm

Figure 3.10 Transition from a saddle-back type (type 2) ST segment to a coved-type (type 1) ST segment at a fast heart rate (during exercise testing) in a carrier of the 1795insD *SCN5A* mutation that enhances intermediate inactivation (see Fig. 3.9). Due to slow recovery from intermediate inactivation, there is cumulation of this inactivation process at short diastolic intervals, i.e., fast heart rates. Accordingly, Na current reduction and the consequent development of coved-type ST elevations are most prominent at fast heart rates. (bpm, beats per minute)

sponsible for the sinus bradycardia. Taken together, patch-clamp studies have provided powerful evidence for the existence of opposing gating defects (enhanced intermediate inactivation and disrupted fast inactivation), that act in concert to reconcile the seemingly contradictory phenotypes of Brugada syndrome ('loss of Na channel function') and LQTS3 ('gain of Na channel function').[18]

Overlap syndromes and modulating factors

Given the pivotal role of Na channels in cardiac excitability, it is not surprising that Na channel dysfunction may cause complex effects on cardiac rate and rhythm. Furthermore, it is becoming increasingly clear that single *SCN5A* mutants may cause a phenotype which combines features of Brugada syndrome, conduction disease, and LQTS3. In addition to 1795insD, careful scrutiny of previously reported mutants and newly discovered ones has revealed that they, too, may engender a mixed phenotype. For instance, the mutants ΔKPQ[75] and D1790G,[76] originally linked to LQTS3, were also found to cause conduction slowing and sinus arrest, while G1406R segregated with isolated conduction disease or Brugada syndrome in different family branches of one larger family.[31] Interestingly, in this

family, Brugada syndrome was found exclusively in males, while 6 of 8 patients afflicted by isolated conduction disease were females.

The emerging notion that one single mutation may cause gating changes with opposing effects highlights that careful clinical phenotyping is of paramount importance, as this may direct patient management. For instance, while the most eye-catching features of 1795insD are signs of Brugada syndrome and LQTS3, its clinical relevance most likely stems from its heart rate slowing effect,[77] that results both from sinus exit block and slowing of the pacemaker firing rate. The explanation for these observations have invoked the hyperpolarizing shift in voltage-dependent inactivation (which results in a slower rate of spontaneous diastolic depolarization of sinus node cells), and the noninactivating Na current (which causes a prolongation of sinus nodal action potential duration).[78] Clinically, long follow-up periods of the large family in whom 1795insD was described revealed that excess mortality, while high in untreated patients, was abolished after pacemaker implantation, indicating that death is related to bradycardia, rather than tachycardia.[77] Holter ECG analysis revealed severe bradycardia episodes (sinus arrest and sinus exit block), but no bradycardia-induced tachycardias such as *torsade de pointes*. Also, ST elevations were attenuated at slow heart rates.[18] Taken together, these observations render it likely that death in 1795insD is due to impediment of excitation and bradycardia, but not (bradycardia induced) VT/VF, unlike other Brugada syndrome or LQTS3 associated *SCN5A* mutants.[59,79] Treatment with a pacemaker rather than an implantable cardioverter-defibrillator, the generally accepted best course for Brugada syndrome patients (see chapter 17), thus appears strongly validated for this particular mutant.[80]

Studies in these overlap syndromes and the observations that there may be large variability in the clinical phenotype among family members who carry the same *SCN5A* mutation all but prove that modulating factors may play a pivotal role. Without any doubt, the most conspicuous modulating factor is gender. While Brugada syndrome has an autosomal dominant mode of inheritance, and both genders thus inherit the genetic predisposition to Brugada syndrome in equal measures, there is a wealth of clinical observations to demonstrate that males more often exhibit the Brugada syndrome phenotype (see chapter 12). An obvious candidate mechanism for this gender disparity are differences in sex hormones. A recent clinical report indicated that testosterone may facilitate the clinical expression of the Brugada syndrome phenotype,[81] while other clinical studies have made it abundantly clear that testosterone may modulate ECG parameters.[82] Biophysical studies, including patch-clamp analysis, to reveal the pathophysiologic basis of these clinical observations are underway. An obvious group of proteins that may harbor the explanation are sarcolemmal ion channels. Accordingly, gender disparities in the expression and function of several sarcolemmal ion channels have been identified.[83] For instance, it is conceivable that the larger current density carried by L-type calcium (Ca) channels (LTCC) in females may be of significance.[84,85] A generalizing electrophysiologic explanation may be that less depolarizing LTCC current in males reduces their 'depolarization reserve', thereby favoring repolarization of the action potential and facilitating the loss of the action potential plateau which is believed to be an important element in the pathophysiology of Brugada syndrome (see chapter 5). Alternatively, gender disparity in the expression of I_{to}, the transient outward current, with females having smaller I_{to}, may protect them from loss of the action potential plateau.[86] Either way, elucidation of the pathophysiologic basis of the gender disparity in phenotypical expression may yield general insights into the function and regulation of proteins involved in cardiac excitability. It is well conceivable that these insights may play a key role in the development of novel treatment strategies for arrhythmias in common acquired disease (e.g., ischemic heart disease, congestive heart failure).

While studies into gender disparity in cardiac electrophysiology and excitability do not, at present, provide leads to guide clinical management (with the possible exception of risk stratification, see chapter 16), a modulating factor that does carry more direct clinical applicability is the temperature sensitivity as observed clinically and confirmed in biophysical analysis of some mutant Na channels. Clinically, the Brugada ECG pattern is often more readily observed during fever.[38,87] Accordingly, patch-clamp studies have revealed that more severe Na current reduction was present when the patch-clamp experiments of the mutant Na channels were conducted at higher temperatures.[48] While the underlying mechanisms of this phenomenon have not yet been elucidated, the implications of these observations may be easily implemented in clinical practice. At present, we advise our Brugada syndrome patients to have an ECG recorded during fever. If this condition should unmask a Brugada ECG pattern, and the ECG at normal temperature reveals a less strongly abnormal ECG (see chapter 6), we advise these patients to take measures to combat fever (antipyretics, e.g., paracetamol, acetaminophen), whenever it occurs. Given that this regime is easily performed and carries no obvious risks, we currently employ it even for patients in whom the underlying molecular genetic defect has not been identified, and patch-clamp studies have not yet confirmed that their particular mutant is temperature-sensitive.

Conclusions

Patch-clamp studies have revealed that the biophysical changes of mutant Na channels implied in Brugada syndrome result in reduced Na current. This is also true for mutant Na channels in isolated cardiac conduction disease. Na current reduction may result from various mechanisms. Dissecting these mechanisms has not only had remarkable success in explaining various aspects of the clinical phenotype, but, more importantly, it is also increasing our insights into the function of the various elements of the Na channel in health and disease. It is anticipated that these insights will facilitate the development of novel therapies for arrhythmias in common disease.

The author was supported by a fellowship grant of the Royal Netherlands Academy of Arts and Sciences (KNAW) and the Netherlands Heart Foundation (2002B191). He is indebted to Dr. Arie O. Verkerk for his assistance in creating the tables.

References

1 Tan HL, Bezzina CR, Smits JPP *et al.* Genetic control of sodium channel function. *Cardiovasc. Res.* 2003; **57**: 961–973.

2 Smits JPP, Eckardt L, Probst V *et al.* Genotype–phenotype relationship in Brugada syndrome: electrocardiographic features differentiate *SCN5A*-related patients from non-*SCN5A*-related patients. *J. Am. Coll. Cardiol.* 2002; **40**: 350–356.

3 Antzelevitch C, Brugada P, Brugada J *et al.* Brugada syndrome: a decade of progress. *Circ. Res.* 2002; **91**: 1114–1118.

4 Weiss R, Barmada MM, Nguyen T *et al.* Clinical and molecular heterogeneity in the Brugada syndrome: a novel gene locus on chromosome 3. *Circulation* 2002; **105**: 707–713.

5 Janse MJ, Wit AL. Electrophysiological mechanisms of ventricular arrhythmias resulting from myocardial ischemia and infarction. *Physiol. Rev.* 1989; **69**: 1049–1169.

6 Greenberg HM, Dwyer EM, Hochman JS *et al.* Interaction of ischaemia and encainide/flecainide treatment: a proposed mechanism for the increased mortality in CAST I. *Br. Heart J.* 1995; **74**: 631–635.

7 Bennett PB, Yazawa K, Makita N *et al.* Molecular mechanism for an inherited cardiac arrhythmia. *Nature* 1995; **376**: 683–685.

8 Bezzina CR, Rook MB, Wilde AAM. Cardiac sodium channel and inherited arrhythmia syndromes. *Cardiovasc. Res.* 2001; **49**: 257–271.

9 Roden DM, Balser JR, George AL *et al.* Cardiac ion channels. *Annu. Rev. Physiol.* 2002; **64**: 431–475.

10 Armstrong CM, Bezzanilla F. Inactivation of the sodium channel. II. Gating current experiments. *J. Gen. Physiol.* 1977; **70**: 567–590.

11 Horn R, Patlak JB, Stevens CF. Sodium channels need not open before they inactivate. *Nature* 1981; **291**: 426–427.

12 Heinemann SH, Terlau H, Stühmer W *et al.* Calcium channel characteristics conferred on the sodium channel by single mutations. *Nature* 1992; **356**: 441–443.

13 Stühmer W, Conti F, Suzuki H *et al.* Structural parts involved in activation and inactivation of the sodium channel. *Nature* 1989; **339**: 597–603.

14 West JW, Patton DE, Scheuer T *et al.* A cluster of hydrophobic amino acid residues required for fast Na(+)-channel inactivation. *Proc. Natl. Acad. Sci. USA* 1992; **89**: 10910–10914.

15 Balser JR. Structure and function of the cardiac sodium channels. *Cardiovasc. Res.* 1999; **42**: 327–338.

16 Balser JR. The cardiac sodium channel: gating function and molecular pharmacology. *J. Mol. Cell. Cardiol.* 2001; **33**: 599–613.

17 Ong BH, Tomaselli GF, Balser JR. A structural rearrangement in the sodium channel pore linked to slow inactivation and use dependence. *J. Gen. Physiol.* 2000; **116**: 653–661.

18 Veldkamp MW, Viswanathan PC, Bezzina C *et al.* Two distinct congenital arrhythmias evoked by a multidysfunctional Na+ channel. *Circ. Res.* 2000; **86**: e91–e97.

19 Viswanathan PC, Bezzina CR, George AL et al. Gating-dependent mechanisms for flecainide action in *SCN5A*-linked arrhythmia syndromes. *Circulation* 2001; **104**: 1200–1205.

20 Rivolta I, Abriel H, Tateyama M *et al.* Inherited Brugada and long QT-3 syndrome mutations of a single residue of the cardiac sodium channel confer distinct channel and clinical phenotypes. *J. Biol. Chem.* 2001; **276**: 30623–30630.

21 Wang DW, Viswanathan PC, Balser JR *et al.* Clinical, genetic, and biophysical characterization of *SCN5A* mutations associated with atrioventricular conduction block. *Circulation* 2002; **105**: 341–346.

22 Wang DW, Makita N, Kitabatake A *et al.* Enhanced sodium channel intermediate inactivation in Brugada syndrome. *Circ. Res.* 2000; **87**: e37–e43.

23 Shirai N, Makita N, Sasaki K *et al.* A mutant cardiac sodium channel with multiple biophysical defects associated with overlapping clinical features of Brugada syndrome and cardiac conduction disease. *Cardiovasc. Res.* 2002; **53**: 348–354.

24 Kasanuki H, Ohnishi S, Ohtuka M *et al.* Idiopathic ventricular fibrillation induced with vagal activity in patients without obvious heart disease. *Circulation* 1997; **95**: 2277–2285.

25 Kanda M, Shimizu W, Matsuo K *et al.* Electrophysiologic characteristics and implications of induced ventricular fibrillation in symptomatic patients with Brugada syndrome. *J. Am. Coll. Cardiol.* 2002; **39**: 1799–1805.

26 Ikeda T, Sakurada H, Sakabe K *et al.* Assessment of noninvasive markers in identifying patients at risk in the Brugada syndrome: insight into risk stratification. *J. Am. Coll. Cardiol.* 2001; **37**: 1628–1634.

27 Nagase S, Fukushima Kusano K, Morita H *et al.* Epicardial

electrogram of the right ventricular outflow tract in patients with the Brugada syndrome: using the epicardial lead. *J. Am. Coll. Cardiol.* 2002; **39**: 1992–1995.

28 Fujiki A, Usui M, Nagasawa H *et al.* ST segment elevation in the right precordial leads induced with class IC antiarrhythmic drugs: insight into the mechanism of Brugada syndrome. *J. Cardiovasc. Electrophysiol.* 1999; **10**: 214–218.

29 Takami M, Ikeda T, Enjoji Y *et al.* Relationship between ST-segment morphology and conduction disturbances detected by signal-averaged electrocardiography in Brugada syndrome. *Ann. Noninvasive Electrocardiol.* 2003; **8**: 30–36.

30 Tan HL, Bink-Boelkens MT, Bezzina CR *et al.* A sodium-channel mutation causes isolated cardiac conduction disease. *Nature* 2001; **409**: 1043–1047.

31 Kyndt F, Probst V, Potet F et al. Novel *SCN5A* mutation leading either to isolated cardiac conduction defect or Brugada syndrome in a large French family. *Circulation* 2001; **104**: 3081–3086.

32 Papadatos GA, Wallerstein PMR, Head CEG *et al.* Slowed conduction and ventricular tachycardia after targeted disruption of the cardiac sodium channel gene *SCN5A*. *Proc. Natl. Acad. Sci. USA* 2002; **99**: 6210–6215.

33 Shaw RM, Rudy Y. Ionic mechanisms of propagation in cardiac tissue: roles of the sodium and L-type calcium currents during reduced excitability and decreased gap junction coupling. *Circ. Res.* 1997; **81**: 727–741.

34 Bezzina CR, Rook MB, Groenewegen WA *et al.* Compound heterozygosity for mutations (W156X and R225W) in *SCN5A* associated with severe cardiac conduction disturbances and degenerative changes in the conduction system. *Circ. Res.* 2003; **92**: 159–168.

35 Vatta M, Dumaine R, Antzelevitch C *et al.* Novel mutations in domain I of *SCN5A* cause Brugada syndrome. *Mol. Gen. Metabol.* 2002; **75**: 317–324.

36 Vatta M, Dumaine R, Varghese G *et al.* Genetic and biophysical basis of sudden unexplained nocturnal death syndrome (SUNDS), a disease allelic to Brugada syndrome. *Hum. Mol. Genet.* 2002; **11**: 337–345.

37 Wan X, Chen S, Sadeghpour A *et al.* Accelerated inactivation in a mutant Na⁺ channel associated with idiopathic ventricular fibrillation. *Am. J. Physiol.* 2001; **280**: H354–H360.

38 Mok NS, Priori SG, Napolitano C *et al.* A newly characterized *SCN5A* mutation underlying Brugada syndrome unmasked by hyperthermia. *J. Cardiovasc. Electrophysiol.* 2003; **14**: 407–411.

39 Potet F, Mabo P, Le Coq G *et al.* Novel Brugada *SCN5A* mutation leading to ST segment elevation in the inferior or the right precordial leads. *J. Cardiovasc. Electrophysiol.* 2003; **14**: 200–203.

40 Baroudi G, Acharfi S, Larouche C *et al.* Expression and intracellular localization of an *SCN5A* double mutant

R1232W/T1620M implicated in Brugada syndrome. *Circ. Res.* 2002; **90**: e11–e16.

41 Wan X, Wang Q, Kirsch GE. Functional suppression of sodium channels by β₁-subunits as a molecular mechanism of idiopathic ventricular fibrillation. *J. Mol. Cell. Cardiol.* 2000; **32**: 1873–1884.

42 Chen Q, Kirsch GE, Zhang D *et al.* Genetic basis and molecular mechanism for idiopathic ventricular fibrillation. *Nature* 1998; **392**: 293–296.

43 Deschênes I, Baroudi G, Berthet M *et al.* Electrophysiological characterization of *SCN5A* mutations causing long QT (E1784K) and Brugada (R1512W and R1432G) syndromes. *Cardiovasc. Res.* 2000; **46**: 55–65.

44 Baroudi G, Pouliot V, Denjoy I *et al.* Novel mechanism for Brugada syndrome: defective surface localization of an *SCN5A* mutant (R1432G). *Circ. Res.* 2001; **88**: e78–e83.

45 Rook MB, Bezzina Alshinawi C, Groenewegen WA *et al.* Human *SCN5A* gene mutations alter cardiac sodium channel kinetics and are associated with the Brugada syndrome. *Cardiovasc. Res.* 1999; **44**: 507–517.

46 Shirai N, Makita N, Sasaki K *et al.* A mutant cardiac sodium channel with multiple biophysical defects associated with overlapping clinical features of Brugada syndrome and cardiac conduction disease. *Cardiovasc. Res.* 2002; **53**: 348–354.

47 Baroudi G, Carbonneau, Pouliot V *et al. SCN5A* mutation (T1620M) causing Brugada syndrome exhibits different phenotypes when expressed in *Xenopus* oocytes and mammalian cells. *FEBS Lett.* 2000; **467**: 12–16.

48 Dumaine R, Towbin JA, Brugada P *et al.* Ionic mechanisms responsible for the electrocardiographic phenotype of the Brugada syndrome are temperature dependent. *Circ. Res.* 1999; **85**: 803–809.

49 Makita N, Shirai N, Wang DW *et al.* Cardiac Na⁺ channel dysfunction in Brugada syndrome is aggravated by β1-subunit. *Circulation* 2000; **101**: 54–60.

50 Akai J, Makita N, Sakurada H *et al.* A novel *SCN5A* mutation associated with idiopathic ventricular fibrillation without typical ECG findings of Brugada syndrome. *FEBS Lett.* 2000; **479**: 29–34.

51 Bezzina C, Veldkamp MW, van den Berg MP et al. A single Na⁺ channel mutation causing both long-QT and Brugada syndromes. Circ. Res. 1999; **85**: 1206–1213.

52 Baroudi G, Chahine M. Biophysical phenotypes of *SCN5A* mutations causing long QT and Brugada syndromes. *FEBS Lett.* 2000; **487**: 224–228.

53 Rivolta I, Abriel H, Tateyama M *et al.* Inherited Brugada and long QT-3 syndrome mutations of a single residue of the cardiac sodium channel confer distinct channel and clinical phenotypes. *J. Biol. Chem.* 2001; **276**: 30 623–30 630.

54 Tan HL, Kupershmidt S, Zhang R *et al.* A calcium sensor in the sodium channel modulates cardiac excitability. *Nature* 2002; **415**: 442–447.

55 Schott JJ, Alshinawi C, Kyndt F *et al.* Cardiac conduction defects associate with mutations in *SCN5A. Nature Genet.* 1999; **23**: 20–21.

56 Probst V, Kyndt F, Potet F *et al.* Haploinsufficiency in combination with aging causes *SCN5A*-linked hereditary Lenègre disease. *J. Am. Coll. Cardiol.* 2003; **41**: 643–652.

57 Wang DW, Viswanathan PC, Balser JR *et al.* Clinical, genetic, and biophysical characterization of *SCN5A* mutations associated with atrioventricular conduction block. *Circulation* 2002; **105**: 341–346.

58 Herfst LJ, Potet F, Bezzina CR *et al.* Na$^+$ channel mutation leading to loss of function and non-progressive cardiac conduction defects. *J. Mol. Cell. Cardiol.* 2003; **35**: 549–557.

59 Priori SG, Napolitano C, Gasparini M *et al.* Natural history of Brugada syndrome: insights for risk stratification and management. *Circulation* 2002; **105**: 1342–1347.

60 Priori SG, Napolitano C, Gasparini M *et al.* Clinical and genetic heterogeneity of right bundle branch block and ST-segment elevation syndrome: a prospective evaluation of 52 families. *Circulation* 2000; **102**: 2509–2515.

61 Perlmutter DH. Misfolded proteins in the endoplasmic reticulum. *Lab. Invest.* 1999; **79**: 623–638.

62 Denning GM, Anderson MP, Amara JF *et al.* Processing of mutant cystic fibrosis transmembrane conductance regulator is temperature-sensitive. *Nature* 1992; **358**: 761–764.

63 Tamarappoo BK, Verkman AS. Defective aquaporin-2 trafficking in nephrogenic diabetes insipidus and correction by chemical chaperones. *J. Clin. Invest.* 1999; **101**: 2257–2267.

64 Morello JP, Petaja-Repo UE, Bichet DG *et al.* Pharmacological chaperones: a new twist on receptor folding. *Trends Pharmacol. Sci.* 2000; **21**: 466–469.

65 Zhou Z, Gong Q, January CT. Correction of defective protein trafficking of a mutant HERG potassium channel in human long QT syndrome: pharmacological and temperature effects. *J. Biol. Chem.* 1999; **274**: 31 123–31 126.

66 Ficker E, Obejero-Paz CA, Zhao S *et al.* The binding site for channel blockers that rescue misprocessed human long QT syndrome type 2 *ether-a-gogo*-related gene (HERG) mutations. *J. Biol. Chem.* 2002; **277**: 4989–4998.

67 Loo TW, Clarke DM. Correction of defective protein kinesis of human P-glycoprotein mutants by substrates and modulators. *J. Biol. Chem.* 1997; **272**: 709–712.

68 Morello JP, Salahpour A, Laperrière A *et al.* Pharmacological chaperones rescue cell-surface expression and function of misfolded V2 vasopressin receptor mutants. *J. Clin. Invest.* 2000; **105**: 887–895.

69 Rajamani S, Anderson CL, Anson BD *et al.* Pharmacological rescue of human K$^+$ channel long-QT2 mutations:

Human Ether-a-go-go-Related Gene rescue without block. *Circulation* 2002; **105**: 2830–2835.

70 Valdivia CR, Ackerman MJ, Tester DJ *et al.* A novel *SCN5A* arrhythmia mutation, M1766L, with expression defect rescued by mexiletine. *Cardiovasc. Res.* 2002; **55**: 279–289.

71 Bezzina CR, Tan HL. Pharmacological rescue of mutant ion channels. *Cardiovasc. Res.* 2002; **55**: 229–232.

72 Priori SG, Napolitano C, Schwartz PJ *et al.* The elusive link between LQT3 and Brugada syndrome: the role of flecainide challenge. *Circulation* 2000; **102**: 945–947.

73 Kambouris NG, Nuss HB, Johns DC *et al.* A revised view of cardiac sodium channel 'blockade' in the long-QT syndrome. *J. Clin. Invest.* 2000; **105**: 1133–1140.

74 Pu J, Balser JR, Boyden PA. Lidocaine action on Na$^+$ currents in ventricular myocytes from the epicardial border zone of the infarcted heart. *Circ. Res.* 1998; **83**: 431–440.

75 Zareba W, Sattari MN, Rosero S *et al.* Altered atrial, atrioventricular, and ventricular conduction in patients with the long QT syndrome caused by the ΔKPQ *SCN5A* sodium channel gene mutation. *Am. J. Cardiol.* 2001; **88**: 1311–1314.

76 Benhorin J, Taub R, Goldmit M *et al.* Effects of flecainide in patients with new *SCN5A* mutation: mutation-specific therapy for Long-QT syndrome? *Circulation* 2000; **101**: 1698–1706.

77 Van den Berg MP, Wilde AAM, Viersma TJW *et al.* Possible bradycardic mode of death and successful pacemaker treatment in a large family with features of long QT syndrome type 3 and Brugada syndrome. *J. Cardiovasc. Electrophysiol.* 2001; **12**: 630–636.

78 Veldkamp MW, Wilders R, Baartscheer A *et al.* Contribution of sodium channel mutations to bradycardia and sinus node dysfunction in LQT3 families. *Circ. Res.* 2003; **92**: 976–983.

79 Lee KL, Lau CP, Tse HF *et al.* Prevention of ventricular fibrillation by pacing in a man with Brugada syndrome. *J. Cardiovasc. Electrophysiol.* 2000; **11**: 935–937.

80 Brugada J, Brugada R, Antzelevitch C *et al.* Long-term follow-up of individuals with the electrocardigraphic pattern of right bundle-branch block and ST-segment elevation in precordial leads V$_1$ to V$_3$. *Circulation* 2002; **105**: 73–78.

81 Matsuo K, Akahoshi M, Seto S *et al.* Disappearance of the Brugada-type electrocardiogram after surgical castration: a role for testosterone and an explanation for the male preponderance. *Pacing Clin. Electrophysiol.* 2003; **26**: 1551–1553.

82 Bidoggia H, Maciel JP, Capalozza N *et al.* Sex differences on the electrocardiographic pattern of cardiac repolarization: possible role of testosterone. *Am. Heart J.* 2000; **140**: 678–683.

83 Pham TV, Rosen MR. Sex, hormones, and repolarization. *Cardiovasc. Res.* 2002; **53**: 740–751.

84 Verkerk AO, Wilders R, Tan HL. Gender differences in cardiac electrophysiology. In: *Proceedings of the 25th Annual International Conference of the IEEE Engineering in Medicine and Biology Society*. 2003: 44–47.

85 Pham TV, Robinson RB, Danilo P *et al*. Effects of gonadal steroids on gender-related differences in transmural dispersion of L-type calcium current. *Cardiovasc. Res.* 2002; **53**: 752–762.

86 DiDiego JM, Cordeiro JM, Goodrow RJ *et al*. Ionic and cellular basis for the predominance of the Brugada syndrome phenotype in males. *Circulation* 2002; **106**: 2004–2011.

87 Saura D, Garcia-Alberola A, Carrillo P *et al*. Brugada-like electrocardiographic pattern induced by fever. *Pacing Clin. Electrophysiol.* 2002; **25**: 856–859.

CHAPTER 4

Molecular genetics of the Brugada syndrome

E. Schulze-Bahr, MD, *L. Eckardt,* MD, *M. Paul,* MD, *T. Wichter,* MD, *G. Breithardt,* MD

Epidemiology of the Brugada syndrome

In approximately 5–10% of survivors of cardiac arrest due to ventricular fibrillation (VF), no structural abnormality of the heart is found after thorough investigation. It has been suggested that Brugada syndrome accounts for approximately 20% of such cases, previously classified as having 'idiopathic VF'.[1–3] A genetic basis of the disease has been suggested because of the description of families with an autosomal dominant mode of inheritance. However, in the majority of patients Brugada syndrome appears to be sporadic.[27] The first cases were reported as early as 50 years ago.[4,5]

Two reports[6,7] have described small series of patients with apparent idiopathic ventricular fibrillation and the distinctive ECG pattern which is now referred to as the Brugada syndrome, a new clinical entity. The typical ECG pattern may be permanent, transient, or latent. In the latter two manifestations, pharmacologic challenge with sodium channel blocking agents may unmask the ECG phenotype.[8–10] Since this effect has been described, an increasing number of patients has been recognized worldwide. A comparable syndrome that is characterized by similar ECG patterns and nocturnal, sudden cardiac death (previously referred to as SUNDS, sudden unexpected nocturnal death syndrome)[11] is one of the leading causes for sudden cardiac death in young males from Southeast Asia. In a series of population-based studies, mostly from Southeast Asia, the frequency of the Brugada ECG pattern in asymptomatic individuals was investigated. In one study, the ECG changes were found in 98 of 13 929 study

subjects (0.70%). However, the diagnostic Type 1 ECG (coved-type ECG in Brugada syndrome)[12] was only found in 0.12% of subjects, predominantly in males, and resulted in a relative frequency of 0.38% in the male population.[13] Similar observations were reported by other Japanese investigators, demonstrating that the disease is rare, but more prevalent than anticipated previously.[14–16] Upon investigation of 4788 Japanese subjects below the age of 50 years, Matsuo *et al.* estimated the prevalence and incidence as 146.2 in 100 000 persons and 14.2 persons per 100 000 person-years, respectively. The incidence in males was nine times higher than in women and the Brugada-type ECG was found in 26% of subjects who died unexpectedly.[14] Taken together, in well-investigated populations, the prevalence of the Type I ECG appears to be between 0.05 and 0.15% in asymptomatic individuals, but population-specific differences may be relevant. Since in these studies, not all patients with the saddleback ECG (Type II ECG) were challenged with sodium channel blocking agents and, thus, conversion into the diagnostic Type I ECG is unknown, the prevalence of Brugada syndrome may be still higher than assumed.

Genetics of the Brugada syndrome

A genetic basis for Brugada syndrome became evident by the detection of mutations in the cardiac sodium channel gene *SCN5A* in familial Brugada syndrome[17] and by the identification of a second disease locus (Fig. 4.1).[18] The first and only gene for Brugada syndrome, *SCN5A*, is predicted to encode for the α subunit of the cardiac sodium channel

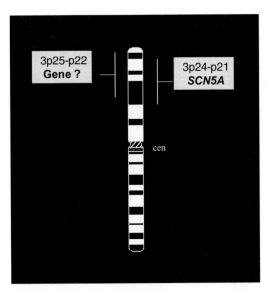

Figure 4.1 Chromosomal loci associated with autosomal dominant Brugada syndrome. Right, BrS-1 locus;[17] left, BrS-2 locus (gene unknown).[44] Despite obvious overlapping, the *SCN5A* gene has been excluded as a candidate for BrS-2 by linkage analysis.[44]

gene.[19] More than 40 mutations in *SCN5A* have been linked to Brugada syndrome since 1998. Interestingly, mutations in *SCN5A* are multiply linked to other arrhythmias, namely the long QT 3 syndrome (Mendelian Inheritance in Man (MIM) entry #603 830),[20] cardiac conduction disease (MIM #113 900, PCCD2, and MIM #115 080),[21,22] and atrial stillstand.[23] Therefore, *SCN5A* mutations may exhibit a variety of electrophysiologic mechanisms in the heart to cause different or overlapping phenotypes of arrhythmias. The observation that *SCN5A* (28 exons, 80 kb on a genomic contig) mutations on chromosome 3p25-p21 are linked to this syndrome[17] supports the hypothesis that it is a channelopathy due to inherited structural defects of cardiac ion channels. Bezzina *et al.* presented a large, eight-generation Dutch family with a specific *SCN5A* mutation (1795insD) and a history of sudden death, most of which had occurred at night.[24,25] Some living members of this family demonstrated ECG features compatible with both Brugada syndrome and QT-prolongation characteristic of LQT-3 syndrome. *SCN5A* gene mutations have also been

found in the Southeast Asian SUNDS, thus confirming the hypothesis that this syndrome[11,26] is in close relationship (or possibly identical) with Brugada syndrome.

Familial Brugada syndrome typically has an autosomal dominant mode of inheritance. Recessive forms have not been reported to date, but may be indistinguishable without further molecular evidence from 'sporadic disease', which is defined as absence of disease in parents and other relatives. Sporadic cases of Brugada syndrome account for 60–70% of patients. Very recently, we were able to demonstrate the absence of a *SCN5A* gene mutation after complete sequencing in 27 unrelated probands with *sporadic* Brugada syndrome.[27] In our study, the disease was familial in 37%, whereas in the majority it was sporadic (63%). Five novel *SCN5A* mutations (three nonsense, one in-frame deletion, one missense mutation) were found and were randomly located in *SCN5A*. Mutation frequencies (*SCN5A+*) differed significantly between familial (38%) and sporadic disease (0%) ($p = 0.001$). Thus, the molecular (or pathophysiologic) basis for Brugada syndrome remains unclear after exclusion of cardiac, non-cardiac, and molecular (*SCN5A* gene) causes for the disease and we proposed that reasons other than genetic reasons also may account for sporadic disease. In addition, no gene mutations have been reported by others in sporadic Brugada syndrome so far. These results are in line with a possible genetic and clinical heterogeneity of Brugada syndrome.

To date, over 60 different *SCN5A* (BrS-1) mutations have been reported and they can be found at http://pc4.fsm.it: 81/cardmoc/. There were no mutational hotspots in the *SCN5A* gene (Fig. 4.2). Moreover, and surprisingly, since the predominant functional mechanisms of *SCN5A* mutations in BS-1 appears to be a reduction in sodium current (I_{Na}) density, causative mutations (resulting in haploinsufficiency) were not clustered to specific functional sodium channel domains. Because they are scattered throughout the gene, a mutation analysis requires the inclusion of the entire coding sequences of *SCN5A*, making a genetic screen time- and cost-consuming. However, gross recombinational events at the *SCN5A* locus or promotor mutations may still be present after careful sequence analysis and cannot be excluded for technical reasons. Mutations (see Table 4.1) include in one-third

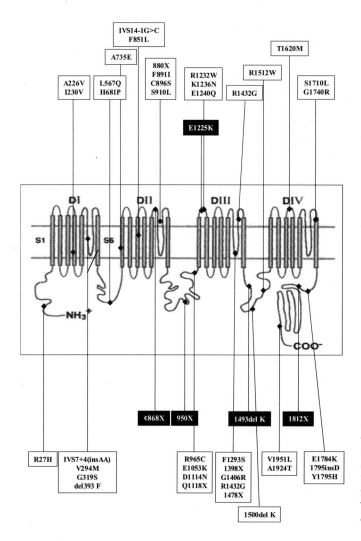

Figure 4.2 Predicted protein structure of the *SCN5A* protein encoding the cardiac Na⁺ ion channel α-subunit. Localization of mutations found in BrS-1. The black boxes show the mutations identified by Schulze-Bahr, Eckardt, Breithardt *et al.*[27] There is an obvious random distribution of disease mutations.

of cases a frameshift, deletion, and other mutations that cause failure of the channel to express, and missense mutations in the remaining cases shift the voltage and time dependence of I_{Na} activation, inactivation, and reactivation. Some mutations appeared to influence sodium channel function in a temperature-dependent manner. This may be related to premature inactivation of the sodium channels being accelerated even further at higher temperature.[28] Clinical manifestations with severe arrhythmias in Brugada syndrome may be uncovered or facilitated during a febrile state in some patients and may lead to specific recommendations for Brugada syndrome patients during fever.

Taken together, more than 20 expressed *SCN5A*

mutants have been studied in heterologous expression systems and resulted in a loss of channel function due either to:

- *quantitative reduction* of functional sodium channels (failure to express, e.g., retention in the endoplasmic reticulum)
- *qualitative alterations* of sodium channel function due to shifts in kinetics (e.g., voltage- and time-dependence of I_{Na} activation, inactivation, reactivation, or access to an intermediate state of inactivation or accelerated inactivation).

Of future interest is the notion of polymorphic sites at the *SCN5A* locus (Table 4.2). To date, over 20 sites are known and only half of them are neutral, i.e., do not change the amino acid composition of the

Table 4.1 Mutations in the cardiac sodium channel gene *SCN5A* associated with BrS-1.

Nucleotide change	Amino acid change	Alteration type	Region	Mutation phenotype
G80A	R27H	Missense	N-terminus	BrS
G253A	G35S	Missense	N-terminus	BrS
G461A	R104Q	Missense	N-terminus	BrS
n.g.	K126E	Missense	DI-S1	BrS
n.g.	E161K	Missense	DI	BrS
C677T	A226V	Missense	DI-S4	BrS
A688G	I230V	Missense	DI-S4	BrS
Ins AAint 7	IVS7DS + 4	Splice error	DI-S5-S6	BrS
G845A	R282H	Missense	DI-S5-S6	BrS
G880A	V294M	Missense	DI-S5-S6	BrS
2581–2582delTT	F861fs950X	Frameshift	DII-5	BrS
G995A	G319S	Missense	DI-S5-S6	BrS
—	G351V	Missense	DI-S5-S6	BrS
G1100A	R367H	Missense	DI-S5-S6	SUNDS
n.g.	R367C	Missense	DI-S5-S6	BrS
n.g.	M369K	Missense	DI-S5-S6	BrS
1177–1179del	393delF	Deletion	DI-S6	BrS
1479del	493delK	Deletion	DI-DII	BrS
n.g.	R535X	Nonsense	DI-DII	BrS
G1663A	E555K	Missense	DI-DII	BrS
T1700A	L567Q	Missense	DI-DII	SIDS
A2042C	H681P	Missense	DI-DII	BrS
n.g.	A735V	Missense	DI-S1	SUNDS
C2204A	A735E	Missense	DI-S1	BrS
IVS14–1G > C	n.g.	Splice Error	DII-S2	BrS
n.g.	G752R	Missense	DII-S2	BrS
T2552C	F851L	Missense	DII-S5	BrS
2602delC	E868X	Nonsense	DII-S5	BrS
2613delC	S871fsX880	Frameshift	DII-S5-S6	BrS
T2674A	F891I	Missense	DII-S5-S6	BrS
T2686A	C896S	Missense	DII-S5-S6	BrS
C2729T	S910L	Missense	DII-S5-S6	BrS
n.g.	D951X	Nonsense	DII-DIII	BrS
C2893T	R965C	Missense	DII-DIII	BrS
G3157A	E1053K	Missense	DII-DIII	BrS
G3340A	D1114N	Missense	DII-DIII	BS/LQT3
C3352T	Q1118X	Nonsense	DII-DIII	BrS
n.g.	E1225K	Missense	DIII-S1	BrS
n.g.	R1232W	Missense	DIII-S1-S2	BrS
G3708T	K1236N	Missense	DIII-S1-S2	BrS
G3718C	E1240Q	Missense	DIII-S2	BrS
3816delG	n.g.	Frameshift	DIII-S3	BrS
T3887C	F1293S	Missense	DIII-S3-S4	BrS
n.g.	G1319V	Missense	DIII-S4-S5	BrS
n.g.	S1382I	Missense	DIII-S5-S6	BrS
4190delA	V1398X	Nonsense	DIII-S5-S6	BrS
n.g.	V1405L	Missense	DIII-S5-S6	BrS
A4372T	G1406R	Missense	DIII-S5-S6	BS/CCD
A1294G	R1432G	Missense	DIII-S5-S6	BrS

continued on p.46

Table 4.1 *Continued*

Nucleotide change	Amino acid change	Alteration type	Region	Mutation phenotype
4402–4406del	G1467fs + 13X	Frameshift	DIII-S6	BrS
4477–4479delAAG	I493delK	Deletion	DIII-DIV	BrS
4498–4500del	K1500del	Deletion	DIII-DIV	BrS/LQT3/CCD
n.g.	G1502S	Missense	DIII-DIV	BrS
C5434T	R1512W	Missense	DIII-DIV	BrS
	T1620M	Missense	DIV-S3-S4	BrS
n.g.	S1710L	Missense	DIV-S5-S6	IVF
IVS21 + 1G > A	n.g.	Splice error	DIV-S5-S6	BrS
G5218A	G1740R	Missense	DIV-S5-S6	BrS
n.g.	G1743E	Missense	DIV-S6	BrS
G5227A	G1743R	Missense	DIV-S6	BrS
G5350A	E1784K	Missense	C-terminus	BrS
Ins TGA 5537	1795 insD	Insertion	C-terminus	BrS/LQT3
C5383C	Y1795H	Missense	C-terminus	BrS
C5425A	S1812X	Nonsense	C-terminus	BrS
n.g.	A1924T	Missense	C-terminus	BrS
G5851T	V1951L	Missense	C-terminus	BrS

n.g., exact information not given/available.

Table 4.2 Polymorphisms and allele frequencies in the cardiac sodium channel gene *SCN5A*.

Nucleotide change	Amino acid change	Mutation type	Region	Allele frequency
G87A	A29A	Neutral	N-terminus	n.g.
C100T	R34C	Missense	N-terminus	0.04
T360G	V120I	Missense	DI-S1	n.g.
n.g.	A180G	Missense	DI-S2	n.g.
T840C	C280C	Missense	N-terminus	n.g.
C1017T	Y339Y	Neutral	DI-S5-S6	n.g.
C1654G	R552G	Missense	DI-DII	n.g.
A1673G	H558R	Missense	DI-DII	0.08–0.16
C1917G	G639G	Neutral	DI-DII	n.g.
A2010C	T670T	Neutral	DI-DII	n.g.
G2182A	V728I	Missense	DII S1	n.g.
A2667C	L889L	Neutral	DII-S5-S6	n.g.
C2961G	H987Q	Missense	DII-DIII	n.g.
A3080G	Q1027R	Missense	DII-DIII	n.g.
C3269T	P1090L	Missense	DII-DIII	0.04
G3578A	R1193Q	Missense	DII-DIII	n.g.
T3723C	Y1241Y	Neutral	DII-S5-S6	n.g.
G3873A	L1291L	Neutral	DIII-S4-S5	n.g.
4299 + 53 T > C	Intron 12	Neutral	DIII-S4-S5	0.27
G4500T	K1500N	Neutral	DIII-DIV	n.g.
C4509T	S1503S	Neutral	DIII-DIV	n.g.
C5454T	A1818A	Neutral	C-terminus	n.g.
C5457T	D1819D	Neutral	C-terminus	0.46
G5851T	V1951L	Missense	C-terminus	0.005

n.g., exact information not given/available.

sodium channel. With the exception of the intron 12, the alterations are non-synonymous and, therefore, change the amino acid residues. However, the use of these polymorphisms, e.g., in the setting of association studies, is unknown because the majority have not been systematically investigated (population specificity, allele frequencies, functional effects). Recently, a possible functional relevance was shown for the H558R variant. This variant had first been reported from a sample of patients with acquired long-QT syndrome (LQTS) in whom it did not appear to alter I_{Na} and to have a role in the acquired LQTS phenotype.[29] The 558R allele was also identified in a family with cardiac conduction disease resulting from the *SCN5A* mutation T512I; co-dominant expression of both mutant alleles suggested a modifying aggravating effect of the 558R.[30] Very recently, the common polymorphism H558R together with the LQT3 mutation M1766L markedly reduced I_{Na} current and the double-mutation M1766L/H558R only in presence of a newly cloned *SCN5A* contig background where the 558R allele naturally occurred.[31] Therefore, it is important to know the exact sequence and function of channels most commonly present in human myocardium. The H558R polymorphism was also studied in context of a shorter 2015 amino acid splice *SCN5A* variant lacking glutamine at position 1077 (Q1077del) (65% of the transcript in human hearts). When H558R was present with Q1077 ([H558R]), current expression was profoundly reduced despite normal trafficking to the cell surface. Thus, four variant sequences of *SCN5A* are commonly present in human myocardium and they exhibit functional differences among themselves and with the previous standard clone. The authors concluded that their results might have implications for the choice of background sequence for experiments with heterologous expression systems, and possibly have implications for electrophysiological function *in vivo* of polymorphisms.[32]

Relationship of Brugada syndrome with other arrhythmogenic syndromes

Idiopathic ventricular fibrillation (IVF) is defined as VF in the setting of an unexplained cardiac arrest in the absence of demonstrable, structural heart disease or other promoting conditions such as drugs, electrolyte disturbances, or metabolic abnormalities. In contrast to Brugada syndrome, the baseline ECG is usually normal. A life-time prevalence of 1 in 20 000 for IVF has been estimated; it accounts for approximately 6–12% of all sudden deaths, particularly in individuals below the age of 40 years. In a review by Viskin and Belhassen, 54 patients fulfilled the criteria for idiopathic VF and over 90% of them had required resuscitation (mean age 36 years, with a gender predominance of males). Available data showed a 69% inducibility of sustained VT/VF and an 11% rate of sudden death within 1 year of diagnosis.[3] The pathogenetic mechanisms of idiopathic VF are scarcely understood. Only a few reports of families with IVF exist that may give evidence for a genetic cause. McRae *et al.* described a family in which three brothers had syncopal attacks and died suddenly at young age. In addition, autopsy in two of them showed no abnormality. A fourth brother had syncopal episodes that proved to be due to paroxysmal ventricular fibrillation induced by stressful emotional stimuli. The mother had also experienced several episodes of syncope precipitated by an emotionally stressful event. Two patients (mother and one son) had a short PR interval in the surface ECG. A gene mutation probably linked to IVF has been reported by Akai *et al.* who recently described a novel missense mutation in the *SCN5A* gene (S1710L) in a sporadical proband with IVF. No typical ECG features of Brugada syndrome or of long-QT syndrome were seen.[33] Heterologously expressed S1710L sodium channels showed a marked acceleration in the I_{Na} current decay together with a large hyperpolarizing shift of steady-state inactivation and depolarizing shift of activation. This observation suggests that mutations in the *SCN5A* gene also may be responsible for IVF in addition to Brugada syndrome or LQT3[33] and that IVF in patients with apparently normal hearts indeed may represent a 'primary electrical disease' of the heart.

Catecholaminergic ventricular tachycardias are a rare form of arrhythmogenic disorders that typically are stress-induced and have a bidirectional or polymorphic pattern (CPVT).[34] These ventricular tachycardias may degenerate into VF. Mutations in the gene encoding the cardiac ryanodine receptor (*RyR2*) or in the *Calsequestrin* gene (*CASQ2*), encoding a calcium-storage protein within the endoplasmic reticulum, were identified in probands affected by the disease.[45,46] A recent study by Priori *et al.* also identified *RyR2* mutations in two of four probands with catecholaminergic IVF, leading to the conclusion that CPVT is clinically and genetically heterogeneous and may manifest severely beyond pediatric age with a spectrum of stress-related ventricular arrhythmias, including IVF.[35]

Beyond altered ion channel function as cause for IVF, other defects may include impairment of cellular, metabolic, or biochemical function, providing a different substrate for electrical instability. In this line, some subtle cardiac abnormalities may be related to minimal structural abnormalities or early disease stages of entities known to be associated with ventricular tachyarrhythmias and sudden cardiac death (i.e., myocarditis or forms of cardiomyopathy). The incidence of such undetermined structural heart disease in cases of so-called 'idiopathic VF' is, however, not known, but subtle morphological alterations may be more frequent and, especially for arrhythmogenic right ventricular cardiomyopathy (ARVC), may cause a similar disease pattern.[36] ARVC is a primary myocardial disorder of unknown origin that is characterized by localized or diffuse replacement by fatty and fibrous tissue predominately in the right ventricular myocardium. It usually manifests with ventricular tachyarrhythmias (left bundle branch block type) and/or sudden cardiac death, frequently before structural abnormalities become apparent (for a review see Ref. 37). A diagnostic scoring system of ARVC, including major and minor criteria, has been proposed by an International Task Force for ARVC.[38] In about 30% the family history will be informative for other individuals with ARVC and a genetic basis can be assumed. So far, a variety of ARVC loci have been reported and, so far, only three genes (autosomal dominant form involving the ARVC2 gene or ryanodine receptor 2 gene; the desmoplakin gene; and an autosomal recessive form involving plakoglobin (Naxos disease)) are known. Of interest, ARVC2 patients presented with an atypical form characterized by catecholaminergic polymorphic VT and only minimal structural abnormalities of the right ventricle.[39,40] Therefore, ARVC2 and CPVT1 are allelic disorders caused by mutations in the *RyR2* gene. It may be difficult on a clinical level to differentiate between these two disorders, since CPVT has no structural cardiac abnor-

malities. Routine genetic testing of ARVC is presently not available, but with further improvements in molecular genetics, genetic testing for disease causing mutations may become part of diagnosis and possibly for risk stratification. Since cardiac imaging techniques as well as endomyocardial biopsies mostly revealed no signs of a structural heart disease, Brugada syndrome is considered to be a 'primary electrical heart disease', but detailed information from thorough morphological evaluation is still sparse. Although there has been a debate whether Brugada syndrome is associated with distinct structural abnormalities of the right ventricle resembling those found in ARVC,[36] no association to any of the ARVC chromosomal loci has been described for Brugada syndrome so far. To date, on the clinical as well as on the molecular level, the two diseases therefore may represent separate entities.

In addition to the related conditions, a role of Brugada syndrome for sudden death in children and, particularly, for the sudden infant death syndrome (SIDS) has been raised by Priori *et al.*[35] who reported on a family with a high incidence of sudden cardiac death with early onset (2–14 months of age). In five children of the same family who died after unexplained cardiac arrest, Brugada syndrome was suspected based on typical electrocardiographic pattern in only one of them. A missense mutation in the *SCN5A* gene was identified in four family members including a 3-year old girl with ventricular fibrillation, suggesting that Brugada syndrome or IVF was the cause for sudden cardiac death in these severely affected children.[35] Independent of this finding, other reports showed that mutations in the cardiac sodium channel gene *SCN5A* are also associated with LQTS and early onset of ventricular tachycardia in neonates.[41]

Value of genetic testing in Brugada syndrome

The opportunity for genetic testing in Brugada syndrome offers additional diagnostic features, but with some limitations. Mutation screening of the *SCN5A* gene in patients with Brugada syndrome may only support a clinical overt or suspicious diagnosis, but obviously cannot make the diagnosis itself. This is directly related to a growing number of observations in genotyped patients with arrhythmogenic disorders that are characterized by:

- variable clinical expressivity (meaning that mutation carriers may have mild to severe signs of disease)
- incomplete penetrance (meaning that mutation carriers may have no phenotypic signs of disease)
- multiple alleles (meaning that mutation carriers may have other arrhythmogenic disease, e.g., progressive cardiac conduction disease or LQT3 syndrome).

Therefore, a positive genetic test result can only be part of the diagnostic approach in Brugada syndrome, as it has to be seen in the complete clinical picture particularly including medical history, electrocardiographic, and electrophysiologic recordings. This limited importance of genetic testing in the diagnostic evaluation for Brugada syndrome is disregarded and genetic testing is widely overscored in the physician's and patient's opinion.

In addition, our own investigations showed that only a minority of patients will be able to be genotyped to date. This refers to the fact that the cardiac sodium channel gene *SCN5A* is the only known gene for Brugada syndrome so far and only 10–15% of all patients will harbour a disease mutation in that gene.[27] Patients with a positive family history for Brugada syndrome have a significantly higher incidence (38%) for identification of an *SCN5A* gene mutation than sporadic probands (having a negative family history) for which we were unable to identify a genetic basis (0%).[27] Since the latter group still represents the majority of cases, a role for genetic testing in sporadic Brugada syndrome is currently not useful and remains a diagnostic challenge for the future.

To our mind, genetic testing of the *SCN5A* gene in Brugada syndrome may be useful:

- to further substantiate the clinical diagnosis
- to differentiate borderline cases (e.g., with an atypical right bundle branch block) or individuals with an overlapping phenotype (cardiac conduction disease or LQT3) from patients with Brugada syndrome
- to identify threatened individuals in high-risk families by advanced genetic testing; in this particular situation, asymptomatic patients having mild or no signs of Brugada syndrome will be accurately recognized and should be further monitored by adult and/or pediatric cardiologists.

For risk stratification in Brugada syndrome, there is currently no need for genotyping. In a study reported by Priori *et al.*, in 200 patients (152 men, 48 women; age, 41 ± 18 years) a genetic analysis was performed and 28 of 130 unrelated probands were *SCN5A+*. During multivariate analysis, it turned out that gender, family history of sudden death, and presence of a *SCN5A* mutation were not associated with a higher risk of cardiac arrest.[42] These results require further confirmation in other study populations. Recently, another study focussed on conduction abnormalities in Brugada syndrome causing distinct genotype–phenotype relations.[43] When ECG features of 23 unrelated Brugada syndrome probands with and 54 unrelated probands without an identified *SCN5A* mutation were compared, *SCN5A+* carriers had a significantly longer PQ interval on the baseline ECG and a significantly longer HV time.[43] A PQ interval of more than 210 ms and an HV interval of more than 60 ms allowed the identification of *SCN5A* carriers. These criteria might be used for stratified genotyping in future.

Supported in part by grants from Deutsche Forschungsgemeinschaft (DFG; Schu1082/3–1), Bonn, Germany and Fondation Leducq, Paris, France.

References

1 Alings M, Wilde A. 'Brugada' syndrome: clinical data and suggested pathophysiological mechanism. *Circulation* 1999; **99**: 666–673.

2 Remme CA, Wever EF, Wilde AA, Derksen R, Hauer RN. Diagnosis and long-term follow-up of the Brugada syndrome in patients with idiopathic ventricular fibrillation. *Eur. Heart J.* 2001; **22**: 400–409.

3 Viskin S, Fish R, Eldar M *et al.* Prevalence of the Brugada sign in idiopathic ventricular fibrillation and healthy controls. *Heart* 2000; **84**: 31–36.

4 Osher H, Wolff L. Electrocardiographic pattern simulating acute myocardial injury. *Am. J. Med. Sci.* 1953; **226**: 541–545.

5 Eideken J. Elevation of RS-T segment, apparent or real in right precordial leads as probale normal variant. *Am. Heart J.* 1954; **48**: 331–339.

6 Nava A, Martini B, Thiene G *et al.* [Arrhythmogenic right ventricular dysplasia. Study of a selected population]. *G. Ital. Cardiol.* 1988; **18**: 2–9.

7 Brugada P, Brugada J. Right bundle branch block, persistent ST segment elevation and sudden cardiac death: a distinct clinical and electrocardiographic syndrome. *J. Am. Coll. Cardiol.* 1992; **20**: 1391–1396.

8 Brugada J, Brugada P. Further characterization of the syndrome of right bundle branch block, ST segment elevation, and sudden cardiac death. *J. Cardiovasc. Electrophysiol.* 1997; **8**: 325–331.

9 Brugada J, Brugada R, Brugada P. Pharmacological and device approach to therapy of inherited cardiac diseases associated with cardiac arrhythmias and sudden death. *J. Electrocardiol.* 2000; **33** Suppl: 41–47.

10 Rolf S, Bruns HJ, Wichter T *et al.* The ajmaline challenge in Brugada syndrome: diagnostic impact, safety, and recommended protocol. *Eur. Heart J.* 2003; **24**: 1104–1112.

11 Nademanee K, Veerakul G, Nimmannit S *et al.* Arrhythmogenic marker for the sudden unexplained death syndrome in Thai men. *Circulation* 1997; **96**: 2595–2600.

12 Wilde AA, Antzelevitch C, Borggrefe M *et al.* Proposed diagnostic criteria for the Brugada syndrome: consensus report. *Circulation* 2002; **106**: 2514–2519.

13 Miyasaka Y, Tsuji H, Yamada K *et al.* Prevalence and mortality of the Brugada-type electrocardiogram in one city in Japan. *J. Am. Coll. Cardiol.* 2001; **38**: 771–774.

14 Matsuo K, Akahoshi M, Nakashima E *et al.* The prevalence, incidence and prognostic value of the Brugada-type electrocardiogram: a population-based study of four decades. *J. Am. Coll. Cardiol.* 2001; **38**: 765–770.

15 Furuhashi M, Uno K, Tsuchihashi K *et al.* Prevalence of asymptomatic ST segment elevation in right precordial leads with right bundle branch block (Brugada-type ST shift) among the general Japanese population. *Heart* 2001; **86**: 161–166.

16 Hermida JS, Lemoine JL, Aoun FB, Jarry G, Rey JL, Quiret JC. Prevalence of the Brugada syndrome in an apparently healthy population. *Am. J. Cardiol.* 2000; **86**: 91–94.

17 Chen Q, Kirsch GE, Zhang D *et al.* Genetic basis and molecular mechanism for idiopathic ventricular fibrillation. *Nature* 1998; **392**: 293–296.

18 Weiss R, Barmada MM, Nguyen T *et al.* Clinical and molecular heterogeneity in the Brugada syndrome: a novel gene locus on chromosome 3. *Circulation* 2002; **105**: 707–713.

19 Gellens ME, George AL, Jr., Chen LQ *et al.* Primary structure and functional expression of the human cardiac tetrodotoxin-insensitive voltage-dependent sodium channel. *Proc. Natl. Acad. Sci. USA* 1992; **89**: 554–558.

20 Wang Q, Shen J, Splawski I *et al.* SCN5A mutations associated with an inherited cardiac arrhythmia, long QT syndrome. *Cell* 1995; **80**: 805–811.

21 Schott JJ, Alshinawi C, Kyndt F *et al.* Cardiac conduction defects associate with mutations in SCN5A. *Nat. Genet.* 1999; **23**: 20–21.

22 Tan HL, Bink-Boelkens MT, Bezzina CR *et al.* A sodium-channel mutation causes isolated cardiac conduction disease. *Nature* 2001; **409**: 1043–1047.

23 Groenewegen WA, Firouzi M, Bezzina CR *et al.* A cardiac sodium channel mutation cosegregates with a rare connexin40 genotype in familial atrial standstill. *Circ. Res.* 2003; **92**: 14–22.

24 Bezzina C, Veldkamp MW, van Den Berg MP *et al* A single Na(+) channel mutation causing both long-QT and Brugada syndromes. *Circ. Res.* 1999; **85**: 1206–1213.

25 Veldkamp MW, Viswanathan PC, Bezzina C, Baartscheer A, Wilde AA, Balser JR. Two distinct congenital arrhythmias evoked by a multidysfunctional Na(+) channel. *Circ. Res.* 2000; **86**: E91–E97.

26 Vatta M, Dumaine R, Varghese G *et al.* Genetic and biophysical basis of sudden unexplained nocturnal death syndrome (SUNDS), a disease allelic to Brugada syndrome. *Hum. Mol. Genet.* 2002; **11**: 337–345.

27 Schulze-Bahr E, Eckardt L, Breithardt G *et al.* Sodium channel gene (SCN5A) mutations in 44 index patients with Brugada syndrome. Different incidences in familial and sporadic disease. *Hum. Mutat.* 2003; Mutation In Brief, #615 (online).

28 Dumaine R, Towbin JA, Brugada P *et al.* Ionic mechanisms responsible for the electrocardiographic phenotype of the Brugada syndrome are temperature dependent. *Circ. Res.* 1999; **85**: 803–809.

29 Yang P, Kanki H, Drolet B *et al.* Allelic variants in long-QT disease genes in patients with drug-associated torsades de pointes. *Circulation* 2002; **105**: 1943–1948.

30 Viswanathan PC, Benson DW, Balser JR. A common SCN5A polymorphism modulates the biophysical effects of an SCN5A mutation. *J. Clin. Invest.* 2003; **111**: 341–346.

31 Ye B, Valdivia CR, Ackerman MJ, Makielski JC. A common human SCN5A polymorphism modifies expression of an arrhythmia causing mutation. *Physiol. Genomics* 2003; **12**: 187–193.

32 Makielski JC, Ye B, Valdivia CR *et al.* A ubiquitous splice variant and a common polymorphism affect heterologous expression of recombinant human SCN5A heart sodium channels. *Circ. Res.* 2003; **93**: 821–828.

33 Akai J, Makita N, Sakurada H *et al.* A novel SCN5A mutation associated with idiopathic ventricular fibrillation without typical ECG findings of Brugada syndrome. *FEBS Lett.* 2000; **479**: 29–34.

34 Leenhardt A, Lucet V, Denjoy I, Grau F, Ngoc DD, Coumel P. Catecholaminergic polymorphic ventricular tachycardia in children. A 7-year follow-up of 21 patients. *Circulation* 1995; **91**: 1512–1519.

35 Priori SG, Napolitano C, Giordano U, Collisani G, Memmi M. Brugada syndrome and sudden cardiac death in children. *Lancet* 2000; **355**: 808–809.

36 Corrado D, Basso C, Buja G, Nava A, Rossi L, Thiene G. Right bundle branch block, right precordial ST-segment elevation, and sudden death in young people. *Circulation* 2001; **103**: 710–717.

37 Wichter T, Schulze-Bahr E, Eckardt L *et al*. Molecular mechanisms of inherited ventricular arrhythmias. *Herz* 2002; **27**: 712–739.

38 McKenna WJ, Thiene G, Nava A *et al*. Diagnosis of arrhythmogenic right ventricular dysplasia/cardiomyopathy. Task Force of the Working Group Myocardial and Pericardial Disease of the European Society of Cardiology and of the Scientific Council on Cardiomyopathies of the International Society and Federation of Cardiology. *Br. Heart J.* 1994; **71**: 215–218.

39 Rampazzo A, Nava A, Erne P *et al*. A new locus for arrhythmogenic right ventricular cardiomyopathy (ARVD2) maps to chromosome 1q42-q43. *Hum. Mol. Genet.* 1995; **4**: 2151–2154.

40 Tiso N, Stephan DA, Nava A *et al*. Identification of mutations in the cardiac ryanodine receptor gene in families affected with arrhythmogenic right ventricular cardiomyopathy type 2 (ARVD2). *Hum. Mol. Genet.* 2001; **10**: 189–194.

41 Wedekind H, Smits JP, Schulze-Bahr E *et al*. De novo muta-

tion in the *SCN5A* gene associated with early onset of sudden infant death. *Circulation* 2001; **104**: 1158–1164.

42 Priori SG, Napolitano C, Gasparini M *et al*. Natural history of Brugada syndrome: insights for risk stratification and management. *Circulation* 2002; **105**: 1342–1347.

43 Smits JP, Eckardt L, Probst V *et al*. Genotype–phenotype relationship in Brugada syndrome: electrocardiographic features differentiate *SCN5A*-related patients from non-*SCN5A*-related patients. *J. Am. Coll. Cardiol.* 2002; **40**: 350–356.

44 Weiss R, Barmada MM, Nguyen T *et al*. Clinical and molecular heterogeneity in the Brugada syndrome: a novel gene locus on chromosome 3. *Circulation* 2002; **105**: 707–709.

45 Priori SG, Napolitano C, Tiso N *et al*. Mutations in the cardiac ryanodine receptor gene (hRyR2) underlie catecholaminergic polymorphic ventricular tachycardia. *Circulation* 2001; **103**: 196–200.

46 Lahat H, Pras E, Olender T *et al*. A missense mutation in a highly conserved region of CASQ2 is associated with autosomal recessive catecholamine-induced polymorphic ventricular tachycardia in Bedouin families from Israel. *Am. J. Hum. Genet.* 2001; **69**: 1378–1384.

CHAPTER 5

Cellular mechanisms underlying the Brugada syndrome

C. Antzelevitch, PhD, *J. M. Fish,* DVM, *J. M. Di Diego,* MD

Introduction

Since its introduction as a new clinical entity in 1992, the Brugada syndrome has attracted great interest because of its high incidence in many parts of the world and its association with high risk for sudden death. The syndrome has also captured the attention of the cardiac electrophysiology community because it serves as a paradigm for our understanding of the role of spatial dispersion of repolarization in the development of cardiac arrhythmias. Recent years have witnessed an exponential rise in the number of reported cases and a striking proliferation of papers serving to define the clinical, genetic, cellular, ionic, and molecular aspects of this disease. In this chapter we review the experimental milestones that have brought us to our current understanding of the cellular mechanisms that underlie the Brugada syndrome.

Brugada syndrome as a paradigm for advancing our understanding of spatial dispersion of repolarization

As with other channelopathies, the emerging concept points to amplification of heterogeneities intrinsic to ventricular myocardium as the principal culprit for the arrhythmogenic substrate underlying the Brugada syndrome. A brief discussion of electrical heterogeneities present in the ventricles of the heart is therefore appropriate.

That repolarization heterogeneities exist within the ventricular myocardium was recognized by Willem Einthoven at the turn of the last century and by the great men of science that followed in his footsteps. Einthoven first recorded the electrocardiogram (ECG) near the turn of the last century, initially using a capillary electrometer and then a string galvanometer.[1,2] Today, nearly a century later, physicians and scientists are still learning how to extract valuable information from the ECG and continue to debate the cellular basis for the various waves of the ECG. Recent reviews have focused on the cellular basis for the repolarization waves of the heart, including the J, T, and U waves of the ECG.[3,4] The J wave and T wave are thought to arise as a consequence of voltage gradients that develop as a result of the electrical heterogeneity that exists within the ventricular myocardium. The basis for the U wave has long been a matter of debate. One theory attributes the U wave to mechano-electrical feedback. A second theory ascribes it to voltage gradients within ventricular myocardium, and a third to voltage gradients between the ventricular myocardium and the His–Purkinje system. In this chapter, our principal focus will be on the J wave since this wave is most pertinent to our understanding of the Brugada syndrome. We begin with a general discussion of the heterogeneities in the electrophysiology and pharmacology of the ventricular myocardium.

Electrical heterogeneity

It was not long ago that ventricular myocardium was thought to be largely homogeneous with respect to its electrical properties and responsiveness to drugs.

Studies from a number of laboratories have advanced evidence in support of the hypothesis that ventricular myocardium is comprised of three electrophysiologically distinct cell types: epicardial, M, and endocardial.[3,5,6] The three ventricular myocardial cell types differ principally with respect to phase 1 and phase 3 repolarization characteristics. Ventricular epicardial and M, but not endocardial, action potentials display a prominent phase 1, due to a prominent 4-aminopyridine (4-AP) sensitive transient outward current (I_{to}), giving rise to a spike and dome or notched configuration. These regional differences in I_{to} have been demonstrated in canine,[7,8] feline,[9] rabbit,[10] rat,[11] and human[12,13] ventricular myocytes. Important differences also exist in the magnitude of I_{to} and the action potential notch between right and left ventricular epicardial and M cells, with right ventricular cells displaying a much greater I_{to}.[14,15] The transmural and interventricular differences in the manifestation of I_{to} have a number of interesting consequences,[14,16–22] including the creation of a transmural voltage gradient responsible for the inscription of the electrocardiographic J wave (Table 5.1).

An I_{to}-mediated spike and dome morphology in epicardium but not endocardium has been shown to lead to different, in some cases opposite, responses to a wide variety of pharmacological agents (Table 5.1).

Epicardium versus endocardium

Endocardium and epicardium respond differently to parasympathetic as well as sympathetic agonists. Acetylcholine (ACh) in concentrations as high as 10^{-5} M exerts essentially no effect on the action potential of canine ventricular endocardium. In contrast, ACh has been shown to either prolong or markedly abbreviate the epicardial action potential,[23] providing support for claims of a direct effect of ACh in the feline and human heart *in vivo*.[24,25] Low concentrations (10^{-7}–10^{-6} M) cause a slowing of the second upstroke, giving rise to a delay in the achievement of peak plateau. The accentuation of the epicardial action potential notch leads to a prolongation of action potential duration. Higher concentrations cause all-or-none repolarization and marked abbreviation of the action potential. These effects of ACh on epicardium are readily reversed with atropine, fail to appear when epicardium is pretreated with the transient outward current blocker 4-AP, are accentuated in the presence of isoproterenol (1×10^{-7} to 5×10^{-6} M; accentuated antagonism), persist in the presence of propranolol and are likely due to inhibition of I_{Ca} and/or activation of $I_{K\text{-}ACh}$.[23] ACh does not influence I_{to}.[26]

The differential responsiveness of epicardium and endocardium to isoproterenol is due to a diminution of the epicardial action potential secondary to a rebalancing of currents flowing during

Table 5.1 Consequences of a prominent I_{to}-mediated action potential notch in epicardium but not endocardium.

Consequence	Reference
J wave (Osborn wave)	16, 19
Differential sensitivity to ischemia & components of ischemia	16, 44, 45, 156
Differential sensitivity to drugs	16, 19, 23, 40, 41, 44, 47, 156
• neurohormones (acetylcholine and isoproterenol)	
• transient outward current blockers	
• calcium channel blockers	
• sodium channel blockers	
• potassium channel openers	
• amiodarone	
Supernormal phase of conduction	16
Phase 2 reentry	20, 41, 44–46
Brugada syndrome	49, 104, 157

the early phases of the action potential. As a consequence, the epicardial action potential abbreviates more than that of endocardium in response to sympathetic stimulation. β adrenergic agonists influence all of the major currents that contribute to phase 1 and phase 3 repolarization, including I_{to}, I_{Ca}, I_K, and calcium- and cAMP-activated I_{Cl}.[27–34] In the presence of pathophysiologically induced abbreviation of the action potential, secondary to loss of the action potential dome, β adrenergic agonists can restore transmural electrical homogeneity by restoring the dome of the epicardial action potential, as discussed below.

Different responses of epicardium and endocardium to calcium channel blockers have been reported in a number of studies. Organic Ca^{2+} channel blockers such as verapamil[35] and nifedipine[36] and inorganic inhibitors such as $MnCl_2$ can cause loss of the action potential dome in canine ventricular epicardium.[37] Exposure to Ca^{2+}-free Tyrode's solution yields similar results.[37] In endocardium, calcium channel blockers cause only a slight abbreviation of the action potential.[38,39]

A variety of sodium channel blockers were found to produce different, and in some cases opposite, effects on canine ventricular epicardium and endocardium.[40,41] Concentrations of tetrodotoxin, propranolol, and flecainide sufficient to reduce the rate of rise of the action potential (V_{max}) by approximately 40–50% abbreviate the action potential in endocardium but prolong it in epicardium. Greater inhibition of I_{Na} leads to a marked abbreviation of the epicardial response due to loss of the action potential dome, while producing only a slight abbreviation of the action potential in endocardium. The paradoxical prolongation of the epicardial action potential is due largely to an accentuation and widening of the action potential notch. With greater inhibition of I_{Na}, termination of phase 1 shifts to more negative potentials at which the availability of I_{Ca} is diminished to a level at which the outward currents may overwhelm the inward currents active at the end of phase 1. This results is an all-or-none repolarization at the end of phase 1, causing loss of the action potential dome and marked abbreviation of the action potential.

As will be discussed later, these actions of ACh and sodium channel blockers, particularly on right ventricular epicardium, facilitate the development of phase 2 reentry, thought to be the trigger for sudden death in patients with the Brugada syndrome.

Not unexpectedly, epicardium and endocardium respond differently to agents that block I_{to}. In relatively low concentrations (0.5–1.0 mM) 4-AP is a fairly selective blocker of I_{to}; higher concentrations also block I_K and I_{K1}.[42,43] As will be discussed in a subsequent section, low concentrations of 4-AP are effective in restoring electrical homogeneity and in abolishing arrhythmias induced by ischemia or drugs and neurohormones that cause dispersion of repolarization and phase 2 reentry (i.e., sodium channel blockers and ACh).[16,44–47] Inhibition of I_{to} by quinidine may contribute to the antiarrhythmic actions of the drug.[48,49]

Chronic administration of amiodarone has been shown to produce very different electrophysiologic effects in canine ventricular epicardium and endocardium.[18,50] Endocardial tissues excised from the hearts of dogs receiving chronic amiodarone (20–25 mg/kg/day over a 5–6 week period) show strong use dependence of V_{max} (30±5.2% decrease with acceleration from a BCL of 2000 to 300 ms) and an action potential duration 16% longer than control. Unlike endocardium, epicardial tissues isolated from amiodarone treated dogs are always markedly depressed (inexcitable) immediately after isolation. The tissue recovered over a period of several hours, showing several distinct phases including: (1) conduction disturbances and (2) acceleration-induced *prolongation* of APD. Neither was seen in endocardium.

M cells

M cells are distinguished by the ability of their action potential to prolong more than other ventricular myocardial cell types in response to a slowing of rate and/or in response to agents with class III actions.[16,51,52] These features of the M cell are due to the presence of a smaller slowly activating delayed rectifier current (I_{Ks}),[53] a larger late sodium current (late I_{Na})[54] and a larger electrogenic sodium–calcium exchange current (I_{Na-Ca}).[55] Electrophysiologically and pharmacologically, M cells appear to be a hybrid between Purkinje and ventricular cells.[3,5,6] M cells displaying the longest action potentials are often localized in the deep subendocardium to midmyocardium in the anterior wall,[56] deep subepicardium to midmyocardium in the lateral wall,[51] and throughout the wall in the region of the right ventricular (RV) outflow tracts.[6] Unlike Purkinje fibers, they are not found in discrete bundles.[57] M cells are also present in the deep layers of endocardial structures, including papillary muscles, trabeculae, and the interventricular septum.[58] Cells with the characteristics of M cells have been described in the canine,[8,51,52,59–62] guinea pig,[63] rabbit,[64] pig,[65] and human[66,67] ventricles.

Transmural distribution of I_{to} as the basis for the J wave of the ECG

The presence of a pronounced action potential notch in epicardium but not endocardium leads to the development of a transmural voltage gradient during ventricular activation that manifests as a late delta wave following the QRS or what more commonly is referred to as a J wave[19] or Osborn wave. The J wave and elevated J point have been described in the ECG of animals and humans[68] since Osborn's observation in the early 1950s.[69] A distinct J wave is commonly observed in the ECG of some animal species, including dogs and baboons, under baseline conditions and is considerably amplified under hypothermic conditions.[70–72] An elevated J point is commonly encountered in humans and some animal species under normal conditions. In humans, a prominent J wave in the ECG is considered pathognomonic of hypothermia,[73–76] hypercalcemia,[77,78] or malignant arrhythmic conditions.[79]

A transmural gradient in the distribution of I_{to} is responsible for the transmural gradient in the magnitude of phase 1 and action potential notch, which gives rise to a voltage gradient across the ventricular wall responsible for the inscription of the J wave or J point elevation in the ECG.[8,17,18,80] Direct evidence in support of the hypothesis that the J wave is caused by a transmural gradient in the magnitude of the I_{to}-mediated action potential notch derives from experiments conducted in the arterially-perfused left ventricular wedge preparation (Fig. 5.1).[19] Data collected from the wedge preparation demonstrated a significant correlation between the amplitude of the epicardial action potential notch and that of the J wave recorded during interventions that alter the appearance of the electrocardiographic J wave, including hypothermia, premature stimulation (restitution), and block of I_{to} by 4-AP (Figs 5.2–5.4).

Ventricular activation from endocardium to epi-

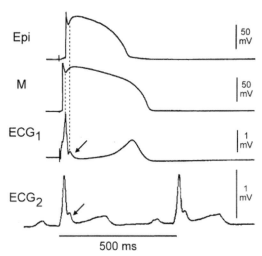

Figure 5.1 Relationship between the spike-and-dome morphology of the epicardial action potential and the appearance of the J wave. ECG_2 is a lead V_5 ECG recorded from the dog *in vivo*. ECG_1 is a transmural ECG recorded across the arterially perfused left ventricular wedge isolated from the heart of the same dog. Both display a prominent J wave at the R-ST junction (arrows). The two upper traces are transmembrane action potentials simultaneously recorded from the epicardial (Epi) and M regions with floating microelectrodes. The preparation was paced at a basic cycle length of 4000 ms. The sinus cycle length at the time ECG_2 was recorded was 500 ms. The J wave is temporally coincident with the notch of the epicardial action potential. Although the M cell action potential also exhibits a prominent notch, it occurs too early to exert an important influence on the manifestation of the J wave. From Ref. 19, with permission.

cardium, with epicardium activated last, is an important prerequisite for the appearance of the J wave. This sequence permits the establishment of a voltage gradient of the early phases of the action potential after activation of the preparation is completed (i.e., after the QRS). Stimulation of the preparation from an epicardial site does not produce a J wave despite the maintenance of cellular differences in the morphology of the action potential; the J wave is buried in the QRS (Fig. 5.5). Although the M cells in the left ventricle possess a prominent action potential notch, it is generally hidden in the QRS, but can be unmasked when the QRS is abbreviated due to removal of the endocardial layer (Fig. 5.6).

Because the right ventricular wall is relatively thin, transmural activation may be so rapid as to

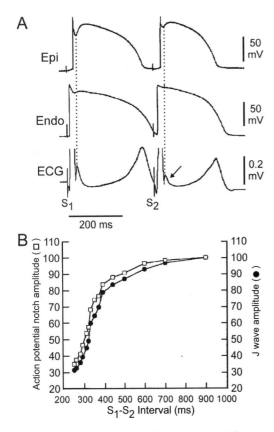

Figure 5.2 Relation between restitution of epicardial action potential notch amplitude and J wave amplitude. **(A)** Simultaneous recording of a transmural ECG and transmembrane action potentials from the epicardial (Epi) and endocardial (Endo) regions of an isolated arterially perfused right ventricular wedge. A significant action potential notch in epicardium is associated with a prominent J wave (arrow) during basic stimulation (S_1–S_2: 4000 ms). Premature stimulation (S_1–S_2: 300 ms) causes a parallel decrease in the amplitude of the epicardial action potential notch and that of the J wave (arrow). **(B)** Plot of the amplitudes of the epicardial action potential notch (□) and J wave (●) as a function of the S_1–S_2 interval. The amplitude of the epicardial action potential notch and that of the J wave are normalized to the value recorded at an S_1–S_2 interval of 900 ms. From Ref. 154, with permission.

bury the J wave generated by the right ventricular epicardium inside the QRS. Thus, although the action potential notch is most prominent in right ventricular epicardium, right ventricular myocardium would be expected to contribute relatively little to the manifestation of the J wave under normal conditions. These observations are consistent with the

manifestation of the J wave in ECG leads in which the mean vector axis is transmurally oriented across the left ventricle and septum. Accordingly, the J wave in the dog is most prominent in leads II, III, aVR, aVF, and mid to left precordial leads V_3 through V_6.[19] A similar picture is seen in the human ECG.[73,76,78] In addition, vector cardiography indicates that the J wave forms an extra loop that occurs at the junction of the QRS and T loops.[81] It is directed leftward and anteriorly, which explains its prominence in leads associated with the left ventricle.

The J wave was first noted in animal experiments involving hypercalcemia conducted in the 1920s.[77] The first extensive description and characterization appeared 30 years later in a study by Osborn involving experimental hypothermia in dogs.[69] As a consequence, this wave, which appears at the R-ST junction, is often referred to as either a J wave or an Osborn wave.

The spike-and-dome morphology of the epicardial action potential is absent in canine neonates, gradually appearing over the first few months of life (Fig. 5.7).[82] The progressive development of the notch is paralleled by the appearance of I_{to}.[82–84] For this reason the J wave is not observed in neonatal dogs.[19]

The appearance of a prominent J wave in the clinic is typically associated with pathophysiological conditions such as hypothermia[73,76] and hypercalcemia.[77,78] A modest J wave is observed in some patients who have recovered from hypothermia.[85,86] The prominent J wave induced by hypothermia is the result of a marked accentuation of the spike-and-dome morphology of the action potential of M and epicardial cells (i.e., an increase in both width and magnitude of the notch), as illustrated in Fig. 5.3. This may be the result of slowing of the kinetics of activation of I_{to} less than the kinetics of the calcium current, I_{Ca}. In addition to inducing a more prominent notch, hypothermia produces a slowing of conduction which allows the epicardial notch to clear the QRS so as to manifest a distinct J wave. Thus, the additional conduction delay from endocardium to epicardium together with the widening of the epicardial action potential notch serve to unmask a latent J wave by moving it out of the QRS complex (Fig. 5.3). The accentuation of the action potential notch is likely due to a temperature-dependent slowing of the kinetics of activation of I_{Ca}

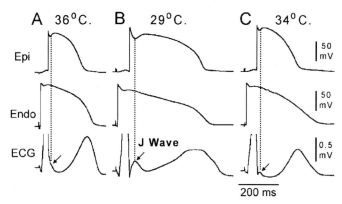

Figure 5.3 Effect of hypothermia on action potential and ECG morphology. Each panel shows transmembrane recordings obtained from the epicardial (Epi) and endocardial (Endo) regions of an isolated arterially perfused canine left ventricular wedge and a transmural ECG recorded simultaneously. **(A)** A small but distinct action potential notch in epicardium but not in endocardium is associated with an elevated J point at the R-ST junction (arrow) under normothermic conditions (36°C). **(B)** A decrease in the temperature of the perfusate and bath to 29°C results in an increase in the amplitude and width of the action potential notch in epicardium but not in endocardium, leading to a prominent J wave on the transmural ECG (arrow). **(C)** Rewarming to a temperature of 34°C is attended by a parallel reduction in the amplitude and width of the J wave and epicardial action potential notch. From Ref. 154, with permission.

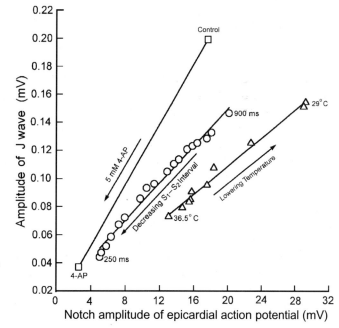

Figure 5.4 Graph showing correlation between amplitude of J wave of transmural ECG and amplitude of epicardial action potential notch recorded at different S_1–S_2 intervals (○) and temperatures (29°C to 36.5°C, △) and in the absence and presence of 5 mmol/L 4-AP (□). Three separate preparations. Basic cycle length was 4000 ms. In the case of the hypothermia and restitution plots, the solid lines were obtained by linear regression ($r^2 = 0.99$ for both). From Ref. 154, with permission.

and decay of I_{to}, thus producing an outward shift of net current during the early phases of the action potential.

Hypercalcemia-induced J waves[77,78,87] may also be explained on the basis of an accentuation of the epicardial action potential notch, possibly as a result of an augmentation of the calcium-activated chloride current and a decrease in I_{Ca}.[45]

The transmural gradient of I_{to} was shown by Rosati and coworkers to be associated with a similar

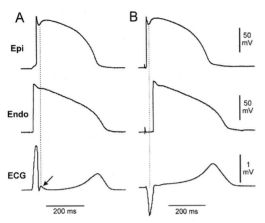

Figure 5.5 Effect of activation sequence on the appearance of the J wave in the ECG. Simultaneous recording of a transmural ECG and transmembrane action potentials from the epicardial (Epi) and endocardial (Endo) regions of an isolated arterially perfused left ventricular wedge are shown. **(A)** The preparation was stimulated from the endocardial surface; a prominent J wave, temporally aligned with the notch of the epicardial action potential, is apparent in the ECG. **(B)** The preparation was stimulated from the epicardial surface; the notch of the epicardial response is coincident with the QRS and a J wave is no longer observed. BCL = 2000 ms. From Ref. 154, with permission.

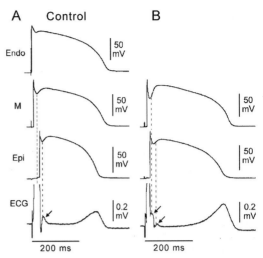

Figure 5.6 The role of M cells in the generation of the J wave. **(A)** A transmural ECG and transmembrane action potentials from endocardial (Endo), M region (M), and epicardial (Epi) sites were simultaneously recorded from an isolated arterially perfused canine left ventricular wedge. The action potential notch in epicardium, but not endo-cardium or M region, was associated with the appearance of a prominent J wave in the ECG (arrow). **(B)** Recordings obtained from the same epicardial and M region sites 1 hour after an approximately 4 mm thick segment of the endocardial surface was excised. Transmural activation time was abbreviated, resulting in a 35% narrower QRS and the appearance of two J waves (arrows). The first J wave is associated with the notch of the action potential recorded from the M region. In the intact preparation (panel **A**), the notch of the M cell is not apparent in the ECG because of its occurrence during the QRS. The second J wave is coincident with the notch of the epicardial response. It is noteworthy that the spike and dome morphology of the M cell action potential is greatly augmented after the endocardium is removed.

gradient in the distribution of mRNA for KChIP2, a calcium-binding protein that co-assembles with Kv4.3 to form the I_{to} channel in dog and human.[88] These authors suggested that KChIP2 expression contributed importantly to the distribution of I_{to} across the ventricular wall. This conclusion was brought into question by Deschenes and coworkers[89] who demonstrated a similar distribution of mRNA and dog and human ventricular myocardium, but found that immunoreactive protein for KChIP2 was equally distributed across the wall. In support of their original hypothesis, Rosati and coworkers using a monoclonal antibody for KChIP2 demonstrated correspondence between mRNA, protein and current transmural gradients.[90]

Phase 2 reentry as a mechanism of extrasystolic activity

Amplification of the intrinsic electrical heterogeneities that characterize the early phases of the action potential among the three principal cell types that make up the ventricular myocardium leads to

accentuation of the J wave and eventually loss of the action potential dome, giving rise to extrasystolic activity in the form of phase 2 reentry. Activation of I_{to} leads to a paradoxical prolongation of APD in canine ventricular tissues,[91] but to the traditional abbreviation of APD in ventricular tissues that normally exhibit brief action potentials (e.g., rat).[92] Pathophysiologic conditions (e.g., ischemia, metabolic inhibition) and some pharmacologic interventions (e.g., I_{Na} or I_{Ca} blockers or I_{K-ATP} activators) can lead to marked abbreviation of the action potential in canine and feline[93] ventricular cells where I_{to} is prominent (Fig 5.8). Under these conditions, canine

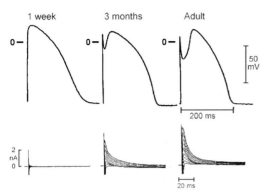

Figure 5.7 Age-related spike and dome morphology and changes in I_{to} in canine ventricular epicardium. Each panel depicts transmembrane activity recorded from right ventricular epicardial tissues (lower trace) and transient outward current (lower trace) recorded from left ventricular epicardial cells isolated from a neonate (5 days of age), a young dog (3 months old), and an adult dog. BCL = 2000 ms; $[K^+] = 4$ mM. The spike and dome configuration of the epicardial action potential and I_{to} density are absent in the neonate, relatively small in the young dog and most prominent in the adult. Reproduced from Ref. 3, with permission.

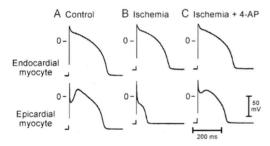

Figure 5.8 Differential effects of ischemia on action potentials recorded from endocardial and epicardial myocytes dissociated from the canine left ventricle. **(A)** Control. **(B)** Responses recorded after 30 min of superfusion with ischemic solution. 'Ischemia' caused a marked abbreviation of APD_{90} in the epicardial cell and a modest shortening in the endocardial cell. **(C)** Responses obtained 5 min after switching to an ischemic solution containing 4-aminopyridine (1 mM). 4-AP reversed the ischemia-induced shortening of APD_{90} in the epicardial myocyte and also prolonged APD_{90} in the endocardial cell. These effects of 4-AP were similar to those observed in syncytial tissue preparations from the corresponding ventricular layer. BCL of 800 ms. From Ref. 46, with permission.

ventricular epicardium exhibits an all-or-none re-polarization as a result of the rebalancing of currents flowing at the end of phase 1 of the action potential. When phase 1 reaches approximately −30 mV, all-

or-none repolarization of the action potential occurs leading to loss of the action potential dome. Failure of the dome to develop occurs at this voltage because the outward currents (principally I_{to}) overwhelm the inward currents (chiefly I_{Ca}). The result is a remarkable (40–70%) abbreviation of the action potential. Loss of the action potential dome usually occurs in a heterogeneous fashion, such that the action potential dome is usually abolished at some epicardial sites but not others, causing a marked dispersion of repolarization within the epicardium. Conduction of the action potential dome from sites at which it is maintained to sites at which it is abolished can cause local re-excitation of the preparation. This mechanism, termed phase 2 reentry, produces extrasystolic beats capable of initiating circus movement reentry[20] (Figs 5.9 and 5.10). Electrical heterogeneity leads to phase 2 reentry in canine epicardium exposed to: (1) K^+ channel openers such as pinacidil;[44] (2) sodium channel blockers such as flecainide;[41] (3) increased $[Ca^{2+}]_o$;[45] (4) metabolic inhibition,[18] and (5) simulated ischemia.[20] Block of I_{to} restores electrical homogeneity and abolishes reentrant activity in all cases.

Phase 2 reentry as a trigger for VT/VF: the Brugada syndrome

Abnormal J waves have long been linked to idiopathic ventricular fibrillation and the Brugada syndrome.[94–97] The Brugada syndrome is characterized by an ST segment elevation (or exaggerated J wave) in the right precordial leads, V_1 to V_3 (unrelated to ischemia, electrolyte abnormalities, or structural heart disease), a normal QT interval, and a high incidence of sudden cardiac death due to ventricular tachycardia or fibrillation (VT/VF).[94] A right bundle branch block configuration of the ECG is observed in many, but not all, cases. Recent data point to similarities between the conditions that predispose to phase 2 reentry and those that attend the appearance of the Brugada syndrome.

Loss of the action potential dome in epicardium, but not endocardium, would be expected to generate a transmural current that manifests on the ECG as an ST segment elevation, similar to that encountered in patients with the Brugada syndrome.[18,19,46] Loss of the dome is caused by an outward shift in the balance of currents active during the early phases of

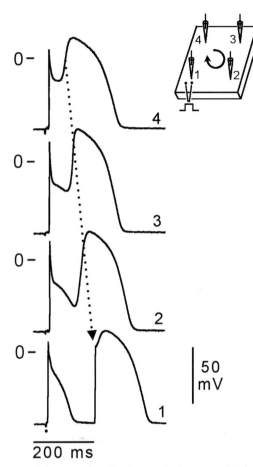

0 –

0 –

0 –

0 –

50
mV

200 ms

Figure 5.9 Phase 2 reentry. Reentrant activity induced by exposure of a canine ventricular epicardial preparation (0.7 cm²) to simulated ischemia. Microelectrode recordings were obtained from 4 sites as shown in the schematic (upper right). After 35 min of ischemia, the action potential dome develops normally at site 4, but not at sites 1, 2, or 3. The dome then propagates in a clockwise direction re-exciting sites 3, 2, and 1 with progressive delays, thus generating a closely coupled reentrant extrasystole (156 ms) at site 1. In this example of phase 2 reentry, propagation of the dome occurs in a direction opposite to that of phase 0, a mechanism akin to reflection. BCL = 700 ms. Modified from Ref. 20, with permission.

the action potential, principally I_{to} and I_{Ca}. Autonomic neurotransmitters like acetylcholine facilitate loss of the action potential dome[23] by suppressing I_{Ca} and/or augmenting potassium current. β adrenergic agonists restore the dome by augmenting I_{Ca}. Sodium channel blockers also facilitate loss of the canine right ventricular action potential dome via a negative shift in the voltage at which

phase 1 begins.[40,41] These findings are consistent with clinical reports of accentuation of the ST segment elevation in patients with the Brugada syndrome following vagal maneuvers or class I antiarrhythmic agents as well as normalization of the ST segment elevation following β adrenergic agents.[19,98] The appearance of an ST segment elevation only in right precordial leads in Brugada patients is consistent with the finding that loss of the action potential dome is much more commonly encountered in right versus left canine ventricular epicardium.[14,18,46] We believe the Brugada syndrome is a right ventricular disease because I_{to} density is intrinsically much greater in right versus left ventricular epicardium.

These observations point to a depressed right ventricular epicardial action potential dome as the basis for the ST segment elevation and to phase 2 reentry as a trigger for episodes of ventricular tachycardia and fibrillation in patients with the Brugada syndrome and other syndromes associated with an ST segment elevation. Direct evidence in support of this hypothesis was recently provided in an arterially perfused canine right ventricular experimental model of the Brugada syndrome (Fig 5.11).[49] The data support the hypothesis that ST segment elevation similar to that observed in patients with the Brugada syndrome results from loss of the action potential dome in right ventricular epicardium, where I_{to} is most prominent. Initiation of VT/VF under these conditions is via phase 2 reentry secondary to heterogeneous loss of the epicardial action potential dome.[49] The VT and VF generated in these preparations is often polymorphic, resembling a very rapid form of *torsade de pointes*. This activity may be mechanistically related to the migrating spiral wave shown to generate a pattern resembling TdP associated with a normal or long QT interval.[99,100]

In recent studies we have established that combined I_{Na} and I_{Ca} block leads to the development of an experimental model of the Brugada syndrome displaying characteristics very similar to those of the clinical syndrome. The ability of combined I_{Na} and I_{Ca} block to cause loss of the epicardial action potential dome and phase 2 reentry in the canine right ventricular wedge preparation is illustrated in Fig. 5.12. High concentrations of terfenadine (5 μM) produce a potent block of I_{Na} and I_{Ca}, leading to

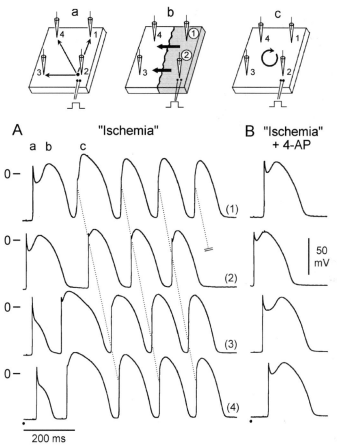

Figure 5.10 Phase 2 reentrant extrasystole triggers circus movement reentry. (**A**) Exposure of a relatively large canine right ventricular epicardial sheet (6.3 cm²) to simulated ischemia results in loss of the dome at sites 3 and 4 but not at sites 1 and 2 (BCL = 1100 ms). Conduction of the basic beat proceeds normally from the stimulation site (site 2; see schematic **a**). Propagation of the action potential dome from the right half of the preparation caused reexcitation of the left half via a phase 2 reentry mechanism (see schematic **b**). The extrasystolic beat generated by phase 2 reentry then initiates a run of tachycardia that is sustained for 4 additional cycles via typical circus movement reentry. The proposed reentrant path is shown in schematic **c**. Note that phase 2 reentry provides an activation front roughly perpendicular to that of the basic beat. This type of cross-field activation has previously been shown to predispose to the development of vortex-like reentry in isolated epicardial sheets. (**B**) Recorded after addition of 1 mM 4-aminopyridine (4-AP), an inhibitor of the transient outward current. In the continued presence of ischemia, 4-AP restored the dome at all epicardial recording sites within 3 min. Thus electrical heterogeneity was restored and all reentrant activity abolished. Modified from Ref. 20, with permission.

accentuation of the epicardial action potential notch following acceleration of the rate from a BCL of 800 ms to 400 ms. The dramatic accentuation of the notch was due to the effect of the drug to depress the phase 0, augment the magnitude of phase 1, and delay the appearance of the second upstroke. The electrocardiographic manifestations of these changes in action potential characteristics include an elevation of J point, augmentation of the J wave, and inversion of the T wave (Figs 5.12A versus 5.12B). With continued rapid pacing, phase 1 became more accentuated, progressing until all-or-none repolarization occurred at the end of phase 1 at some epicardial sites but not others, leading to the development of both epicardial (EDR) and transmural (TDR) dispersion of repolarization (Fig. 5.12C). Propagation of the dome from the region where it was maintained to the region at which it was

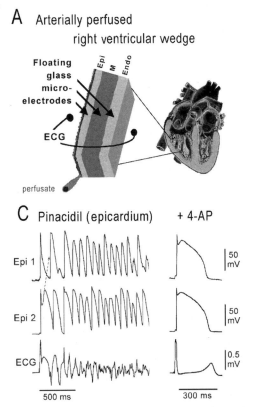

A   Arterially perfused
right ventricular wedge

Floating
glass
micro-
electrodes

ECG

perfusate

Epi   M   Endo

B   Local pressure epicardium

M Cell

Epi 1

Epi 2

ECG

$\begin{vmatrix} 50 \\ mV \end{vmatrix}$

$\begin{vmatrix} 50 \\ mV \end{vmatrix}$

$\begin{vmatrix} 50 \\ mV \end{vmatrix}$

$\begin{vmatrix} 2 \\ mV \end{vmatrix}$

200 ms

C   Pinacidil (epicardium)   + 4-AP

Epi 1

Epi 2

ECG

$\begin{vmatrix} 50 \\ mV \end{vmatrix}$

$\begin{vmatrix} 50 \\ mV \end{vmatrix}$

$\begin{vmatrix} 0.5 \\ mV \end{vmatrix}$

500 ms   300 ms

D   Pinacidil (2.5 µM, perfusate)   + 4-AP

Endo

Epi 1

Epi 2

ECG

$\begin{vmatrix} 50 \\ mV \end{vmatrix}$

$\begin{vmatrix} 50 \\ mV \end{vmatrix}$

$\begin{vmatrix} 50 \\ mV \end{vmatrix}$

$\begin{vmatrix} 1.0 \\ mV \end{vmatrix}$

300 ms   200 ms

Figure 5.11 ECG and arrhythmias with typical features of the Brugada syndrome recorded from canine right ventricular wedge preparations (see inset – top left). **(A)** Schematic of arterially perfused right ventricular wedge preparation. **(B)** Pressure–induced phase 2 reentry and VT. Shown are transmembrane action potentials simultaneously recorded from two epicardial (Epi 1 and Epi 2) and one M region (M) sites, together with a transmural ECG. Local application of pressure near Epi 2 results in loss of the action potential dome at that site but not at Epi 1 or M sites. The dome at Epi 1 then re-excites Epi 2 giving rise to a phase 2 reentrant extrasystole which triggers a short run of ventricular tachycardia. Note the ST segment elevation due to loss of the action potential dome in a segment of epicardium. **(C)** Polymorphic VT/VF induced by local application of the potassium channel opener pinacidil (10 µM) to the epicardial surface of the wedge. Action potentials from two epicardial sites (Epi 1 and Epi 2) and a transmural ECG were simultaneously recorded. Loss of the dome at Epi 1 but not Epi 2 creates a marked dispersion of repolarization, giving rise to a phase 2 reentrant extrasystole. The extrasystolic beat then triggers a long episode of ventricular fibrillation (22 s). Right panel: Addition of 4-aminopyridine (4-AP, 2 mM), a specific I_{to} blocker, to the perfusate restored the action potential dome at Epi 1, thus reducing dispersion of repolarization and suppressing all arrhythmic activity. BCL = 2000 ms. **(D)** Phase 2 reentry gives rise to VT following addition of pinacidil (2.5 µM) to the coronary perfusate. Transmembrane action potentials form 2 epicardial sites (Epi 1 and Epi 2) and one endocardial site (Endo) as well as a transmural ECG were simultaneously recorded. Right panel: 4-AP (1 mM) markedly reduces the magnitude of the action potential notch in epicardium, thus restoring the action potential dome throughout the preparation and abolishing all arrhythmic activity. **(D)** is from Ref. 49, with permission.

lost resulted in the development of local phase 2 reentry (Fig. 5.12D).

Figure 5.13 shows the ability of terfenadine-induced phase 2 reentry to generate an extrasystole, couplet and polymorphic VT/VF. Figure 5.13D illustrates an example of programmed electrical stimulation to initiate VT/VF under similar conditions.

Mibefradil is another agent capable of potently blocking both I_{Ca} and I_{Na}. Figure 5.14 shows the effect of mibefradil to induce an acquired form of the Brugada syndrome.

The cellular mechanisms responsible for the development of the Brugada syndrome have gradually come into better focus. The electrocardiographic

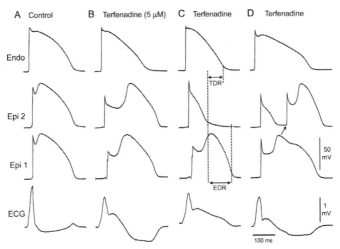

Figure 5.12 Terfenadine-induced ST segment elevation, T wave inversion, transmural and endocardial dispersion of repolarization and phase 2 reentry. Each panel shows transmembrane action potentials from one endocardial (top) and two epicardial sites together with a transmural ECG recorded from a canine arterially perfused right ventricular wedge preparation. (**A**) Control (BCL = 400 ms). (**B**) Terfenadine (5 μM) accentuated the epicardial action potential notch creating a transmural voltage gradient that manifests as an ST segment elevation or exaggerated J wave in the ECG. First beat recorded after changing from BCL = 800 ms to BCL = 400 ms. (**C**) Continued pacing at BCL = 400 ms results in all-or-none repolarization at the end of phase 1 at some epicardial sites but not others, creating a local epicardial dispersion of repolarization (EDR) as well as a transmural dispersion of repolarization (TDR). (**D**) Phase 2 reentry occurs when the epicardial action potential dome propagates from a site where it is maintained to regions where it has been lost. Modified from Ref. 155, with permission.

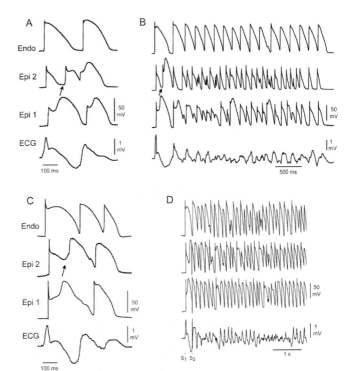

Figure 5.13 Spontaneous and programmed electrical stimulation-induced polymorphic VT in RV wedge preparations pretreated with terfenadine (5–10 μM). (**A**) Phase 2 reentry in epicardium gives rise to a closely coupled extrasystole. (**B**) Phase 2 reentrant extrasystole triggers a brief episode of polymorphic VT. (**C**) Extrastimulus (S$_1$–S$_2$ = 250 ms) applied to epicardium triggers a polymorphic VT (part **D**). Modified from Ref. 155, with permission.

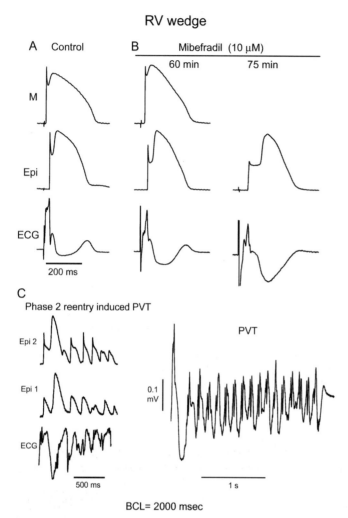

Figure 5.14 Mibefradil-induced Brugada syndrome. Time-dependent decrease in the amplitude of phase 0 in a RV wedge preparation exposed to 10 µM mibefradil (BCL = 2000 ms). (A) Control recordings. (B) Effect of 10 µM mibefradil after 60 and 75 min of perfusion. (C) RV epicardial heterogeneity leads to phase 2 reentry and polymorphic VT.

manifestations of the syndrome have been attributed to one of two basic mechanisms: (1) conduction delay in the right ventricular epicardial free wall in the region of the outflow tract (RVOT) or (2) premature repolarization of the right ventricular epicardial action potential secondary to loss of the action potential dome.

A schematic representation of the cellular changes believed to underlie the Brugada phenotype in hypothesis 2 is shown in Fig. 5.15.[101,102] Under normal conditions, the J wave is relatively small, in large part reflecting the left ventricular action potential notch, since that of right ventricular epicardium is usually buried in the QRS complex. The ST segment is isoelectric because of the absence of transmural voltage gradients at the level of the action potential plateau (Fig. 5.15A). Accentuation of the right ventricular notch under pathophysiologic conditions leads to exaggeration of transmural voltage gradients and thus to accentuation of the J wave or to J point elevation. This would be expected to give rise to a saddleback configuration of the repolarization waves (Fig. 5.15B). The development of a prominent J wave under these conditions is indistinguishable from an ST segment elevation. Under these conditions, the T wave remains positive because epicardial repolarization precedes repolarization of the cells in the M and endocardial regions. Further accentuation of the notch may be accompanied by a prolongation of the epicardial action potential such that the direction of repolarization across the right ventricular wall and transmural voltage gradients are reversed, leading to the development of a coved-type ST segment elevation and

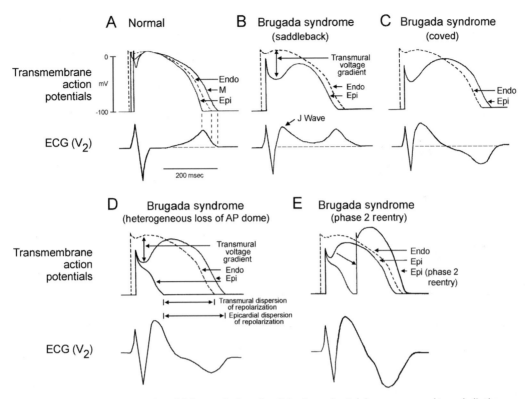

Figure 5.15 Schematic representation of right ventricular epicardial action potential changes proposed to underlie the electrocardiographic manifestation of the Brugada syndrome. Modified from Ref. 101, with permission.

inversion of the T wave (Fig. 5.15C), typically observed in the ECG of Brugada patients. A delay in epicardial activation may also contribute to inversion of the T wave. The down-sloping ST segment elevation, or accentuated J wave, observed in the experimental wedge models often appears as an R′, suggesting that the appearance of a RBBB morphology in Brugada patients may be due at least in part to early repolarization of right ventricular (RV) epicardium, rather than to impulse conduction block in the right bundle. Indeed a rigorous application of RBBB criteria reveals that a large majority of RBBB-like morphologies encountered in cases of Brugada syndrome do not fit the criteria for RBBB.[103] Moreover, attempts by Miyazaki and coworkers to record delayed activation of the RV in Brugada patients met with failure.[98] Although the typical Brugada morphology is present in Figs 15B and 15C, the substrate for reentry is not present. We believe that the arrhythmogenic substrate arises when a further shift in the balance of current leads to loss of the action potential dome at some epicardial sites but not others (Fig. 5.15D). Loss of the action potential dome in

epicardium but not endocardium results in the development of a marked transmural dispersion of repolarization and refractoriness, responsible for the development of a vulnerable window during which a premature impulse or extrasystole can induce a reentrant arrhythmia. Loss of the action potential dome in epicardium is usually heterogeneous, leading to the development of epicardial dispersion of repolarization (Fig. 5.15D). Conduction of the action potential dome from sites at which it is maintained to sites at which it is lost causes local re-excitation via a phase 2 reentry mechanism, leading to the development of a very closely coupled extrasystole, which captures the vulnerable window across the wall, thus triggering a circus movement reentry in the form of VT/VF (Fig. 15E).[20,49] The phase 2 reentrant beat fuses with the negative T wave of the basic response. Because the extrasystole originates in epicardium, the QRS complex is largely comprised of a Q wave, which serves to accentuate the negative deflection of the inverted T wave, giving the ECG a more symmetrical appearance. This morphology is often observed in the clinic preceding the

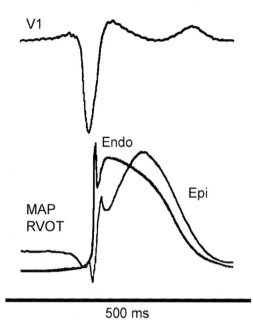

Figure 5.16 Monophasic action potential (MAP) recordings from endocardium (Endo) and epicardium (Epi) of the right ventricular outflow tract of a Brugada patient. A prominent action potential notch is apparent in the epicardial MAP, but not in the endocardial MAP, coincident with the appearance of the accentuated J wave or ST segment elevation in the ECG (V₁). Modified from Ref. 104, with permission.

onset of polymorphic VT. Support for these hypotheses derives from experiments involving the arterially perfused right ventricular wedge preparation[49] and from recent studies by Kurita *et al.* in which monophasic action potential (MAP) electrodes where positioned on the epicardial and endocardial surfaces of the right ventricular outflow tract (RVOT) in patients with the Brugada syndrome (Fig. 5.16).[104,105]

Cellular basis for late potentials in patients with the Brugada syndrome

These characteristics of the action potential of ventricular epicardium suggest that activation forces, generated by the second upstroke of the right ventricular epicardial action potential and/or phase 2 reentry, may extend beyond the QRS in Brugada patients. Indeed, signal averaged ECG (SAECG) recordings have demonstrated late potentials in patients with the Brugada syndrome, especially in the

anterior wall of the right ventricular outflow tract (RVOT).[106,107] The basis for these late potentials, commonly ascribed to delayed conduction within the ventricle, are largely unknown. Endocardial recordings have been unrevealing. Nagase and coworkers[108] introduced a guide wire into the conus branch of the right coronary artery to record signals from the epicardial surface of the anterior wall of the RVOT in patients with the Brugada syndrome. The unipolar recordings displayed delayed potentials, which coincided with late potentials recorded in the SAECG. The study also demonstrated extension of the delayed unipolar potentials and electrocardiographic late potentials further into diastole following the administration of class IC antiarrhythmic agents. The authors conclude that recordings from the conus branch of the right coronary artery can identify an 'epicardial abnormality' in the RVOT which is accentuated in the presence of IC agents, thus uncovering part of the arrhythmogenic substrate responsible for VT/VF in Brugada syndrome, which may be related to the second upstroke or a concealed phase 2 reentrant beat. While late potentials are commonly regarded as being representative of delayed activation of the myocardium, in the case of the Brugada syndrome other possibilities exist as discussed above. For example, the second upstroke of the epicardial action potential, thought to be greatly accentuated in Brugada syndrome[109] might be capable of generating late potentials when RVOT activation is otherwise normal. Moreover, the occurrence of phase 2 reentry, especially when concealed (i.e., when it fails to trigger transmural reentry), may contribute to the generation of delayed unipolar and late SAECG potentials (Fig. 5.17).

How then can we discriminate between the two? One approach is to examine the rate-dependence of the ECG sign. If the Brugada ECG sign is due to delayed conduction in the RVOT, acceleration of the rate would be expected to further aggravate conduction and thus accentuate the ST segment elevation and the RBBB morphology of the ECG. If, on the other hand, the Brugada sign is secondary to accentuation of the epicardial action potential notch, at some point leading to loss of the action potential dome, acceleration of the rate would be expected to normalize the ECG, by restoring the action potential dome and reducing the notch. This occurs because the transient outward current, which is at the heart

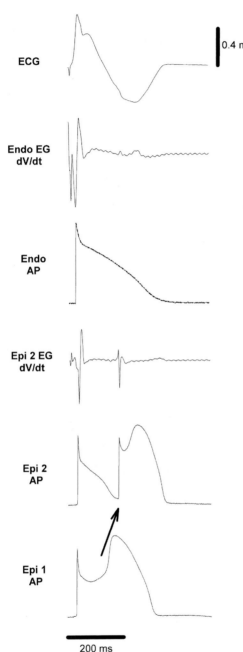

Figure 5.17 Delayed potential observed in unipolar electrogram recorded from epicardium but not endocardium. Phase 2 reentry occurs as the action potential dome is propagated from the site where it is maintained (Epi 1 AP) to the site where it has been lost (Epi 2 AP), but this reentry fails to propagate to the endocardium to generate a closely coupled extrasystole. This local reentry within the epicardium is observed as a second V_{min} on the first derivative of the unipolar electrogram recorded near the Epi 2 AP (Epi 2 EG dV/dt) but not in the endocardium (Endo EG dV/dt). Recorded in the presence of 5 μM terfenadine at BCL = 800 ms.

of this mechanism, is slow to recover from inactivation and is less available at faster rates. The fact of the matter is that Brugada patients usually display a normalization of their ECG or no change when heart rate is increased, thus favoring the second hypothesis (Fig. 5.15). Further evidence in support of this hypothesis derives from the recent observations of Shimizu and coworkers.[110] Using a unipolar catheter introduced into the great cardiac vein, they recorded unipolar activation recovery intervals (ARI), a measure of local action potential duration, from the epicardial surface of the RVOT in a 53-year-old Brugada patient. ARI in the RVOT was observed to abbreviate dramatically whenever the ST segment was elevated in V_2 following a pause or the administration of a sodium channel blocker. Thus, the available data, both experimental and clinical, point to transmural voltage gradients that develop secondary to accentuation of the epicardial notch and loss of the action potential dome as being in large part responsible for the Brugada ECG signature.

Gender and other modulating factors

The ECG sign of the Brugada syndrome is dynamic and often concealed, but can be unmasked by potent sodium channel blockers such as ajmaline, flecainide, procainamide, disopyramide, propafenone, and pilsicainide.[111–113] In addition to sodium channel blockers, a febrile state, vagotonic agents, α adrenergic agonists, β adrenergic blockers, tricyclic antidepressants, first generation antihistaminics (dimenhydrinate), alcohol intoxication, insulin, glucose, and cocaine toxicity can unmask the Brugada syndrome or lead to accentuation of ST segment elevation in patients with the syndrome.[98,111,114–120]

Despite equal genetic transmission of the mutation between the sexes, the clinical phenotype is 8 to 10 times more prevalent in males than in females. The basis for this sex-related distinction was recently shown to be due to a more prominent transient outward current (I_{to})-mediated action potential notch in the right ventricular (RV) epicardium of males versus females[121] (Figs 5.18 and 5.19). The more prominent I_{to} causes the end of phase 1 of the RV epicardial action potential to repolarize to more negative potentials in tissue and arterially perfused wedge preparations from males, facilitating loss of

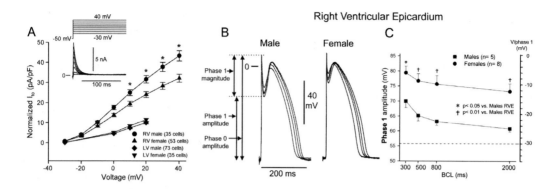

Figure 5.18 Sex-based and interventricular differences in I_{to}. **(A)** Mean I–V relationship for Ito recorded from RV epicardial cells isolated from hearts of male and female dogs. Inset, Representative Ito current traces and voltage protocol. I_{to} density was significantly greater in male versus female RV epicardial cells. No sex differences were observed in LV. **(B)** Transmembrane action potentials recorded from isolated canine RV epicardial male and female tissue slices. BCLs 300, 500, 800, and 2000 ms. **(C)** Rate dependence of phase 1 amplitude and voltage at end of phase 1 (V/phase 1, mV) in males (solid squares) versus females (solid circles). Modified from Ref. 121, with permission.

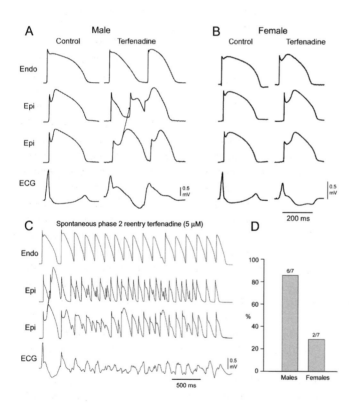

Figure 5.19 Terfenadine induces Brugada phenotype more readily in male than female RV wedge preparations. Each panel shows action potentials recorded from 2 epicardial sites and 1 endocardial site, together with a transmural ECG. Control recordings were obtained at BCL = 2000 ms, whereas terfenadine data were recorded at BCL = 800 ms after a brief period of pacing at BCL = 400 ms. **(A)** Terfenadine (5 μM)-induced, heterogeneous loss of action potential dome, ST segment elevation, and phase 2 reentry (arrow) in a male RV wedge preparation. **(B)** Terfenadine fails to induce Brugada phenotype in a female RV wedge preparation. **(C)** Polymorphic VT triggered by spontaneous phase 2 reentry in a male preparation. **(D)** Incidence of phase 2 reentry in male (6 of 7) versus female (2 of 7) RV wedge preparations when perfused with 5 μM terfenadine for up to 2 hours. Modified from Ref. 121, with permission.

the action potential dome and the development of phase 2 reentry and polymorphic VT. A rebalancing of currents active at the end of phase 1 underlies the unmasking of the syndrome in response to drugs. Vagotonic agents, I_{K-ATP} activators and hypokalemia achieve this by augmenting outward currents, whereas sodium channel blockers, β blockers, cocaine, antidepressants, and antihistamines like terfenadine are likely to accomplish this by reducing inward currents.

Temperature dependence

The sensitivity to sodium channel blockers is consistent with linkage of the syndrome to a defect in the sodium channel gene. The only gene thus far linked is that encoding for the α subunit of the cardiac sodium channel gene, *SCN5A*,[122–127] the same gene implicated in the LQT3 form of the long QT syndrome and in progressive conduction disease. Bezzina and coworkers[127] uncovered a mutation in *SCN5A* (1795InsD) capable of producing both the Brugada and LQT3 phenotypes and Kyndt and coworkers[128] have recently reported an *SCN5A* gene mutation capable of producing both the Brugada syndrome and progressive conduction disease. *SCN5A* mutations linked to the Brugada syndrome cause a reduction in the availability of I_{Na} secondary to: (1) failure of the sodium channel to express; (2) a shift in the voltage- and time-dependence of I_{Na} activation, inactivation, or reactivation; (3) entry of the channel into an intermediate inactivation state from which it recovers more slowly; and/or (4) acceleration of the inactivation of the sodium channel.[122,124,125,127,129–137]

Accelerated inactivation of the sodium channel can be temperature sensitive.[124] A rise of temperature beyond the physiological range dramatically reduces the charge carried by the sodium channel current (I_{Na}) with the T1620M missense mutation. This finding led us to suggest that a febrile state may unmask the Brugada syndrome and/or exacerbate ST segment elevation and arrhythmogenesis.[109,124] A number of case reports of fever-induced Brugada symptoms have appeared over the past couple of years.[138–142] In the report by Porres and coworkers, fever arising secondary to tonsillitis is shown to unmask the Brugada sign and to precipitate episodes of polymorphic VT in a 66-year-old male Brugada patient. In the case of Kum *et al.*, fever developing secondary to lobar pneumonia is shown to unmask the Brugada sign in a 39-year-old male.

The mechanism responsible for the unmasking of the Brugada syndrome and the precipitation of polymorphic VT is thought to involve an effect of fever to reduce I_{Na}. This can occur as a result of a progressively more premature closing of the sodium channel at high temperatures as in the case of the T1620M mutation[124] or as a result of the failure of channel to express at high temperatures as suggested by the study of Wan *et al.* involving the T1620M/R1342W double mutant.[129]

Early repolarization syndrome

The early repolarization syndrome (ERS) is characterized by an upward ST segment concavity ending in a positive T wave in V_2–$V_{4(5)}$. The syndrome is generally regarded to be benign. Clinical interest in ERS has been rekindled due to similarities with the electrocardiographic manifestations of the highly arrhythmogenic Brugada syndrome and the potential for misdiagnosis. The benign nature of the syndrome may be due to the fact that a transmural voltage gradient develops due to depression, but not to loss, of the epicardial action potential dome. Because final repolarization is not affected, a vulnerable window does not develop. In experimental models, the ECG signature of ERS can be converted to that of the Brugada syndrome, raising the possibility that ERS may not be as benign as generally thought, and that under certain conditions known to predispose to ST segment elevation (including acute ischemia), ERS patients may be at greater risk. Further clinical and experimental data are required to test these hypotheses. The characteristics of ERS need to be more fully delineated within the framework of what has been learned about the Brugada syndrome in recent years. It is tempting to speculate that similar mechanisms may be involved in the two syndromes, but that a marked dispersion of repolarization occurs in the Brugada syndrome due to the presence of an intrinsically high level of I_{to} in RV (V_1–V_3) than in septal or LV regions (V_2–V_5) which permits loss of the action potential dome at sites with intrinsically large I_{to}. It follows that ERS may be more likely to occur when the balance of currents in the early phases of the action potential is shifted outward (due to a decrease in inward currents or an increase in outward currents) in hearts with an intrinsically weak I_{to}. A similar shift in outward current in hearts with intrinsically prominent I_{to} might be expected to display characteristics of the Brugada syndrome rather than of the early repolarization syndrome.

Ischemia

The electrocardiographic manifestations of the

Brugada syndrome are similar to those encountered during ischemia. As such, the Brugada syndrome may represent a stable (non-ischemic) model of the cellular changes that occur during acute ischemic injury as well as of other syndromes associated with an ST segment elevation. The presence of an additional outward current (i.e., I_{to}) in ventricular epicardium predisposes to loss of the action dome during ischemia, thus leading to amplification of transmural heterogeneities and the development of phase 2 reentry and VT/VF.

Cellular and ionic mechanism underlying the Brugada syndrome

The proposed cellular mechanism for the Brugada syndrome is summarized in Fig. 5.20. The available data support the hypothesis that the Brugada syndrome results from amplification of heterogeneities intrinsic to the early phases of the action potential among the different transmural cell types. The amplification is secondary to a rebalancing of currents active during phase 1, including a decrease in I_{Na} or I_{Ca} or augmentation of any one of a number of outward currents. ST segment elevation similar to that observed in patients with the Brugada syndrome occurs as a consequence of the accentuation of the action potential notch, eventually leading to loss of the action potential dome in right ventricular epicardium, where I_{to} is most prominent. Loss of the dome gives rise to both a transmural as well as epicardial dispersion of repolarization. The transmural dispersion is responsible for the development of ST segment elevation and the creation of a vulnerable

window across the ventricular wall, whereas the epicardial dispersion gives rise to phase 2 reentry which provides the extrasystole that captures the vulnerable window, thus precipitating VT/VF. The VT generated is usually polymorphic, resembling a very rapid form of *torsade de pointes*.

Rationale for pharmacologic approach to therapy

Despite important strides in the identification and characterization of the Brugada syndrome since the mid-1990s, progress relative to therapy has been less impressive. The various device and pharmacologic therapies tested clinically or suggested based on experimental evidence are listed in Table 5.2. ICD implantation is the only proven effective treatment for the disease.[143,144] This, however, is not an adequate solution for infants and young children or for adults residing in regions of the world where an ICD is unaffordable. Although arrhythmias and sudden death generally occur during sleep or at rest and have been associated with bradycardic states, a potential therapeutic role for pacing remains largely unexplored.

The pharmacologic approach to therapy has been tailored to a rebalancing of currents active during the early phases of the epicardial action potential in the right ventricle so as to reduce the magnitude of the action potential notch and/or restore the action potential dome. Antiarrhythmic agents such as amiodarone and β blockers have been shown to be ineffective.[145] Class IC antiarrhythmic drugs such as flecainide and propafenone are clearly contraindi-

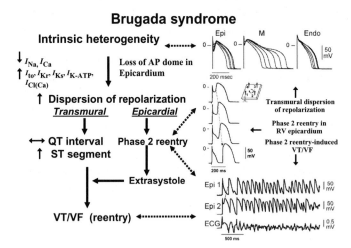

Figure 5.20 Proposed mechanism for the Brugada syndrome. A shift in the balance of currents serves to amplify existing heterogeneities by causing loss of the action potential dome at some epicardial sites, but not endocardial sites. A vulnerable window develops as a result of the dispersion of repolarization and refractoriness within epicardium as well as across the wall. Epicardial dispersion leads to the development of phase 2 reentry, which provides the extrasystole that captures the vulnerable window and initiates VT/VF via a circus movement reentry mechanism. Modified from Ref. 102, with permission.

Table 5.2 Device and pharmacologic considerations for therapy in the Brugada syndrome.

Devices
✓ ICD – only established effective therapy
? Pacemaker
? Ablation or cryosurgery

Pharmacologic
✗ Amiodarone – does not protect[145]
✗ β Blockers – do not protect[145]
✓ β Adrenergic agonists – Isoproterenol[98,149]
✓ Phosphodiesterase inhibitors – cilostazol[153]
✗ Class IC antiarrhythmics – flecainide, propafenone – contraindicated
Class IA antiarrhythmics
✗ Procainamide, disopyramide – contraindicated
✓ Quinidine[49,147,148,152]
? Tedisamil
✓ I_{to} blockers – cardioselective and ion channel specific

cated for reasons previously discussed. Class IA agents such as procainamide and disopyramide are contraindicated for similar reasons. Other class IA agents, such as quinidine and tedisamil, however, may exert a therapeutic action. Because the presence of a prominent transient outward current, I_{to}, is at the heart of the mechanism underlying the Brugada syndrome, any agent that inhibits this current may be protective. Cardioselective and I_{to}-specific blockers are not currently available. The only agent on the market in the United States with significant I_{to} blocking properties is quinidine. It is for this reason that we suggested several years ago that this agent may be of therapeutic value in the Brugada syndrome.[146] Experimental studies have since shown quinidine to be effective in restoring the epicardial action potential dome, thus normalizing the ST segment and preventing phase 2 reentry and polymorphic VT in experimental models of the Brugada syndrome.[49] Clinical evidence of the effectiveness of quinidine in normalizing ST segment elevation in patients with the Brugada syndrome has been reported,[147,148] although clinical trials designed to assess the efficacy of this agent are not available. Agents that boost the calcium current, such as isoproterenol, may be useful as well.[49,109] Both types of agents have been shown to be effective in normalizing ST segment elevation in patients with the Brugada syndrome and in controlling electrical

storms, particularly in children.[147–151] Other than the study by Belhassen and coworkers involving quinidine, none have as yet demonstrated long-term efficacy in the prevention of sudden death.[147,152] The most recent addition to the pharmacologic armamentarium is the phospodiesterase III inhibitor, cilostazol,[153] which normalizes the ST segment most likely by augmenting calcium current (I_{Ca}) as well as by reducing I_{to} secondary to an increase in heart rate. Finally, an experimental antiarrhythmic agent, tedisamil, with potent actions to block I_{to}, among other outward currents, has been suggested as a therapeutic candidate.[109] Tedisamil may be more potent than quinidine because it lacks the relatively strong inward current blocking actions of quinidine. The development of a cardioselective and I_{to}-specific blocker would be a most welcome addition to the limited therapeutic armamentarium currently available to combat this disease. One potential candidate is an agent recently reported to be a selective I_{to} and I_{Kur} blocker, AVE0118. Appropriate clinical trials are needed to establish the effectiveness of all of the above pharmacologic agents as well as the possible role of pacemakers.

Supported by grants from the National Institutes of Health (HL 47678), the American Heart Association, New York State Affiliate, and the Masons of New York State and Florida.

References

1 Einthoven W. The galvanometric registration of the human electrocardiogram, likewise a review of the use of the capillary electrometer in physiology. *Pflugers Arch.* 1903; **99**: 472–480.

2 Einthoven W. Uber die Deutung des Electrokardio-gramms. *Pflugers Arch.* 1912; **149**: 65–86.

3 Antzelevitch C, Dumaine R. Electrical heterogeneity in the heart: physiological, pharmacological and clinical implications. In: Page E, Fozzard HA, Solaro RJ, eds. *Handbook of Physiology. The Heart.* New York: Oxford University Press, 2002: 654–692.

4 Antzelevitch C, Zygmunt AC, Dumaine R. Electrophysiology and pharmacology of ventricular repolarization. In: Gussak I, Antzelevitch C, eds. *Cardiac Repolarization. Bridging Basic and Clinical Sciences.* Totowa, NJ: Humana Press, 2003: 63–90.

5 Antzelevitch C. Heterogeneity of cellular repolarization in LQTS. The role of M cells. *Eur. Heart J.* 2001; **Suppl. 3**: K-2–K-16.

6 Antzelevitch C, Shimizu W, Yan GX et al. The M cell. Its contribution to the ECG and to normal and abnormal electrical function of the heart. *J. Cardiovasc. Electrophysiol.* 1999; **10**: 1124–1152.

7 Antzelevitch C, Nesterenko VV. Contribution of electrical heterogeneity of repolarization to the ECG. In: Gussak I, Antzelevitch C, eds. *Cardiac Repolarization. Bridging Basic and Clinical Science.* Totowa, NJ: Humana Press, 2003: 111–126.

8 Liu DW, Gintant GA, Antzelevitch C. Ionic bases for electrophysiological distinctions among epicardial, midmyocardial, and endocardial myocytes from the free wall of the canine left ventricle. *Circ. Res.* 1993; **72**: 671–687.

9 Furukawa T, Myerburg RJ, Furukawa N et al. Differences in transient outward currents of feline endocardial and epicardial myocytes. *Circ. Res.* 1990; **67**: 1287–1291.

10 Fedida D, Giles WR. Regional variations in action potentials and transient outward current in myocytes isolated from rabbit left ventricle. *J. Physiol. (Lond.)* 1991; **442**: 191–209.

11 Clark RB, Bouchard RA, Salinas-Stefanon E et al. Heterogeneity of action potential waveforms and potassium currents in rat ventricle. *Cardiovasc. Res.* 1993; **27**: 1795–1799.

12 Wettwer E, Amos GJ, Posival H et al. Transient outward current in human ventricular myocytes of subepicardial and subendocardial origin. *Circ. Res.* 1994; **75**: 473–482.

13 Nabauer M, Beuckelmann DJ, Uberfuhr P et al. Regional differences in current density and rate-dependent properties of the transient outward current in subepicardial and subendocardial myocytes of human left ventricle. *Circulation* 1996; **93**: 168–177.

14 Di Diego JM, Sun ZQ, Antzelevitch C. I_{to} and action potential notch are smaller in left vs. right canine ventricular epicardium. *Am. J. Physiol.* 1996; **271**: H548–H561.

15 Volders PG, Sipido KR, Carmeliet E et al. Repolarizing K^+ currents ITO1 and IKs are larger in right than left canine ventricular midmyocardium. *Circulation* 1999; **99**: 206–210.

16 Antzelevitch C, Sicouri S, Litovsky SH et al. Heterogeneity within the ventricular wall: electrophysiology and pharmacology of epicardial, endocardial and M cells. *Circ. Res.* 1991; **69**: 1427–1449.

17 Antzelevitch C, Sicouri S, Lukas A et al. Regional differences in the electrophysiology of ventricular cells: physiological and clinical implications. In: Zipes DP, Jalife J, eds. *Cardiac Electrophysiology: From Cell to Bedside.* Philadelphia: W.B. Saunders Co., 1995: 228–245.

18 Antzelevitch C, Sicouri S, Lukas A et al. Clinical implications of electrical heterogeneity in the heart: the electrophysiology and pharmacology of epicardial, M and endocardial cells. In: Podrid PJ, Kowey PR, eds. *Cardiac Arrhythmia: Mechanism, Diagnosis and Management.* Baltimore, MD: William & Wilkins, 1995: 88–107.

19 Yan GX, Antzelevitch C. Cellular basis for the electrocardiographic J wave. *Circulation* 1996; **93**: 372–379.

20 Lukas A, Antzelevitch C. Phase 2 reentry as a mechanism of initiation of circus movement reentry in canine epicardium exposed to simulated ischemia. The antiarrhythmic effects of 4-aminopyridine. *Cardiovasc. Res.* 1996; **32**: 593–603.

21 Antzelevitch C, Di Diego JM, Sicouri S et al. Selective pharmacological modification of repolarizing currents. Antiarrhythmic and proarrhythmic actions of agents that influence repolarization in the heart. In: Breithardt J, ed. *Antiarrhythmic Drugs: Mechanisms of Antiarrhythmic and Proarrhythmic Actions.* Berlin: Springer-Verlag, 1995: 57–80.

22 Lukas A, Antzelevitch C. The contribution of K^+ currents to electrical heterogeneity across the canine ventricular wall under normal and ischemic conditions. In: Dhalla NS, Pierce GN, Panagia V, eds. *Pathophysiology of Heart Failure.* Boston: Academic Publishers, 1996: 440–456.

23 Litovsky SH, Antzelevitch C. Differences in the electrophysiological response of canine ventricular subendocardium and subepicardium to acetylcholine and isoproterenol. A direct effect of acetylcholine in ventricular myocardium. *Circ. Res.* 1990; **67**: 615–627.

24 Blair RW, Shimizu T, Bishop VS. The role of vagal afferents in the reflex control of the left ventricular refractory period in the cat. *Circ. Res.* 1980; **46**: 378–386.

25 Prystowsky EN, Jackman WM, Rinkenberger RL et al. Effect of autonomic blockade on ventricular refractoriness and atrioventricular nodal conduction in man. Evidence

supporting a direct cholinergic action on ventricular muscle refractoriness. *Circ. Res.* 1981; **49**: 511–518.

26 Mubagwa K, Carmeliet E. Effects of acetylcholine on electrophysiological properties of rabbit cardiac Purkinje fibers. *Circ. Res.* 1983; **53**: 740–751.

27 Trautwein W, Kameyama M. Intracellular control of calcium and potassium currents in cardiac cells. *Jpn. Heart J.* 1986; **27** Suppl 1: 31–50.

28 Nakayama T, Fozzard HA. Adrenergic modulation of the transient outward current in isolated canine Purkinje cells. *Circ. Res.* 1988; **62**: 162–172.

29 Harvey RD, Hume JR. Isoproterenol activates a chloride current, not the transient outward current, in rabbit ventricular myocytes. *Am. J. Physiol.* 1989; **257**: C1177–C1181.

30 Zygmunt AC, Gibbons WR. Calcium-activated chloride current in rabbit ventricular myocytes. *Circ. Res.* 1991; **68**: 424–437.

31 Zygmunt AC, Gibbons WR. Properties of the calcium-activated chloride current in heart. *J. Gen. Physiol.* 1992; **99**: 391–414.

32 Zygmunt AC. Intracellular calcium activates chloride current in canine ventricular myocytes. *Am. J. Physiol.* 1994; **267**: H1984-H1995.

33 Takano M, Noma A. Distribution of the isoprenaline-induced chloride current in rabbit heart. *Pflugers Arch.* 1992; **420**: 223–226.

34 Hume JR, Harvey RD. Chloride conductance pathways in heart. *Am. J. Physiol.* 1991; **261**: C399–C412.

35 Saeki Y, Kamiyama A. Possible mechanism of rate-dependent change of contraction in dog ventricular muscle: relation to calcium movements. In: Kobayashi T, Sano R, Dhalla NS, eds. *Recent Advances in Studies on Cardiac Structure and Metabolism*, Vol. II. Baltimore, MD: University Park Press, 1978: 131–135.

36 Kimura S, Nakaya H, Kanno M. Electrophysiological effects of diltiazem, nifedipine and Ni^{2+} on the subepicardial muscle cells of canine heart under the condition of combined hypoxia, hyperkalemia and acidosis. *Naunyn Schmiedebergs Arch. Pharmacol.* 1983; **324**: 228–232.

37 Kamiyama A, Saeki Y. Myocardial action potentials of right- and left-subepicardial muscles in the canine ventricle and effects of manganese ions. *Proc. Jap. Acad.* 1974; **50**: 771–774.

38 Gilmour RF, Jr., Zipes DP. Different electrophysiological responses of canine endocardium and epicardium to combined hyperkalemia, hypoxia, and acidosis. *Circ. Res.* 1980; **46**: 814–825.

39 Kimura S, Bassett AL, Kohya T *et al.* Regional effects of verapamil on recovery of excitability and conduction time in experimental ischemia. *Circulation* 1987; **76**: 1146–1154.

40 Krishnan SC, Antzelevitch C. Sodium channel blockade produces opposite electrophysiologic effects in canine ventricular epicardium and endocardium. *Circ. Res.* 1991; **69**: 277–291.

41 Krishnan SC, Antzelevitch C. Flecainide-induced arrhythmia in canine ventricular epicardium: phase 2 reentry? *Circulation* 1993; **87**: 562–572.

42 Jochim K, Katz LN, Mayne W. The monophasic electrogram obtained from the mammalian heart. *Am. J. Physiol.* 1935; **111**: 177–186.

43 Van Bogaert PP, Snyders DS. Effects of 4-aminopyridine on inward rectifing and pacemaker currents of cardiac purkinje fibers. *Pflugers Arch.* 1982; **394**: 230–238.

44 Di Diego JM, Antzelevitch C. Pinacidil-induced electrical heterogeneity and extrasystolic activity in canine ventricular tissues: does activation of ATP-regulated potassium current promote phase 2 reentry? *Circulation* 1993; **88**: 1177–1189.

45 Di Diego JM, Antzelevitch C. High $[Ca^{2+}]$-induced electrical heterogeneity and extrasystolic activity in isolated canine ventricular epicardium: phase 2 reentry. *Circulation* 1994; **89**: 1839–1850.

46 Lukas A, Antzelevitch C. Differences in the electrophysiological response of canine ventricular epicardium and endocardium to ischemia: role of the transient outward current. *Circulation* 1993; **88**: 2903–2915.

47 Antzelevitch C, Di Diego JM. The role of K^+ channel activators in cardiac electrophysiology and arrhythmias. *Circulation* 1992; **85**: 1627–1629.

48 Imaizumi Y, Giles WR. Quinidine-induced inhibition of transient outward current in cardiac muscle. *Am. J. Physiol.* 1987; **253**: H704–H708.

49 Yan GX, Antzelevitch C. Cellular basis for the Brugada syndrome and other mechanisms of arrhythmogenesis associated with ST segment elevation. *Circulation* 1999; **100**: 1660–1666.

50 Sicouri S, Moro S, Litovsky SH *et al.* Chronic amiodarone reduces transmural dispersion of repolarization in the canine heart. *J. Cardiovasc. Electrophysiol.* 1997; **8**: 1269–1279.

51 Sicouri S, Antzelevitch C. A subpopulation of cells with unique electrophysiological properties in the deep subepicardium of the canine ventricle: the M cell. *Circ. Res.* 1991; **68**: 1729–1741.

52 Anyukhovsky EP, Sosunov EA, Rosen MR. Regional differences in electrophysiologic properties of epicardium, midmyocardium and endocardium: In vitro and in vivo correlations. *Circulation* 1996; **94**: 1981–1988.

53 Liu DW, Antzelevitch C. Characteristics of the delayed rectifier current (I_{Kr} and I_{Ks}) in canine ventricular epicardial, midmyocardial and endocardial myocytes: a weaker I_{Ks} contributes to the longer action potential of the M cell. *Circ. Res.* 1995; **76**: 351–365.

54 Eddlestone GT, Zygmunt AC, Antzelevitch C. Larger late sodium current contributes to the longer action potential of the M cell in canine ventricular myocardium. *Pacing Clin. Electrophysiol.* 1996; **19**: No.4, Part 2: 569 (Abstract).

55 Zygmunt AC, Goodrow RJ, Antzelevitch C. $I_{Na\text{-}Ca}$ contributes to electrical heterogeneity within the canine ventricle. *Am. J. Physiol.* 2000; **278**: H1671–H1678.

56 Yan GX, Shimizu W, Antzelevitch C. Characteristics and distribution of M cells in arterially-perfused canine left ventricular wedge preparations. *Circulation* 1998; **98**: 1921–1927.

57 Sicouri S, Fish J, Antzelevitch C. Distribution of M cells in the canine ventricle. *J. Cardiovasc. Electrophysiol.* 1994; **5**: 824–837.

58 Sicouri S, Antzelevitch C. Electrophysiologic characteristics of M cells in the canine left ventricular free wall. *J. Cardiovasc. Electrophysiol.* 1995; **6**: 591–603.

59 Weissenburger J, Nesterenko VV, Antzelevitch C. Transmural heterogeneity of ventricular repolarization under baseline and long QT conditions in the canine heart in vivo. Torsades de Pointes develops with halothane but not pentobarbital anesthesia. *J. Cardiovasc. Electrophysiol.* 2000; **11**: 290–304.

60 Rodriguez-Sinovas A, Cinca J, Tapias A *et al.* Lack of evidence of M-cells in porcine left ventricular myocardium. *Cardiovasc. Res.* 1997; **33**: 307–313.

61 El-Sherif N, Caref EB, Yin H *et al.* The electrophysiological mechanism of ventricular arrhythmias in the long QT syndrome: tridimensional mapping of activation and recovery patterns. *Circ. Res.* 1996; **79**: 474–492.

62 Balati B, Varro A, Papp JG. Comparison of the cellular electrophysiological characteristics of canine left ventricular epicardium, M cells, endocardium and Purkinje fibres. *Acta Physiol. Scand.* 1998; **164**: 181–190.

63 Sicouri S, Quist M, Antzelevitch C. Evidence for the presence of M cells in the guinea pig ventricle. *J. Cardiovasc. Electrophysiol.* 1996; **7**: 503–511.

64 McIntosh MA, Cobbe SM, Smith GL. Heterogeneous changes in action potential and intracellular Ca^{2+} in left ventricular myocyte sub-types from rabbits with heart failure. *Cardiovasc. Res.* 2000; **45**: 397–409.

65 Stankovicova T, Szilard M, De Scheerder I *et al.* M cells and transmural heterogeneity of action potential configuration in myocytes from the left ventricular wall of the pig heart. *Cardiovasc. Res.* 2000; **45**: 952–960.

66 Drouin E, Charpentier F, Gauthier C *et al.* Electrophysiological characteristics of cells spanning the left ventricular wall of human heart: evidence for the presence of M cells. *J. Am. Coll. Cardiol.* 1995; **26**: 185–192.

67 Li GR, Feng J, Yue L *et al.* Transmural heterogeneity of action potentials and Ito1 in myocytes isolated from the human right ventricle. *Am. J. Physiol.* 1998; **275**: H369–H377.

68 Gussak I, Bjerregaard P, Egan TM *et al.* ECG phenomenon called the J wave. History, pathophysiology, and clinical significance. *J. Electrocardiol.* 1995; **28**: 49–58.

69 Osborn JJ. Experimental hypothermia: respiratory and blood pH changes in relation to cardiac function. *Am. J. Physiol.* 1953; **175**: 389–398.

70 Hugo N, Dormehl IC, Van Gelder AL. A positive wave at the J-point of electrocardiograms of anaesthetized baboons. *J. Med. Primatol.* 1988; **17**: 347–352.

71 West TC, Frederickson EL, Amory DW. Single fiber recording of the ventricular response to induced hypothermia in the anesthetized dog. Correlation with multicellular parameters. *Circ. Res.* 1959; **7**: 880–888.

72 Santos EM, Frederick KC. Electrocardiographic changes in the dog during hypothermia. *Am. Heart J.* 1957; **55**: 415–420.

73 Clements SD, Hurst JW. Diagnostic value of ECG abnormalities observed in subjects accidentally exposed to cold. *Am. J. Cardiol.* 1972; **29**: 729–734.

74 Thompson R, Rich J, Chmelik F *et al.* Evolutionary changes in the electrocardiogram of severe progressive hypothermia. *J. Electrocardiol.* 1977; **10**: 67–70.

75 Dillon SM, Allessie MA, Ursell PC *et al.* Influences of anisotropic tissue structure on reentrant circuits in the epicardial border zone of subacute canine infarcts. *Circ. Res.* 1988; **63**: 182–206.

76 Eagle K. Images in clinical medicine. Osborn waves of hypothermia. *N. Engl. J. Med.* 1994; **10**: 680.

77 Kraus F. Ueber die wirkung des kalziums auf den kreislauf. *Dtsch. Med. Wochenschr.* 1920; **46**: 201–203.

78 Sridharan MR, Horan LG. Electrocardiographic J wave of hypercalcemia. *Am. J. Cardiol.* 1984; **54**: 672–673.

79 Yan GX, Lankipalli RS, Burke JF *et al.* Ventricular repolarization components on the electrocardiogram: cellular basis and clinical significance. *J. Am. Coll. Cardiol.* 2003; **42**: 401–409.

80 Litovsky SH, Antzelevitch C. Transient outward current prominent in canine ventricular epicardium but not endocardium. *Circ. Res.* 1988; **62**: 116–126.

81 Emslie-Smith D, Sladden GE, Stirling GR. The significance of changes in the electrocardiogram in hypothermia. *Br. Heart J.* 1959; **21**: 343–351.

82 Antzelevitch C, Sicouri S. Clinical relevance of cardiac arrhythmias generated by afterdepolarizations: The role of M cells in the generation of U waves, triggered activity and torsade de pointes. *J. Am. Coll. Cardiol.* 1994; **23**: 259–277.

83 Jeck CD, Boyden PA. Age-related appearance of outward currents may contribute to developmental differences in ventricular repolarization. *Circ. Res.* 1992; **71**: 1390–1403.

84 Pacioretty LM, Gilmour RF, Jr. Developmental changes in the transient outward potassium current in canine epicardium. *Am. J. Physiol.* 1995; **268**: H2513–H2521.

85 Phillipson EA, Herbert FA. Accidental exposure to freezing: clinical and laboratory observations during convalescence from near-fatal hypothermia. *Can. Med. Assoc. J.* 1967; **97**: 786–792.

86 Okada M, Nishimura F, Yoshino H *et al.* The J wave in accidental hypothermia. *J. Electrocardiol.* 1983; **16**: 23–28.

87 Sridharan MR, Johnson JC, Horan LG *et al.* Monophasic action potentials in hypercalcemic and hypothermic 'J' waves – a comparative study. *Am. Fed. Clin. Res.* 1983; **31**: 219.

88 Rosati B, Pan Z, Lypen S *et al.* Regulation of KChIP2 potassium channel beta subunit gene expression underlies the gradient of transient outward current in canine and human ventricle. *J. Physiol.* 2001; **533**: 119–125.

89 Deschenes I, DiSilvestre D, Juang GJ *et al.* Regulation of Kv4.3 current by KChIP2 splice variants: a component of native cardiac *I*(to)? *Circulation* 2002; **106**: 423–429.

90 Rosati B, Grau F, Rodriguez S *et al.* Concordant expression of KChIP2 mRNA, protein and transient outward current throughout the canine ventricle. *J. Physiol.* 2003; **548**: 815–822.

91 Litovsky SH, Antzelevitch C. Rate dependence of action potential duration and refractoriness in canine ventricular endocardium differs from that of epicardium: the role of the transient outward current. *J. Am. Coll. Cardiol.* 1989; **14**: 1053–1066.

92 Kilborn MJ, Fedida D. A study of the developmental changes in outward currents of rat ventricular myocytes. *J. Physiol. (Lond.)* 1990; **430**: 37–60.

93 Furukawa T, Kimura S, Cuevas J *et al.* Role of cardiac ATP-regulated potassium channels in differential responses of endocardial and epicardial cells to ischemia. *Circ. Res.* 1991; **68**: 1693–1702.

94 Brugada P, Brugada J. Right bundle branch block, persistent ST segment elevation and sudden cardiac death: a distinct clinical and electrocardiographic syndrome: a multicenter report. *J. Am. Coll. Cardiol.* 1992; **20**: 1391–1396.

95 Aizawa Y, Tamura M, Chinushi M *et al.* Catheter ablation with radiofrequency current of ventricular tachycardia originating from the right ventricle. *Am. Heart J.* 1993; **126**: 1473–1474.

96 Aizawa Y, Tamura M, Chinushi M *et al.* An attempt at electrical catheter ablation of the arrhythmogenic area in idiopathic ventricular fibrillation. *Am. Heart J.* 1992; **123**: 257–260.

97 Bjerregaard P, Gussak I, Kotar Sl *et al.* Recurrent synocope in a patient with prominent J-wave. *Am. Heart J.* 1994; **127**: 1426–1430.

98 Miyazaki T, Mitamura H, Miyoshi S *et al.* Autonomic and antiarrhythmic drug modulation of ST segment elevation in patients with Brugada syndrome. *J. Am. Coll. Cardiol.* 1996; **27**: 1061–1070.

99 Pertsov AM, Davidenko JM, Salomonsz R *et al.* Spiral waves of excitation underlie reentrant activity in isolated cardiac muscle. *Circ. Res.* 1993; **72**: 631–650.

100 Asano Y, Davidenko JM, Baxter WT *et al.* Optical mapping of drug-induced polymorphic arrhythmias and torsade de pointes in the isolated rabbit heart. *J. Am. Coll. Cardiol.* 1997; **29**: 831–842.

101 Antzelevitch C. The Brugada syndrome: ionic basis and arrhythmia mechanisms. *J. Cardiovasc. Electrophysiol.* 2001; **12**: 268–272.

102 Antzelevitch C. The Brugada syndrome. diagnostic criteria and cellular mechanisms. *Eur. Heart J.* 2001; **22**: 356–363.

103 Gussak I, Antzelevitch C, Bjerregaard P *et al.* The Brugada syndrome: clinical, electrophysiological and genetic aspects. *J. Am. Coll. Cardiol.* 1999; **33**: 5–15.

104 Antzelevitch C, Brugada P, Brugada J *et al.* Brugada syndrome: a decade of progress. *Circ. Res.* 2002; **91**: 1114–1118.

105 Kurita T, Shimizu W, Inagaki M *et al.* The electrophysiologic mechanism of ST-segment elevation in Brugada syndrome. *J. Am. Coll. Cardiol.* 2002; **40**: 330–334.

106 Futterman LG, Lemberg L. Brugada. *Am. J. Crit. Care* 2001; **10**: 360–364.

107 Fujiki A, Usui M, Nagasawa H *et al.* ST segment elevation in the right precordial leads induced with class IC antiarrhythmic drugs: insight into the mechanism of Brugada syndrome [see comments]. *J. Cardiovasc. Electrophysiol.* 1999; **10**: 214–218.

108 Nagase S, Kusano KF, Morita H *et al.* Epicardial electrogram at the right ventricular outflow tract in patients with Brugada syndrome using epicardial lead. *J. Am. Coll. Cardiol.* 2002; **39**: 1992–1995.

109 Antzelevitch C. The Brugada syndrome: ionic basis and arrhythmia mechanisms. *J. Cardiovasc. Electrophysiol.* 2001; **12**: 268–272.

110 Shimizu W, Aiba T, Kurita T *et al.* Paradoxic abbreviation of repolarization in epicardium of the right ventricular outflow tract during augmentation of Brugada-type ST segment elevation. *J. Cardiovasc. Electrophysiol.* 2001; **12**: 1418–1421.

111 Brugada R, Brugada J, Antzelevitch C *et al.* Sodium channel blockers identify risk for sudden death in patients with ST-segment elevation and right bundle branch block but structurally normal hearts. *Circulation* 2000; **101**: 510–515.

112 Shimizu W, Antzelevitch C, Suyama K *et al.* Effect of sodium channel blockers on ST segment, QRS duration, and corrected QT interval in patients with Brugada syndrome. *J. Cardiovasc. Electrophysiol.* 2000; **11**: 1320–1329.

113 Priori SG, Napolitano C, Gasparini M *et al.* Clinical and genetic heterogeneity of right bundle branch block and ST-segment elevation syndrome: a prospective evalua-

tion of 52 families [In Process Citation]. *Circulation* 2000; **102**: 2509–2515.

114 Brugada P, Brugada J, Brugada R. Arrhythmia induction by antiarrhythmic drugs. *Pacing Clin. Electrophysiol.* 2000; **23**: 291–292.

115 Babaliaros VC, Hurst JW. Tricyclic antidepressants and the Brugada syndrome: an example of Brugada waves appearing after the administration of desipramine. *Clin. Cardiol.* 2002; **25**: 395–398.

116 Goldgran-Toledano D, Sideris G, Kevorkian JP. Overdose of cyclic antidepressants and the Brugada syndrome. *N. Engl. J. Med.* 2002; **346**: 1591–1592.

117 Tada H, Sticherling C, Oral H et al. Brugada syndrome mimicked by tricyclic antidepressant overdose. *J. Cardiovasc. Electrophysiol.* 2001; **12**: 275.

118 Pastor A, Nunez A, Cantale C et al. Asymptomatic Brugada syndrome case unmasked during dimenhydrinate infusion. *J. Cardiovasc. Electrophysiol.* 2001; **12**: 1192–1194.

119 Ortega-Carnicer J, Bertos-Polo J, Gutierrez-Tirado C. Aborted sudden death, transient Brugada pattern, and wide QRS dysrrhythmias after massive cocaine ingestion. *J. Electrocardiol.* 2001; **34**: 345–349.

120 Nogami A, Nakao M, Kubota S et al. Enhancement of J-ST-segment elevation by the glucose and insulin test in Brugada syndrome. *Pacing Clin. Electrophysiol.* 2003; **26**: 332–337.

121 Di Diego JM, Cordeiro JM, Goodrow RJ et al. Ionic and cellular basis for the predominance of the Brugada syndrome phenotype in males. *Circulation* 2002; **106**: 2004–2011.

122 Chen Q, Kirsch GE, Zhang D et al. Genetic basis and molecular mechanisms for idiopathic ventricular fibrillation. *Nature* 1998; **392**: 293–296.

123 Rook MB, Alshinawi CB, Groenewegen WA et al. Human SCN5A gene mutations alter cardiac sodium channel kinetics and are associated with the Brugada syndrome. *Cardiovasc. Res.* 1999; **44**: 507–517.

124 Dumaine R, Towbin JA, Brugada P et al. Ionic mechanisms responsible for the electrocardiographic phenotype of the Brugada syndrome are temperature dependent. *Circ. Res.* 1999; **85**: 803–809.

125 Deschenes I, Baroudi G, Berthet M et al. Electrophysiological characterization of SCN5A mutations causing long QT (E1784K) and Brugada (R1512W and R1432G) syndromes. *Cardiovasc. Res.* 2000; **46**: 55–65.

126 Priori SG, Napolitano C, Glordano U et al. Brugada syndrome and sudden cardiac death in children. *Lancet* 2000; **355**: 808–809.

127 Bezzina C, Veldkamp MW, van Den Berg MP et al. A single Na($^+$) channel mutation causing both long-QT and Brugada syndromes. *Circ. Res.* 1999; **85**: 1206–1213.

128 Kyndt F, Probst V, Potet F et al. Novel SCN5A mutation leading either to isolated cardiac conduction defect or Brugada syndrome in a large French family. *Circulation* 2001; **104**: 3081–3086.

129 Wan X, Wang Q, Kirsch GE. Functional suppression of sodium channels by beta(1)-subunits as a molecular mechanism of idiopathic ventricular fibrillation [In Process Citation]. *J. Mol. Cell. Cardiol.* 2000; **32**: 1873–1884.

130 Wang DW, Makita N, Kitabatake A et al. Enhanced Na($^+$) channel intermediate inactivation in Brugada syndrome. *Circ. Res.* 2000; **87**: E37–E43.

131 Balser JR. Sodium 'channelopathies' and sudden death. Must you be so sensitive? *Circ. Res.* 1999; **85**: 872–874.

132 Baroudi G, Pouliot V, Denjoy I et al. Novel mechanism for Brugada syndrome: defective surface localization of an SCN5A mutant (R1432G). *Circ. Res.* 2001; **88**: E78–E83.

133 Baroudi G, Acharfi S, Larouche C et al. Expression and intracellular localization of an SCN5A double mutant R1232W/T1620M implicated in Brugada syndrome. *Circ. Res.* 2002; **90**: E11–E16.

134 Vatta M, Dumaine R, Varghese G et al. Genetic and biophysical basis of sudden unexplained nocturnal death syndrome (SUNDS), a disease allelic to Brugada syndrome. *Hum. Mol. Genet.* 2002; **11**: 337–345.

135 Viswanathan PC, Bezzina CR, George AL, Jr. et al. Gating-dependent mechanisms for flecainide action in SCN5A-linked arrhythmia syndromes. *Circulation* 2001; **104**: 1200–1205.

136 Gima K, Rudy Y. Ionic current basis of electrocardiographic waveforms: a model study. *Circ. Res.* 2002; **90**: 889–896.

137 Bezzina CR, Rook MB, Wilde AA. Cardiac sodium channel and inherited arrhythmia syndromes. *Cardiovasc. Res.* 2001; **49**: 257–271.

138 Madle A, Kratochvil Z, Polivkova A. [The Brugada syndrome]. *Vnitr. Lek.* 2002; **48**: 255–258.

139 Gonzalez Rebollo G, Madrid H, Carcia A et al. Reccurrent ventricular fibrillation during a febrile illness in a patient with the Brugada syndrome. *Rev. Esp. Cardiol.* 2000; **53**: 755–757.

140 Saura D, Garcia-Alberola A, Carrillo P et al. Brugada-like electrocardiographic pattern induced by fever. *Pacing Clin. Electrophysiol.* 2002; **25**: 856–859.

141 Porres JM, Brugada J, Urbistondo V et al. Fever unmasking the Brugada syndrome. *Pacing Clin. Electrophysiol.* 2002; **25**: 1646–1648.

142 Kum L, Fung JWH, Chan WWL et al. Brugada syndrome unmasked by febrile illness. *Pacing Clin. Electrophysiol.* 2002; **25**: 1660–1661.

143 Brugada J, Brugada R, Brugada P. Pharmacological and device approach to therapy of inherited cardiac diseases associated with cardiac arrhythmias and sudden death. *J. Electrocardiol.* 2000; **33** Suppl: 41–47.

144 Brugada P, Brugada R, Brugada J et al. Use of the prophylactic implantable cardioverter defibrillator for patients with normal hearts. Am. J. Cardiol. 1999; **83**: 98D–100D.

145 Brugada J, Brugada R, Brugada P. Right bundle-branch block and ST-segment elevation in leads V_1 through V_3. A marker for sudden death in patients without demonstrable structural heart disease. Circulation 1998; **97**: 457–460.

146 Antzelevitch C, P Brugada, J Brugada, R Brugada, K Nademanee, JA Towbin. The Brugada Syndrome. Armonk, NY: Futura Publishing Company, Inc., 1999: 1–99.

147 Belhassen B, Viskin S, Antzelevitch C. The Brugada syndrome: is ICD the only therapeutic option? Pacing Clin. Electrophysiol. 2002; **25**: 1634–1640.

148 Alings M, Dekker L, Sadee A et al. Quinidine induced electrocardiographic normalization in two patients with Brugada syndrome. Pacing Clin. Electrophysiol. 2001; **24**: 1420–1422.

149 Shimizu W, Matsuo K, Takagi M et al. Body surface distribution and response to drugs of ST segment elevation in Brugada syndrome: clinical implication of eighty-seven-lead body surface potential mapping and its application to twelve-lead electrocardiograms. J. Cardiovasc. Electrophysiol. 2000; **11**: 396–404.

150 Suzuki H, Torigoe K, Numata O et al. Infant case with a malignant form of Brugada syndrome. J. Cardiovasc. Electrophysiol. 2000; **11**: 1277–1280.

151 Tanaka H, Kinoshita O, Uchikawa S et al. Successful prevention of recurrent ventricular fibrillation by intravenous isoproterenol in a patient with Brugada syndrome. Pacing Clin. Electrophysiol. 2001; **24**: 1293–1294.

152 Belhassen B, Viskin S, Fish R et al. Effects of electrophysiologic-guided therapy with class IA antiarrhythmic drugs on the long-term outcome of patients with idiopathic ventricular fibrillation with or without the Brugada syndrome [see comments]. J. Cardiovasc. Electrophysiol. 1999; **10**: 1301–1312.

153 Tsuchiya T, Ashikaga K, Honda T et al. Prevention of ventricular fibrillation by cilostazol, an oral phosphodiesterase inhibitor, in a patient with Brugada syndrome. J. Cardiovasc. Electrophysiol. 2002; **13**: 698–701.

154 Yan GX, Antzelevitch C. Cellular basis for the electrocardiographic J wave. Circulation 1995; **92**: 1–71 (Abstract).

155 Fish JM, Antzelevitch C. Role of sodium and calcium channel block in unmasking the Brugada syndrome. Heart Rhythm 2004; **1**: 210–217.

156 Antzelevitch C, Litovsky SH, Lukas A. Epicardium vs. endocardium. Electrophysiology and pharmacology. In: Zipes DP, Jalife J, eds. Cardiac Electrophysiology, From Cell to Bedside. New York: W.B. Saunders, 1990: 386–395.

157 Antzelevitch C, Brugada P, Brugada J et al. Brugada syndrome: 1992–2002. A historical perspective. J. Am. Coll. Cardiol. 2003; **41**: 1665–1671.

CHAPTER 6

Brugada syndrome: diagnostic criteria

A. A. M. Wilde, MD, PhD

Introduction

In 1992 Pedro and Josep Brugada described eight successfully resuscitated patients with a comparable characteristic ECG.[1] These ECG characteristics were described in the title of this landmark study: 'Right bundle branch block, persistent ST segment elevation and sudden cardiac death, a distinct clinical and electrocardiographic syndrome'. All ECGs showed an ST segment elevation in the right precordial leads of >0.1 mV (of the coved type, see below). Although the ECG had been described as early as in 1953,[2] these authors first described it as a distinct clinical entity associated with a high risk of sudden cardiac death with, because of the absence of structural heart disease in all patients, a functional basis for the ECG changes.[1]

In later years, the syndrome of right bundle branch block, ST segment elevation in V_1–V_3, and sudden death, named Brugada syndrome from 1996 onward,[3] has received a lot of attention. The syndrome appeared to be a familial disease with an autosomal dominant mode of transmission with incomplete penetrance. Heterogeneity has been shown with as yet only *SCN5A*, the gene encoding for the α subunit of the sodium channel, causally involved.[4] There seems a male predominance and arrhythmic events tend to appear from the 4th decade onward, with notable exceptions at both ends of the age spectrum (range: 2 to 77 years).[1,5] Sudden unexplained death syndrome (SUDS), a major cause of death of young Southeast Asian men appeared largely similar to Brugada syndrome, including the typical electrophysiological characteristics and the genetic basis.[6]

In different regions of the world the incidence varies markedly. Furthermore, there is considerable discussion as to the prognostic significance of several electrocardiographic and clinical characteristics. In part these controversies may be caused by the criteria applied to reach the diagnosis of Brugada syndrome. Indeed, it has been shown that the number of idiopathic ventricular patients diagnosed as having the Brugada syndrome is a sensitive function of the diagnostic criteria applied.[7] This led to an attempt to come to a consensus report on 'Diagnostic criteria for the Brugada syndrome' published in late 2002 simultaneously in the journals of the American Heart Association and the European Society of Cardiology.[8,9] In 2001, an alternative classification scheme had been published based on major and minor criteria.[10] Instead, by virtue of the lack of sensitive data on risk stratification, a quantitative approach was considered premature and the consensus report chose to provide descriptions of different clinical and electrocardiographic characteristics.

Clinical presentations/ symptomatology

Frequently (aborted) sudden cardiac death is the one and only symptom in a patient with Brugada syndrome. Upon monitoring such patients, it has become clear that rapid polymorphic VTs are the underlying cause. Self-terminating episodes, actually a typical feature of Brugada syndrome, may lead to (repeated) syncope. By carefully analyzing stored electrograms of ICDs, it has been shown that two-thirds of VF episodes were preceded by premature ventricular complexes which closely resembled the initiating PVC of VF.[11] These initiating PVCs appeared in the terminal part of the T wave and only rarely a long-short sequence was observed.[11] Rarely monomorphic VTs are observed.[12,13] Sudden death and documented arrhythmias predominantly occur in the early morning hours.[14,62] There appears to be an increased prevalence of atrial arrhythmias, including AV nodal reentry, atrial flutter, and atrial fibrillation.[16,17]

Both in patients with and without the typical ECG at baseline (see below), the presence of symptoms is very important with respect to prognosis.[18,19] The mean age of symptoms in affected individuals is in the third to fourth decade. However, among the first patients described, a symptomatic twin of 2 years of age and an individual with his first symptom at an age of 77 years were included.[1] Recently other pediatric cases have been reported.[5,20] There is a strong male preponderance of the ECG pattern[19,21,22] for which recently an elegant pathophysiologic basis has been suggested. Because surgical castration has been shown to normalize the ECG, a role for testosterone has also been suggested.[15] Electrocardiographically affected males are more readily inducible than females[19] and have a slight excess of events on follow-up.[18] The family history is very important and is often positive for sudden cardiac death at a young age. In particular, nocturnal death of a male family member should alert physicians.

The ECG

There is little doubt that ECG characteristics, including both repolarization as well as depolarization abnormalities, constitute the hallmark of Brugada syndrome (Fig. 6.1). Since a number of structural heart diseases might lead to identical electrocardiographic abnormalities (see below), a prerequisite for the diagnosis of Brugada syndrome is no evidence for structural cardiac abnormalities whatsoever. Extensive non-invasive as well as invasive routine diagnostic cardiologic investigations are required to decide on the absence of structural heart disease.

We have recognized three types of repolarization patterns in the right precordial leads (Fig. 6.2).[8,9]
- Type 1 is the one described in the 1992 paper, i.e., a high take-off ST segment elevation: J point elevation or ST segment elevation of ≥2 mm giving rise

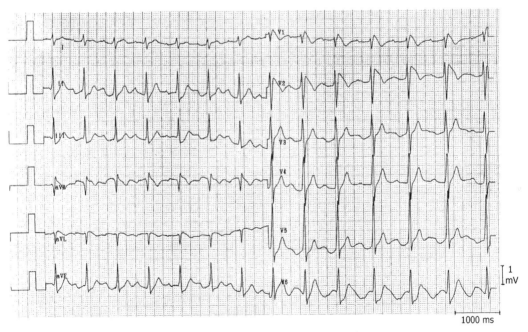

Figure 6.1 12 lead ECG of a 40-year-old resuscitated male. The ECG shows typical repolarization as well as depolarization abnormalities. The former consist of ST segment elevation in leads V₁ and V₂ (of the coved type: Type 1). Depolarization abnormalities are present as PQ prolongation (270 ms), prolonged QRS width (120 ms) and S waves in leads I, II, and III. P wave duration is also wide.

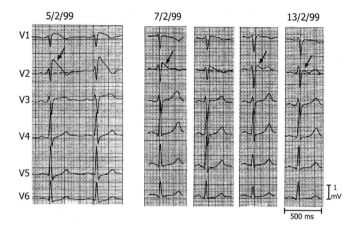

Figure 6.2 Precordial leads of a resuscitated patient. Within a couple of days the ECG changed from Type 1 (5/2/99) to Type 2 and 3 (far right panels 13/2/99). On 7/2/99 the ECG pattern is Type 2-like. Such dynamic changes are typically seen in Brugada patients. Calibrations are given. The arrows denote the J wave.

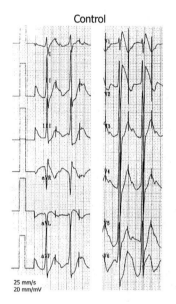

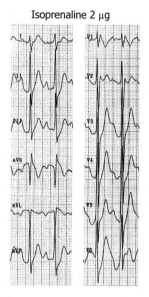

Figure 6.3 12 lead ECG of the same patient as in Fig. 6.1, with and without isoproterenol. In the left panel the atrium is paced with 100 bpm. ST elevation in leads V_1 and V_2 is obvious. In the right panel isoproterenol is infused (2 mg/kg/min), and ST elevation has almost disappeared.

to a coved type ST segment, in electrical continuity with a negative T wave and without a separating isoelectric track.

- Type 2 also has a high take-off ST segment elevation. In this variant, the J point elevation (≥ 2 mm) gives rise to a gradually descending elevated ST segment (remaining ≥ 1 mm above the baseline) and a positive or biphasic T wave. This ST-T segment morphology is referred to as the saddleback type.
- Type 3 is the coved or saddleback type with <1 mm ST elevation.

In all types, the QT interval itself does not need special requirements. A slight prolongation is often observed[21] and, of note, in distinct families ST segment elevation coincides with QT prolongation.[23,24]

In the interpretation of these ECG descriptions a few considerations are of importance.

1 The ECG pattern is dynamic and often concealed. In individual patients all patterns can be encountered (Fig. 6.2). Sodium channel blockers, α-adrenoceptor stimulation, and cholinergic stimulation augment the ST segment elevation, whereas α-adrenoceptor blockade and β-adrenoceptor stimulation mitigate the abnormalities (Fig. 6.3).[25] Body temperature also influences the ECG patterns, with fever provoking the characteristic features.[26,27]

2 The influence of the absolute amplitude of the ECG complex on the magnitude of the ST segment elevation has been stressed by Surawicz.[28] Hence, in the presence of a low amplitude QRS complex less ST segment elevation might be sufficient.

3 The descriptions are based on correct placement of the right precordial leads (i.e., the 4th intercostal space for leads V_1 and V_2 and the 5th intercostal space for V_3). Placement in a superior intercostal space (up to the 2nd intercostal space) has been advocated to increase sensitiveness of the ECG with or without drug testing (Fig. 6.4).[29,30] Whereas in individuals with a high clinical suspicion (see below) the arrhythmic substrate might indeed be unmasked in superior placed leads, it should be realized, however, that these positions are not that widely validated.

4 Frequently, the initiating event in Brugada patients is ventricular fibrillation, for which resuscitation and/or DC shock is required. ECG recordings in the first hours after resuscitation or immediately after DC shock should be interpreted with great caution.[8,9]

Upper inter-costal space

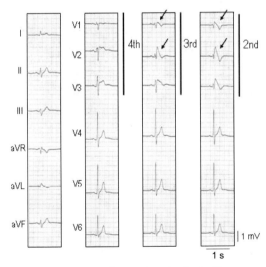

Figure 6.4 Four traces of a resuscitated patient with Brugada syndrome. The left two panels demonstrate the 12 lead ECG at conventional position of the precordial leads (fourth intercostal space). The right two panels are the precordial leads in the third and second intercostal space. Note the presence of a Type 2 ECG in lead V_2 in the fourth intercostal space and Type 1 ECG in leads V_2 and V_3 in the third and second intercostal spaces. (Courtesy of Dr Wataru Shimizu).

Depolarization abnormalities are frequently observed (Fig. 6.1) and include prolongation of the P wave duration, the PR interval, and of the QRS complex. It is likely that PR prolongation reflects HV conduction delay which usually is slight but may be pronounced.[21] PR prolongation (and HV conduction delay) is particularly observed in patients with *SCN5A* involvement.[31] Ventricular conduction delay varies from specific, pointing to involvement of a particular part of the conduction system (i.e., the right bundle or the left anterior bundle), to nonspecific. In the extremity leads I, II and III a broad S, giving rise to left or extreme axis deviation, is often encountered. Right bundle branch block (RBBB) was initially described as part of the syndrome,[1] but nowadays it is well recognized that RBBB is often suggested by the high take-off right precordial ST segment. However, true RBBB requires terminal broad negativity in the left lateral leads and the absence of it precludes right ventricular conduction delay. It has been suggested that pronounced delay in the terminal part of the right precordial S-wave indicates a vulnerable arrhythmogenic substrate.[32]

Brugada syndrome seems rare in pediatric patients. The electrocardiographic diagnosis is difficult because of the different chest morphology and the age-dependent predominance of right ventricular forces. In addition, control data is lacking. Described patients with arrhythmic events at a very young age are characterized by pronounced conduction disease.[5,24] Hence, in pediatric patients with suspect symptoms and typical electrocardiographic and other relevant features (family history, etc), the diagnosis should be considered.

Drug testing

In the section above, we indicated that the ECG pattern is dynamic and often concealed. Intravenous administration of certain drugs may modify the ECG pattern. Particularly ajmaline (1 mg/kg body weight; 10 mg/min), flecainide (2 mg/kg, max. 150 mg; in 10 min) and procainamide (10 mg/kg; 100 mg/min) have successfully been used to exaggerate the ST segment elevation or unmask it when it is initially absent (Fig. 6.5). Sensitivity (with genetic data as the golden standard) varies between 100%,[33] 71%,[18] and 35%.[22] It should be realized that the first study is particularly small with only 8 mutation car-

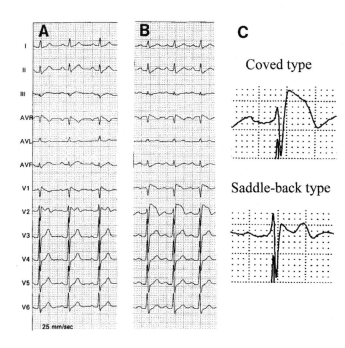

Coved type

Saddle-back type

Figure 6.5 Another resuscitated patient with Brugada syndrome. Type 2 ECG pattern (**B**) is converted into Type 1 by ajmaline (1 mg/kg body weight; 10 mg/min) (**A**). The test result is considered positive (see text). (**C**) Enlargements from lead V_2 before (lower panel) and after ajmaline (upper panel).

riers (one family),[33] and the last study is also small with 17 mutation carriers in 4 families.[22] Reproducibility of the drug challenge has not been tested for all drugs, but in the case of flecainide it was 100% in a small series.[34] Earlier preliminary data indicated only 50% reproducibility.[22] There is consensus that procainamide is not the most potent drug. Safety has been reported to be high for ajmaline with malignant ventricular arrhythmias in only 1.3% of patients.[35] Both patients that did develop arrhythmias had a type I ECG in whom the drug test does not add to diagnostic valve (see below). For flecainide safety might be lower. In 4 out of 22 patients serious ventricular arrhythmias occurred.[34] In this latter study the ECG type before testing is not given, but interestingly carriers of an *SCN5A* mutation seem to be at increased risk.[34]

In light of the above observations concerning safety, it is strongly recommended to monitor the patient continuously (12 lead ECG and blood pressure) during drug testing. CPR facilities should be at hand. Drug infusion should be stopped when the test is positive (see below), on preset values regarding QRS widening (≥30%) or when arrhythmias appear. In patients with Type 1 ECGs the drug test does not add to diagnostic value. When these criteria were applied, ajmaline did not evoke any ventricular ar-

rhythmias.[35] Monitoring is recommended until the ECG has normalized. With the use of flecainide this may require 24 hours. Isoproterenol is one of the only (if not the only) drug(s) that has been shown to successfully suppress ventricular arrhythmias in this setting.[20,36]

The definition of a positive test is an increase in the absolute J wave amplitude of >2 mm with or without RBBB (lead V_1 and/or V_2 and/or V_3) in the case of a negative baseline ECG. The test is considered positive upon an increase in the ST segment elevation by >2 mm in lead V_1 and/or V_2 and/or V_3 with or without RBBB.[29] In patients with Types 2 and 3 ECGs, where the test is recommended to clarify the diagnosis, a change into a Type 1 ECG is considered positive. An increase of more than 2 mm in ST elevation is also considered significant. A change of Type 3 into Type 2 ECG is considered inconclusive.[29]

Electrophysiological testing

Whereas an electrophysiological study is helpful in establishing the diagnosis, its value is debated as far as risk stratification is concerned. For diagnostic relevance a protocol using two stimulation sites (right ventricular apex (RVA), right ventricular outflow tract (RVOT)), 3 CL (600, 430, 330) and 1, 2 and 3 extrastimuli (minimal coupling interval 200 ms) is suggested. 50 to 70% of patients are inducible.[18,19,37,61] When only stimulation from the RVA is performed inducibility rate drops; [37,61] stimulation at the RVOT is particularly arrhythmogenic.[37] Atrial vulnerability is also enhanced and atrial fibrillation is more readily induced.[17] The clinical relevance of repeating EPS after class I drug treatment is not known.

A complete electrophysiological study is recommended in all symptomatic patients, but in VF survivors with a typical ECG it is of no diagnostic value. In asymptomatic patients with an abnormal baseline ECG, Brugada et al. recommend an EPS as well because inducibility identifies patients at risk for future events.[19] In contrast, Priori et al.[18] concluded that EPS in general is not able to quantify the risk for future events. In this study, a subdivision on ECG pattern was not made however. At present, asymptomatic patients without an abnormal ECG at baseline should probably not be tested. It is important to note, however, that the ECG pattern may be intermittently absent.

Molecular genetics

The role of molecular genetics in reaching the diagnosis Brugada syndrome is limited at present. The only causal gene known so far is *SCN5A*, encoding for the alpha subunit of the cardiac sodium channel. Mutations are identified in many individual patients and small families. Linkage data are limited to one large family in which ST segment elevation is combined with bradycardia-related QT prolongation.[23] The location of the mutations is throughout the gene.[38] By different mechanisms all mutations give rise to a reduction of available sodium current.[38] *SCN5A* mutations are identified in 15 to 30% of patients. Its identification in a single patient does not necessarily prove a causal relationship. In such cases biophysical studies of the mutant may underscore a causal relationship. With regard to screening of relatives, a 'proven' mutation in the proband could enable better follow-up and possibly treatment of presently asymptomatic family members.

Further causal genes are to be awaited. One of them will be found in a region on chromosome 3 next to the region of *SCN5A*.[39]

The differential diagnosis

In the above sections it has been stressed that Brugada syndrome can only be diagnosed reliably in the absence of other factors that can cause or contribute to the electrocardiographic alterations. In healthy young men some degree of right precordial ST elevation, mimicking a Type 2 or 3 Brugada ECG pattern, might be physiological. Also the early repolarization syndrome with often some J wave elevation in the left precordial leads is considered physiologic. A drug challenge might be of help in reaching the proper diagnosis.

A particularly difficult differential diagnosis is arrhythmogenic right ventricular cardiomyopathy (ARVC).[8] In some patients with ARVC right precordial ST elevation may be dynamic and in patients/families with ST elevation sudden death also occurs predominantly at rest or during sleep.[40] These features are remarkably similar to Brugada syndrome. Also in these cases a drug challenge may be needed to reach the proper diagnosis. In the near future, when more causal genes for both entities will have been identified, molecular genetics might differentiate between these conditions.

Other differential diagnostic considerations include: right or left bundle branch block and left ventricular hypertrophy,[41] acute myocardial infarction,[42,43] or right ventricular infarction,[44] acute myocarditis,[45] dissecting aortic aneurysm,[46] acute pulmonary thromboemboli,[47] various central and autonomic nervous system abnormalities,[48,49] heterocyclic antidepressant overdose,[50,51] cocaine intoxication,[52,53] Duchenne muscular dystrophy,[54] Friedreich's ataxia,[55] thiamine deficiency,[56,63] electrolyte disorders among which hypercalcemia,[57] hyperkalemia[58] and hypokalemia,[59] mediastinal tumor compressing RVOT,[60] high body temperature,[26,27] and arrhythmogenic right ventricular dysplasia/cardiomyopathy.[40]

The diagnosis of Brugada syndrome

The consensus report concluded that Brugada syndrome should be strongly considered in the following cases:[8]

- Type 1, i.e., coved type ECG in more than one right precordial lead (V_1–V_3), spontaneously present or drug induced (with or without associated phenomena in the ECG) and/or documented fibrillation, self-terminating polymorphic ventricular tachycardia, a family history positive for SCD (<45 years), coved type ECGs in family members, EP inducibility, syncope, or nocturnal agonal respiration. There should be no other abnormality that can cause the ECG changes (see previous paragraph).

- The exclusive presence of the ECG features, i.e., without clinical symptoms, is referred to as an idiopathic Brugada ECG pattern (not Brugada syndrome). The terminology 'asymptomatic Brugada syndrome' for these individuals should be discouraged (see also Refs 28 and 51).

- Type 2 'saddleback type' ECG: a drug challenge that transfers the saddleback type ECG into a coved type ECG is considered similar to a spontaneously present coved type ECG. Also an increase of more than 2 mm ST segment elevation upon drugs should raise the possibility of Brugada syndrome, when one or more clinical criteria are present (see above). A patient with a negative drug test (i.e., no change in the ST segment) is not considered to have the Brugada syndrome.

- Type 3 ECG: a patient with a Type 3 ECG and a positive drug test (change to Type 1) should be screened according to the above criteria. A change into Type 2 is considered inconclusive and absence of change in the ECG is considered to be negative for the Brugada syndrome.

References

1 Brugada P, Brugada J. Right bundle branch block, persistent ST segment elevation and sudden cardiac death: a distinct clinical and electrocardiographic syndrome: a multicenter report. *J. Am. Coll. Cardiol.* 1992; **20**: 1391–1396.

2 Osher HL, Wolff L. Electrocardiographic pattern simulating acute myocardial injury. *Am. J. Med. Sci.* 1953; **226**: 541–545.

3 Yan GX, Antzelevitch C. Cellular basis for the electrocardiographic J wave. *Circulation* 1996; **93**: 372–379.

4 Chen Q, Kirsch GE, Zhang et al. Genetic basis and molecular mechanisms for idiopathic ventricular fibrillation. *Nature* 1998; **392**: 293–296.

5 Priori SG, Napolitano C, Giordano U, Collisani G, Memmi M. Brugada syndrome and sudden cardiac death in children. *Lancet* 2000A; **355**: 808–809.

6 Vatta M, Dumaine R, Varghese G et al. Genetic and biophysical basis of sudden unexplained nocturnal death syndrome (SUNDS), a disease allelic to Brugada syndrome. *Hum. Mol. Genet.* 2002; **11**: 337–345.

7 Remme CA, Wever EFD, Wilde AAM, Derksen R, Hauer RNW. Diagnosis and long-term follow-up of Brugada syndrome in patients with idiopathic ventricular fibrillation. *Eur. Heart J.* 2001; **22**: 400–409.

8 Wilde AAM, Antzelevitch C, Borggrefe M et al. for the study group on the molecular basis of arrhythmias of the European Society of Cardiology. Diagnostic Criteria for the Brugada Syndrome. A Consensus Report. *Circulation* 2002; **106**: 2514–2519.

9 Wilde AAM, Antzelevitch C, Borggrefe M et al. for the study group on the molecular basis of arrhythmias of the European Society of Cardiology. Diagnostic Criteria for the Brugada Syndrome. A Consensus Report. *Eur. Heart J.* 2002; **23**: 1648–1654.

10 Gussak I, Bjerregaard P, Hammill SC. Clinical diagnosis and risk stratification in patients with Brugada syndrome. *J. Am. Coll. Cardiol.* 2001; **37**: 1635–1638.

11 Kakishita M, Kurita T, Matsuo K et al. Mode of onset of ventricular fibrillation in patients with Brugada syndrome detected by implantable cardioverter defibrillator therapy. *J. Am. Coll. Cardiol.* 2000; **36**: 1646–1653.

12 Shimada M, Miyazaki T, Miyoshi S et al. Sustained monomorphic ventricular tachycardia in a patient with Brugada syndrome. *Jpn. Circ. J.* 1996; **60**: 364–370.

13 Boersma LVA, Jaarsma W, Jessurun ER et al. Brugada syndrome: a case report of monomorphic ventricular tachycardia. *Pacing Clin. Electrophysiol.* 2001; **24**: 112–115.

14 Nademanee K, Veerakul G, Nimmannit S et al. Arrhythmogenic marker for the sudden unexplained death syndrome in Thai men. *Circulation* 1997; **96**: 2595–2600.

15 Matsuo K, Akahoshi M, Seto S, Yano K. Disappearance of the Brugada-type electrocardiogram after surgical castration: a role for testosterone and an explanation for the male preponderance? *Pacing Clin. Electrophysiol.* 2003; **26**[Pt. I]: 1551–1553.

16 Eckardt L, Kirchhof P, Loh P et al. Brugada syndrome and supraventricular tachyarrhythmias: a novel association? *J. Cardiovasc. Electrophysiol.* 2001; **12**: 680–685.

17 Morita H, Kusano-Fukushima K, Nagase S et al. Atrial fibrillation and atrial vulnerability in patients with Brugada syndrome. *J. Am. Coll. Cardiol.* 2002; **40**: 1437–1444.

18 Priori SG, Napolitano C, Gasparini M et al. Natural history of Brugada Syndrome. Insights for risk stratification and management. *Circulation* 2002; **105**: 1342–1347.

19 Brugada P, Brugada R, Mont L, Rivero M, Geelen P, Brugada J. Natural history of Brugada syndrome: the prognostic value of programmed electrical stimulation of the heart. *J. Cardiovasc. Electrophysiol.* 2003; **14**: 455–457.

20 Suzuki H, Torigoe K, Numata O et al. Infant case with a malignant form of Brugada syndrome. *J. Cardiovasc. Electrophysiol.* 2000; **11**: 1277–1280.

21 Alings M, Wilde A. 'Brugada' syndrome: clinical data and suggested pathophysiological mechanism. *Circulation* 1999; **99**: 666–673.

22 Priori SG, Napolitano C, Gasparini M *et al.* Clinical and genetic heterogeneity of right bundle branch block and ST-segment elevation syndrome. A prospective evaluation of 52 families. *Circulation* 2000; **102**: 2509–2515.

23 Bezzina C, Veldkamp MW, Van den Berg MP *et al.* A single Na⁺ channel mutation causing both long-QT and Brugada syndromes. *Circ. Res.* 1999; **85**: 1206–1213.

24 Priori SG, Napolitano C, Schwartz PJ *et al.* The elusive link between LQT3 and Brugada syndrome: the role of flecainide challenge. *Circulation* 2000; **102**: 945–947.

25 Miyazaki T, Mitamura H, Miyoshi S *et al.* Autonomic and antiarrhythmic drug modulation of ST segment elevation in patients with BS. *J. Am. Coll. Cardiol.* 1996; **27**: 1061–1070.

26 Saura D, García-Alberola A, Carrillo P, Pascular D, Martínez-Sánchez J, Valdés M. Brugada-like electrocardiographic pattern induced by fever. *Pacing Clin. Electrophysiol.* 2002; **25**: 856–859.

27 Mok NS, Priori SG, Napolitano C, Chan NY, Chahine M, Baroudi G. A newly characterized *SCN5A* mutation underlying Brugada Syndrome unmasked by hyperthermia. *J. Cardiovasc. Electrophysiol.* 2003; **14**: 407–411.

28 Surawicz B. Brugada syndrome: manifest, concealed, 'asymptomatic', suspected and simulated. Editorial comment. *J. Am. Coll. Cardiol.* 2001; **38**: 775–777.

29 Shimizu W, Matsuo K, Takagi M *et al.* Body surface distribution and response to drugs of ST segment elevation in Brugada syndrome: clinical implication of eighty-seven-lead body surface potential mapping and its application to twelve-lead electrocardiograms. *J. Cardiovasc. Electrophysiol.* 2000; **11**: 396–404.

30 Sangwatanaroi S, Prechawat S, Sunsaneewitayakul B, Sitthisook S, Tosukhowong P, Tungsanga K. New electrocardiographic leads and the procainamide test for the detection of the Brugada sign in sudden unexplained death syndrome survivors and their relatives. *Eur. Heart J.* 2001; **22**: 2290–2296.

31 Smits JPP, Eckardt L, Probst V *et al.* Genotype–phenotype relationship in Brugada Syndrome: electrocardiographic features differentiate *SCN5A*-related patients from non-*SCN5A*-related patients. *J. Am. Coll. Cardiol.* 2002; **40**: 350–356.

32 Atarashi H, Ogawa S, for the Idiopathic Ventricular Fibrillation Investigators: New criteria for high-risk Brugada syndrome. *Circulation J.* 2003; **67**: 8–10.

33 Brugada R, Brugada J, Antzelevitch C *et al.* Sodium channel blockers identify risk for sudden death in patients with ST-segment elevation and right bundle branch block but structurally normal hearts. *Circulation* 2000; **101**: 510–515.

34 Gasparini M, Priori SG, Mantica M *et al.* Flecainide test in Brugada syndrome: a reproducible but risky tool. *Pacing Clin. Electrophysiol.* 2003; **26** [Pt. II]: 338–341.

35 Rolf S, Bruns HJ, Wichter T *et al.* The ajmaline challenge in Brugada syndrome: diagnostic impact, safety, and recommended protocol. *Eur. Heart J.* 2003; **24**: 1104–1112.

36 Tanaka H, Kinoshita O, Uchikawa S *et al.* Successful prevention of recurrent ventricular fibrillation by intravenous isoproterenol in a patient with Burgada syndrome. *Pacing Clin. Electrophysiol.* 2001; **23**: 1293–1294.

37 Morita H, Fukushima-Kusano K, Nagase S *et al.* Site-specific arrhythmogenesis in patients with Brugada syndrome. *J. Cardiovasc. Electrophysiol.* 2003; **14**: 373–379.

38 Tan HL, Bezzina CR, Smits JPP, Verkerk AO, Wilde AAM. Genetic control of sodium channel function. *Cardiovasc. Res.* 2003; **57**: 961–973.

39 Weiss R, Barmada MM, Nguyen T *et al.* Clinical and molecular heterogeneity in the Brugada syndrome. A novel gene locus on chromosome 3. *Circulation* 2002; **105**: 707–713.

40 Corrado D, Basso C, Buja G *et al.* Right bundle branch block, right precordial ST-segment elevation and sudden death in young people. *Circulation* 2001; **103**: 710–717.

41 Rowlands DJ. *Clinical Electrocardiography.* Philadelphia, PA: JB Lippincott Company, 1991.

42 Goldberger AL. *Myocardial Infarction: Electrocardiographic Differential Diagnosis*, 4th edn. St. Louis, MO: Mosby-Year Book Inc., 1991.

43 Kobayashi H, Tsuchihashi K, Hashimoto A *et al.* Exercise-induced STV1 elevation: a sign of right ventricular dysfunction in recent inferior myocardial infarction. *Can. J. Cardiol.* 1994; **10**: 355–362.

44 Andersen HR, Falk E, Nielsen D. Right ventricular infarction. The evolution of ST-segment elevation and Q wave in right chest leads. *J. Electrocardiol.* 1989; **22**: 181–186.

45 Spodick DH, Greene TO, Saperia G. Acute myocarditis masquerading as acute myocardial infarction. *Circulation* 1995; **91**: 1886–1887.

46 Myers GB. Other QRS-T pattern that may be mistaken for myocardial infarction. IV. Alterations in blood potassium: myocardial ischemia; subepicardial myocarditis; distortion associated with arrhythmias. *Circulation* 1950; **2**: 75–93.

47 Sreeram N, Cheriex EC, Smeets JL, Gorgels AP, Wellens HJ. Value of the 12-lead electrocardiogram at hospital admission in the diagnosis of pulmonary embolism. *Am. J. Cardiol.* 1994; **73**: 298–303.

48 Abbott JA, Cheitlin MD. The nonspecific camel-hump sign. *JAMA* 1976; **235**: 413–144.

49 Hersch C. Electrocardiographic changes in head injuries. *Circulation* 1961; **23**: 853–860.

50 Bolognesi R, Tsialtas D, Vasini P, Contu M, Manca C. Abnormal ventricular repolarization mimicking myocardial

infarction after heterocyclic antidepressant overdose. *Am. J. Cardiol.* 1997; **79**: 242–245.

51 Littmann L, Monroe MH, Kerns WP, Svenson RH, Gallagher JJ. Brugada syndrome and 'Brugada sign': clinical spectrum with a guide for the clinician. *Am. Heart J.* 2003; **145**: 768–778.

52 Lipski J, Stimmel B, Donoso E. The effect of heroin and multiple drugs abuse on the electrocardiogram. *Am. Heart J.* 1973; **86**: 663–668.

53 Littmann L, Monroe MH, Svenson RH. Brugada-type electrocardiographic pattern induced by cocaine. *Mayo Clin. Proc.* 2000; **75**: 845–849.

54 Perloff JK, Henze E, Schelbert HR. Alterations in regional myocardial metabolism, perfusion, and wall motion in Duchenne muscular dystrophy studied by radionuclide imaging. *Circulation* 1984; **69**: 33–42.

55 Grauer K. Bizarre ECG in a young adult. *Intern. Med. Alert* 1997; **19**: 56.

56 Read DH, Harrington DD. Experimentally induced thiamine deficiency in beagle dogs: clinical observations. *Am. J. Vet. Res.* 1981; **42**: 984–991.

57 Douglas PS, Carmichael KA, Palvsky PM. Extreme hypercalcemia and electrocardiographic changes. *Am. J. Cardiol.* 1984; **54**: 674–675.

58 Levine HD, Wanzer SH, Merrill JP. Dialyzable currents of injury in potassium intoxication resembling acute myocardial infarction or pericarditis. *Circulation* 1956; **13**: 29–36.

59 Araki T, Konno T, Itoh H, Ino H, Shimizu M. Brugada Syndrome with ventricular tachycardia and fibrillation related to hypokalemia. *Circ. J.* 2003; **67**: 93–95.

60 Tarin N, Farre J, Rubio JM, Tunon J, Castro-Dorticos J. Brugada-like electrocardiographic pattern in a patient with a mediastinal tumor. *Pacing Clin. Electrophysiol.* 1999; **22**: 1264–1266.

61 Eckardt L, Kirchhof P, Schulze-Bahr E *et al.* Electrophysiologic investigation in Brugada syndrome. Yield of programmed ventricular stimulation at two ventricular sites with up to three premature beats. *Eur. Heart J.* 2002; **23**: 1394–1401.

62 Matsuo K, Kurita T, Inagaki M *et al.* The circadian pattern of the development of ventricular fibrillation in patients with Brugada syndrome. *Eur. Heart J.* 1999; **20**: 465–470.

63 Hundley JM, Ashburn LL, Sebrell WH. The electrocardiogram in chronic thiamine deficiency in rats. *Am. J. Physiol.* 1954; **144**: 404–414.

CHAPTER 7

Value of 12 lead electrocardiogram and derived methodologies in the diagnosis of Brugada disease

A. R. Perez Riera, MD, *C. Ferreira,* MD, PhD, *E. Schapachnik,* MD

Introduction

The association of right bundle branch block (RBBB) with J point and ST segment elevation in the right precordial leads (V_1 and V_2) with a normal QTc interval (although minor QTc prolongation is observed in some patients),[1] occurring predominantly in males of Southeast Asian origin in the productive age of life, free of structural heart disease, raises the suspicion of Brugada syndrome (BS).

The classical 12 lead electrocardiogram (ECG) is an invaluable tool in the diagnosis of this and many other arrhythmic syndromes. Recent studies indicate that modified precordial leads at higher intercostal space positions in the second and third intercostal space increase diagnostic sensitivity.[2–8] The vectorcardiogram (VCG) is valuable for the differential diagnosis in cases of extreme deviation of QRS axis on the frontal plane in the top left quadrant, present in approximately 9.5% of the cases in BS. The method can differentiate a dromotropic disorder in the region of the right ventricular outflow tract (RVOT) or block of superior division of right bundle branch (SDRBBB) from a left anterior fascicular block (LAFB). The first one (SDRBBB) indicates that the dromotropic disorder is in a distal position, in the free wall of the right ventricle in one of the right branch divisions, without necessarily affecting the HV interval.

VCG has also allowed us to verify that in BS there are cases without incomplete or complete RBBB.[9] Ikeda *et al.*[10,11] demonstrated that the signal-averaged ECG (SAECG) in BS has a high sensitivity (89%), a 50% specificity, 70% positive predictive value, and 77% negative predictive value for the presence of late potentials (LP).

QT-interval dispersion[12–14] and T-wave alternans (TWA) did not appear to be significant markers of mortality; however, class IA (procainamide) and class IC (pilsicainide) antiarrhythmic drugs are known to induce TWA in patients with BS. Exercise stress testing is often accompanied by normalization of the ST segment elevation, as a consequence of an increase in sympathetic tone, with an aggravation of ST segment elevation during the recovery period, due to vagal predominance during this phase.[13,15–18]

Ambulatory electrocardiography permits the assessment of right precordial J point and ST segment alterations caused by the increase of vagal tone and a concomitant decrease of sympathetic tone,[19] and it can record the trigger of polymorphic ventricular tachycardia (PVT), often by a closely coupled extrasystole. Patients with BS have a low heart rate variability (HRV) at night, which may predispose to the occurrence of PVT/ventricular fibrillation (VF) episodes.[20]

Body surface mapping (BSM) is a method created with the goal of improving the capacity for identifying cardiac electric activity in relation to the classical 12 lead ECG and VCG (higher sensitivity). It requires a great number of electrodes (usually 87), besides the classical 12 lead ECG and the X, Y and Z orthogonal leads of VCG. The method shows a correlation between the area of ST segment elevation, and the presence of LP in SAECG and inducibility in programmed electrical stimulation (PES).[21]

This chapter aims to discuss the value of these electrocardiographic methods.

The BS was the last clinical-cardiologic entity to be identified in the 20th century.[22,23] It is considered a distinct form of idiopathic VF and it displays clinical and electrocardiographic diagnostic criteria.[24] It is part of the so-called congenital ion channel disorders, channel-related diseases, or channelopathies.[25–28] Additionally, the entity is considered a primary electrical disease because of a lack of demonstrable structural heart disease.[29] It is a hereditary, autosomal dominant, heterogeneous, polygenic disorder with nearly five dozen different mutations identified, located in the *SCN5A* gene that encodes the α subunit of the sarcolemmal Na^+ channel located on chromosome 3. There are references of sporadic cases.[30] Like the long QT syndrome (LQTS), acquired forms of BS are described, caused by a series of drugs and conditions capable of producing transient J point and ST segment elevation in leads V_1 to V_2 or V_3 and with a higher tendency to sudden cardiac death (SCD).

The entity is characterized by an electrocardiographic pattern of complete RBBB or incomplete RBBB, associated with J point and ST segment elevation in the right precordial leads (V_1 and V_2) or in the anteroseptal wall (V_1 to V_3). Dynamic changes of repolarization are frequent and substantially modified over time. The RBBB pattern is frequently atypical (without wide, shallow terminal S wave in leads DI, aVL V_5–V_6), having been called 'pseudo RBBB' or 'RBBB like'.

The first European Consensus about the syndrome[24] classified the repolarization disorders that occurred in the right precordial leads (V_1 and V_2) or in the anteroseptal wall (V_1 to V_3) into three types:

- Type 1: ST segment elevation coved to the top ('coved type') ≥2 mm (0.2 mV), and followed by negative T wave (Brugada phenotype) (Fig. 7.1).
- Type 2: J point and ST segment elevation ≥2 mm (0.2 mV) with saddleback appearance, followed by positive T wave (Fig. 7.2).
- Type 3: J point and ST segment elevation <1 mm and with variable shape: whether coved type or saddleback appearance (Fig. 7.3).

These patterns could be observed spontaneously and sequentially in the same patient or after the administration of certain drugs that block the fast Na^+ channel, such as the class IA antiarrhythmic

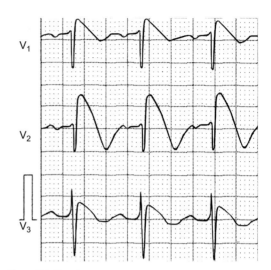

Figure 7.1 Type 1.

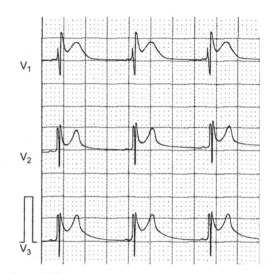

Figure 7.2 Type 2.

agents ajmaline and procainamide and the IC class drugs flecainide and pilsicainide.

The electrocardiographic association of complete or incomplete RBBB with J point and coved-type ST segment elevation from V_1 to V_2 or V_3 constitutes the key for the diagnosis, and is known as the 'Brugada sign' (idiopathic J wave). In rare cases, this wave could be observed also or exclusively in the inferior wall. The syndrome carrier has a high risk of PVT, with very short coupling of the first extra-systole, which frequently degenerates into VF.[31]

The existing electrical instability does not possess

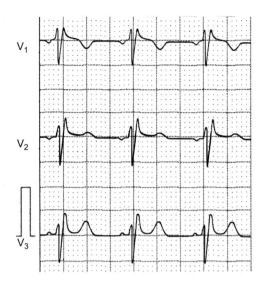

Figure 7.3 Type 3.

a demonstrable underlying organic substrate, such as atherosclerotic or vasospastic coronary heart disease, electrolytic disorder, cardiomyopathy, or any other. The clinical presentation includes syncope and circulatory arrest secondary to PVT/VF that occurs predominantly during night sleep or at rest (85%); however, in 15% of the patients it occurs during physical activity.[32] The nocturnal predominance of the events suggests that the increase in vagal activity and the decrease in sympathetic tone that happens during the sleep play an important role.[33]

The cause for the male predominance of the syndrome has been recently demonstrated.[34] Testosterone may also play a significant role in the ECG pattern.[35] Surgical castration eliminates the typical ECG manifestations.[36] It is believed that the entity could be responsible for 4 to 12% of all SCD and approximately 20% of the deaths of patients without structural heart disease.[37] From all cases of VF, 85% present with structural heart disease and only 15% appear without it. From the last set, at least 60% is classified as idiopathic VF and probably 30% of them are BS.[38]

BS is a major health problem for residents of rural Northeast Thailand. This disorder may be the leading cause of natural death among young men in the poverty-stricken northeast of Thailand. The annual mortality rate in this group was said to be as high as 26–38: 100 000 in one study[39] or 1: 2500 in another.[40]

ECG is a simple and useful method to identify cases with potential risk. Recently, a publication pointed out that the spontaneous presence of the typical ECG pattern is associated with a high risk of SCD[41] and had a worse prognosis than those cases where the typical ECG manifests only after pharmacologic tests.

The term 'idiopathic Brugada pattern' is used to indicate those asymptomatic patients with the classical ECG pattern present only spontaneously or after pharmacologic tests without positive family history of SCD in first-degree relatives under 45 years of age, not inducible with PES, and without genetic verification.

Takenaka et al., in 11 patients with Brugada-type ECG without family history of SCD and an average follow-up of 43 months, showed a similar clinical evolution compared to the general population.[42]

12 lead ECG and derived methodologies in diagnosis of Brugada syndrome

12 lead electrocardiogram
Rhythm

Sinus rhythm is the rule; however, supraventricular arrhythmias may be present in 10–25% of cases since the arrhythmogenic substrate is not limited to the ventricles. Atrial fibrillation was mentioned in the initial publication by the Brugada brothers,[43] and by Brazilian[44] and Japanese authors.[45] The latter pointed out that paroxysmal atrial fibrillation is observed in 30% of cases. Eckardt et al.[46] found supraventricular arrhythmias in 29% of cases, described in association with atrioventricular junctional rhythms episodes, and with the Wolff–Parkinson–White syndrome.[47]

Heart rate

There are no special features.

P wave

Smits et al. mentioned the eventual prolongation of P wave duration.[48]

PR interval

The PR interval of ECG has a maximal normal value in adults of 200 ms for rates between 70 and 90 bpm and is comprised in the His bundle electrogram (HBE) recordings of:

1 PA interval (30–50 ms);

2 AH interval (which reflects conduction time through the AV node to the bundle of His or supra-Hisian AV conduction time: normal value: 60–125 ms);

3 HV interval (which reflects conduction time between the His spike and the onset of ventricular deflections or septal activation: normal value: 35–55 ms) (Fig. 7.4).

In BS the PR interval is prolonged in approximately 50% of cases. This prolongation of the PR interval is observed predominantly in cases where the SCN5A gene mutation is demonstrated (carriers).[48] In these cases the HV interval is prolonged by nearly 100 ms.[49] The presence of a prolonged HV interval is possible in HBE by the existence of intra-His or infra-His blockade.

QRS axis on frontal plane

In BS the QRS axis on the frontal plane is within the normal range in 90.5% of cases; however, in 9.5% a marked left QRS axis deviation is observed according to a prospective 3 year follow-up study of a population of workers in the Tokyo area.[50] A marked left QRS axis deviation could be the consequence of a LAFB or of SDRBBB. This set of fibers of the right bundle division in the free wall of the right ventricle is situated within the RVOT; a location electrophysiologically affected in BS.

Both dromotropic disorders can be easily differentiated through electro-vectorcardiography, as we will see below.

QRS duration and morphology

The QRS complex represents the duration of ventricular activation (QRSD). The mean QRSD in BS is between 90 and 130 ms (110 ± 2 ms).[51] Pharmacologic tests with fast Na^+ current blockers prolong QRS duration in carriers of a SCN5A mutation.

J point and ST segment

Incomplete RBBB or complete RBBB are associated with J point and ST segment elevation, usually convex to the top ('coved type') in the leads V_1 and V_2 or anteroseptal leads from V_1 to V_3 'Brugada sign' and rarely in the inferior wall. Besides BS, other conditions can cause ST segment elevation in the right precordial leads:

1 early repolarization syndrome (ERS)[52]

2 juvenile pattern

3 asthenia habit

4 technical problems with the recording device

5 arrhythmogenic right ventricular cardiomyopathy/dysplasia

6 acute phase of myocardial infarction

7 acute myocardial ischemia

8 vasospastic angina or Prinzmetal angina.

ECG manifestations of BS could be similar to the ones found during variant angina. In both, ST segment elevation is observed, although with different causes: in variant angina it is due to transient vasospasm of the subepicardial vessels, whereas in BS it is caused by an increase in electrical heterogeneity in the right ventricular (RV) epicardium. The coexistence of both entities in the same patients has been described.[53] In these, coronary angiography did not reveal organic stenosis. The patients presented with

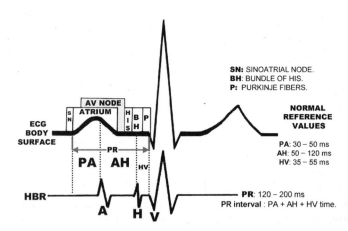

Figure 7.4 PR interval and His bundle recordings.

ST segment elevation that coincided with pain episodes, or intracoronary injection of acetylcholine. The ECG recorded without pain displayed the typical Brugada pattern including RBBB and ST segment elevation in right precordial leads, with augmentation of repolarization abnormalities with class I antiarrhythmic drugs and inducibility in PES. The authors concluded that susceptibility to develop VF could be modulated by an interaction of coronary vasospasm with BS. Table 7.1 summarizes the principal differences between BS and vasospastic angina.

Other causes of ST segment elevation are:
- LQTS 3 variant
- mediastinum tumor that compresses the RVOT
- hyperkalemia
- hypercalcemia
- Duchenne–Erb paralysis or Duchenne muscular dystrophy
- Friederiech's ataxia
- myotonic muscular dystrophy (Steinert's disease)
- acute pulmonary embolism
- acute myocarditis
- aortic aneurysm dissection
- autonomic nervous system (ANS) abnormalities
- disease of the central nervous system, e.g., subarachnoid and intracranial bleeding
- B1 vitamin deficit
- left or right bundle branch block
- ventricular enlargement
- athlete's heart
- ventricular aneurysm
- acute pericarditis
- acute cor pulmonale
- myocardial injury
- ventricular trauma
- hypothermia: J wave, Osborn wave, delta (δ) late wave, camel-hump sign, hump-like deflection or injury lesion potential
- following cardioversion
- antiarrhythmic drugs: class IA and IC agents
- cocaine abuse (recently a case has been reported about a patient that massively consumed this drug, and in whom a dysrhythmic episode with long QRS was observed, aborted cardiac arrest and transitory Brugada pattern)[55]
- pectus excavatum.[56]

In exceptional cases, J point and ST segment elevation may occur in inferior leads in the absence of hypothermia, ischemia or electrolyte imbalance. This possibility is called 'atypical Brugada pattern'.[57] Figure 7.5 shows such an atypical case.

Changes in the degree of J point and ST segment elevation could be triggered by the following.

1 Fever. The Na^+ channel and other channels modify their functional state depending on temperature, which alters their permeability.[58]

2 Drugs. Anti-malarial agents, antidepressants (particularly excessive doses of tricyclic antidepressants),[59] class IA (ajmaline, procainamide, and disopyramide) and IC (flecainide,[61,62] propafenone, and pilsicainide) antiarrhythmic agents, and recently prajmalium bitartrate.[60] Fast Na^+ channel blockers are used to bring out the concealed forms of the syndrome.[63,64] These drugs identify the patients with risk of SCD, who present with ST segment elevation and RBBB without structural heart disease.[65] They are used to assess inducibility during PES both in apparent and concealed forms of BS.

3 Hyperglycemia.[66,67]

4 Bradycardia.

5 Alcohol.

Catecholamines decrease ST elevation in some patients with BS.[68] Thus, adrenergic medications such as dobutamine, isoprenaline, and isoproterenol speed up ventricular repolarization and decrease J point and ST segment elevation. Isoproterenol is used for the treatment of the so-called 'electrical storms' (ES).[69] This event consists of the appearance of recurrent and multiple VF or VT episodes, and is sometimes observed in BS. The infusion of isoproterenol associated with general anesthesia and cardiopulmonary bypass is effective in decreasing ST segment elevation in right precordial leads and aborting ES crises.[70]

There is a single reference to the need of orthotopic transplantation as a heroic measure[71] and to the efficacy of endovenous amiodarone in this type of event.[72] The latter was not considered as protecting in the second consensus on BS held in Lake Placid, NY, in 2003. Dobutamine has been used as a pharmacologic test to identify patients at risk, asymptomatic carriers, and relatives of BS carriers. The test, called 'ajmaline and dobutamine test,' consists of an initial infusion of ajmaline, and if the patient develops the typical ECG pattern, dobutamine is immediately administered. If the ECG alterations

Table 7.1 Differential characteristics between Brugada syndrome and vasospastic angina.

	Brugada syndrome	Vasospastic angina
Precordial pain	No	Yes
Tendency to VT/VF	High	High
Structural heart disease	Absent	Could exist
Response to nitrates and nitroglycerine	Null	Improves or suppresses clinical/electrocardiographic manifestations
Permanence of ST segment elevation	Persistent (or fluctuating) and without pain	Brief, transitory and accompanied by pain
Cause	Na^+ channel genetic aberrances	Possible alteration in nitrous oxide production in vascular wall
Presence of image in mirror or reciprocal in ECG	Could be present	Present
Topography of ST elevation	Right precordial leads from V_1 to V_3. Rarely, it could be observed in inferior wall. It is triggered or increased by class IC and IA antiarrhythmic agents[54]	Variable. It could alternate between precordial and inferior leads. It could be triggered by hyperventilation
Dromotropic disorders	First-degree AV block by H-V prolongation in Hissian electrogram, particularly in carriers of the mutation	They could occur transitorily up to a high degree of AV block during the episode, and they are associated to a higher risk of arrhythmia and SCD
Persistent T wave inversion	Negative T wave in precordial leads from V_1 to V_3, characteristic of type 1	Inverted and deep T waves from V_1 to V_4 associated to anterior hypokinesia, suggesting myocardial 'stunning' that indicates critical lesion of the anterior descending artery: 'LAD-T wave pattern.
Presence of transitory Q wave	No	Could happen
Stress test	Elevation could be normalized during effort	Variable response
Myocardial scintigraphy with thallium 201	Normal	Transitory transmural hypoperfusion
Response to endovenous ergonovine maleate test in a 0.05–0.40 mg dose (alpha adrenergic and serotoninergic receptor stimulant)	There could be a mild and diffuse reduction of caliber without spasm when doses ≥0.40 mg are used	Intense coronary spasm accompanied by pain and ST segment elevation on ECG. Eventually cardiac block, asystole, and VT
Response to hyperventilation	Does not modify	Severe spasm and reproduction of clinical and electrocardiographic manifestations
Response to intracoronary acetylcholine, with each dose administered in a time longer than 1 minute in 10 µg, 25 µg, 50 µg and 100 µg doses, in 5-minute intervals	It may worsen ST elevation with paradoxical dilatation of coronary vessels	Severe spasm and reproduction of clinical and electrocardiographic manifestations
Response to magnesium sulphate	Not mentioned	It suppresses events induced by hyperventilation and exercise
Treatment	ICD in association with quinidine or cilostazol, drugs that contribute to decrease the number of shocks. Isoproterenol prescribed in 'electrical storms' associated to general anesthesia and cardiopulmonary 'bypass'	Calcium antagonists such as nifedipine, diltiazem, verapamil, and felodipine associated to nitrates. There are references of benefits with prazosin

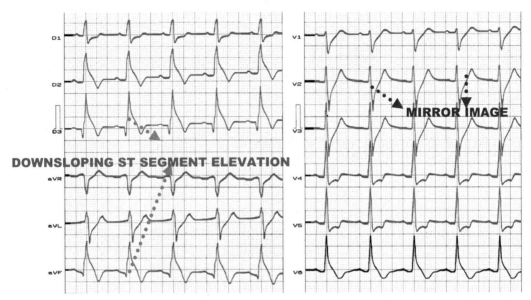

Figure 7.5 Brugada syndrome with atypical ECG: Name: Y. A. S. Sex: Male. Age: 26 years old. Race: Yellow. Weight: 64 kg. Height: 1.68 m. Date: 05/03/2002. Downsloping ST segment elevation is present in inferior leads (idiopathic J waves or Osborn wave). Mirror image observed in anterior wall. Absence of hypothermia, ischemia or electrolytic disorders.

disappear, the test is considered positive and indicates the need for PES.[73]

T wave

The T wave can have a variable configuration: bifid, alternate, or enigmatic polarity,[74] negative in the terminal portion from V_1 to V_3 and with intermittent normalization. J point and ST segment elevation ≥2 mV followed by negative T wave in right precordial leads V_1 to V_2 or from V_1 to V_3 could be found both in arrhythmogenic right ventricular cardiomyopathy/dysplasia, and in BS (type 1 pattern); however, in the first one it is permanent whereas in BS it could vary with time.

Characteristics of ventricular tachycardia
Very fast PVTs (from 260 to 352 bpm) are frequent with very short onset extrasystole coupling (388 ± 28 ms), they are generally preceded by premature ventricular contractions (PVCs) identical to the beat that starts PVT. Specific PVCs trigger spontaneous episodes of VF in patients with BS.[75]

Arrhythmic events occur in 93% of cases during sleep or at dawn, and in 92% of cases in the presence of a significant ST segment elevation. The degree of ST segment elevation may be responsible for arrhythmias.

These forms resemble fast *torsade de pointes* (TdP) observed in patients with normal QTc; nevertheless, there are clear differences between both tachyarrhythmias, which are displayed in Table 7.2.

In exceptional cases, bursts of spontaneous monomorphic ventricular tachycardia (MVT) occur;[76] observed principally when drug induced although it has been reported in the absence of drugs.[77,78] There are references about spontaneous MVT appearance after the administration of ajmaline.[79] An automatic mechanism mediated by the beta-receptor seems to hold an important role in the spontaneous MVTs that originate in the RVOT. The origin of the event could be very close to the lesion that causes ST elevation.[80] In these cases in which MVT is inducible by drugs, an automatic mechanism is suggested as an electrophysiologic substrate, triggered by late after-depolarization located in the RVOT.[81]

Figure 7.6 shows a typical polymorphic ventricular tachycardia in Brugada syndrome.

Table 7.2 Main differences between *torsades de pointes* (TDP) and true PVT observed in Brugada syndrome.

	TdP	*True PVT*
Heart rate of PVT	200 to 250 bpm	260 to 352 bpm
Electrolyte abnormalities	Frequent	No
Coupling of first PVC	Long	Short: 388 ± 28 ms
QTc	Long	Normal (slightly long in V_1–V_3)
Treatment	Beta-blockers in high doses, mexiletine, stellectomy, pacing, ICD, and associations	ICD + drugs: quinidine, cilostazol Electrical storms: isoproterenol, + general anesthesia + cardiopulmonary bypass

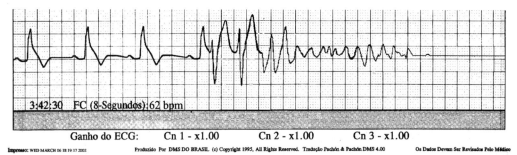

Figure 7.6 Long-term (Holter) eletrocardiographic recording. Typical polymorphic tachycardia. Name: Y. A. S. Sex: Male. Age: 26 years old. Race: Yellow. Weight: 64 kg. Height: 1.68 m. Date: 03/05/2002. Time: 3:42:30 AM. Patient sleeping. Sudden cardiac death by IPVT/IVF with short coupling ending in cardiac arrest.

QTc interval

The QTc interval is normal in BS; however, prolongation of QTc interval of around 500 ms is possible after a PVT.[82] This fact indicates a relationship between BS and its mirror allelic image: the LQT3 variant of LQTS. In a large family of patients of carriers of mixed manifestations, intrinsic dysfunction of the SA node and dromotropic alterations were detected. Pacemaker implantation turned out to be an effective prevention for SCD, suggesting that the mechanism of lethal tachyarrhythmias in BS may rarely be associated to bradycardia.[83] In some patients, minor QTc prolongation is observed.[1]

Modified precordial leads: right precordial leads at higher intercostal space positions: V_{1H}–V_{2H}–V_{3H}

Several studies have concluded that 12 lead ECG sensitivity increases by using accessory leads located in the high right precordial area (V_{1H}–V_{2H}), over the 3rd or 2nd intercostal space, just to the right (V_{1H}) or left (V_{2H}) of the sternum. In certain cases, the Brugada sign was not observed using only the 12 conven-

tional leads, but is now visualized. The procedure is based on the fact that modified precordial leads on right precordial leads (V_{1H}–V_{2H}) or on anteroseptal wall (V_{1H} to V_{3H}) at higher intercostal space positions are located exactly opposite to the RVOT.[2–8]

Figure 7.7 shows the right ventricle regions and their corresponding leads. The right ventricle has five regions that are better detected by the following leads:

1 V_2 and V_3: trabecular area
2 V_3–V_4: low right paraseptal area
3 V_1 to V_4: free wall
4 aVF, V_4R, and V_5R: right ventricle inflow tract (RVIT)
5 aVR, V_{1H}, V_{2H}, V_{3H}: RVOT: the area affected in BS.

Figure 7.8 shows the regions of RV and the corresponding leads.

Vectorcardiogram (VCG)

The diagnosis of RBBB cannot be made without broad terminal S wave on left leads DI, aVL, V_5 and V_6. This element, essential for an accurate diagnosis of RBBB can be observed in some cases of BS. The phenomenon originated terms such as 'pseudo RBBB', 'RBBB-like', or 'atypical RBBB'. The ECG in Figs 7.9–7.11 is a typical example of this situation.

According to the guidelines for rest ECG from the Brazilian Society of Cardiology, the diagnostic criteria for incomplete RBBB and complete RBBB are:[84]

1 QRS duration ≥120 ms (complete RBBB) or between 100 and 120 ms (incomplete RBBB);

2 triphasic pattern in right precordial leads (V_1 and V_2) of the rSr', rsr', rsR', rSR' or 'M' complex type. The final R' wave usually displays a greater voltage and duration than onset r or R. In incomplete RBBB the most common pattern is rSr';

3 occasionally a wide and notched final R wave in leads V_1, V_2 and aVR;

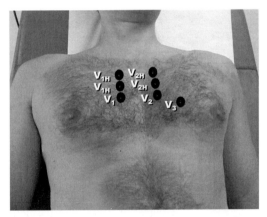

Figure 7.7 Right ventricle regions and their corresponding leads. V_1—over the 4th intercostal space, just to the right of the sternum. V_2—over the 4th intercostal space, just to the left of the sternum. V_3—midway between V_2 and V_4. V_{1H}—over the 3rd or 2nd intercostal space, just to the right of the sternum. V_{2H}—over the 3rd or 2nd intercostal space, just to the left of the sternum.

4 negative final S wave, wide and deep on left leads: DI, aVL and V_5 V_6;

5 the intermittence of the phenomenon, as well as its evolution into complete RBBB, is important because it indicates the presence of a dromotropic disorder, and not right ventricular hypertrophy, crista supraventricularis hypertrophy, or any other of the possible pattern determinants.

The basic VCG criteria for RBBB diagnosis are:

1 right end conduction delay (RECD) (after 60 ms) visible at least in two planes;

2 terminal appendage of QRS loop with delay (tears very close together) (Fig. 7.12);

3 in the frontal plane: RECD superior, middle, or inferior in localization;

4 in the horizontal plane: RECD: terminal finger-like appendage in 'glove finger' with delay located in the right anterior (tears very close together) (complete RBBB) or right posterior (incomplete RBBB) quadrant.

The right His system (Fig. 7.13) is comprised of:

(A) on the interventricular septum, the right portion of the His bundle:

1 right penetrating portion;

2 right branching portion;

then the right bundle-branch, which is composed of three portions:

3 trunks, proximal or of membranous septum;

4 middle, intramyocardial, or mimetic;

5 inferior, distal, or moderator band;

(B) on the free wall of the right ventricle:

6 divisional portion of right bundle on free wall of right ventricle, which is where the three divisions in the right ventricle free wall Purkinje fibers start:

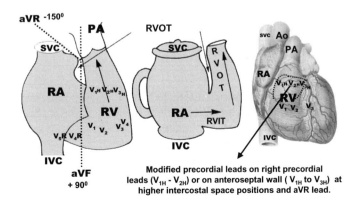

Figure 7.8 Regions of the right ventricle and the corresponding leads.

Modified precordial leads on right precordial leads (V_{1H} - V_{2H}) or on anteroseptal wall (V_{1H} to V_{3H}) at higher intercostal space positions and aVR lead.

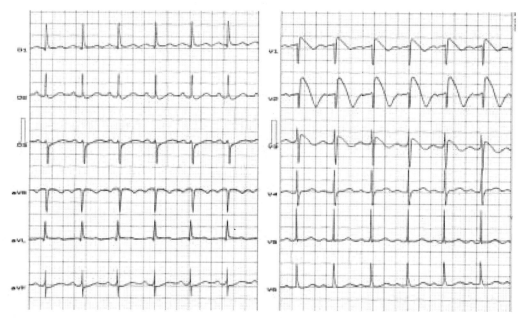

Figure 7.9 Typical type 1 Brugada pattern of repolarization: Name: ESR. Sex: Male. Age: 37 years old. Race: Caucasian. Weight: 72 kg. Height: 1.75 m. Date: 02/01/2003. Case Number: 322. J point and ST elevation coved to the top and negative T wave V$_1$–V$_3$. There is no negative final broad S wave on left leads: DI, aVL and V$_6$. There is no final R wave on unipolar aVR limb lead; the QRS duration is normal: 104 ms. Conclusion: Type 1 Brugada pattern. There is no RBBB.

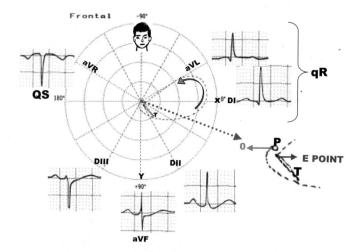

Figure 7.10 ECG/VCG correlation in the frontal plane. Name: ESR. Sex: Male. Age: 37 years old. Race: Caucasian. Weight: 72 kg. Height: 1.75 m. Date: 02/01/2003. Case Number: 322. In this plane, ECG/VCG completely rules out the RBBB diagnosis: The QRS loop does not present right end conduction delay (RECD) to the end of the QRS loop; the unipolar aVR limb lead shows QS pattern without broad terminal R wave as it would be seen in a RBBB. In the enhanced image to the right, we observe that the 0 point (start of QRS loop) does not coincide with the E point (end of QRS loop).

  I superior division of right bundle branch;
 II inferior division of right bundle branch;
III middle division of right bundle branch.
- Blocks at levels 1, 2 and 3 are called proximal.
- Blocks at levels 4 and 5 are called peripheral.
- Blocks at level 6 (on the free wall of the right ventricle), when they involve the three divisions at the same time, are called global divisional blocks of right bundle (GDRB). We find a typical example post-operatively following the total repair of Fallot's tetralogy and the ventricular septal defect that had a free wall of right ventricle approach (right ventriculotomy). The surgical incision tackles globally the parietal Purkinje of the right bundle

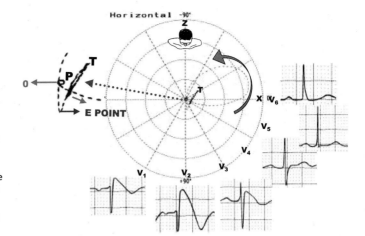

Figure 7.11 ECG/VCG correlation in the horizontal plane. In this plane, we observe Brugada pattern Type 1. The VCG completely rules out RBBB: absence of RECD. The 0 point (start of QRS loop) does not coincide with the E point (end of QRS loop). This is located opposite to the 0 point.

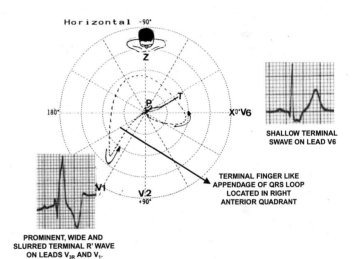

Figure 7.12 Typical QRS loop of RBBB on horizontal or transversal plane.

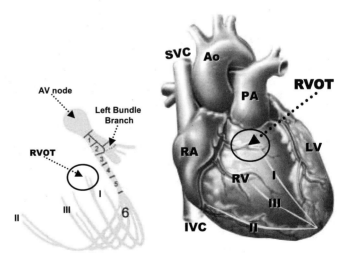

Figure 7.13 The right His system components.

branch, causing in 80 to 95% of the cases typical complete RBBB pattern: GDRB.

The isolated block of one of the three right branch divisions: (6 I, II, or III) is generically called right end conduction delay (RECD). In BS, because it electrophysiologically affects the area corresponding to the RVOT, it could involve conduction in the superior division of right bundle branch and cause the so-called blockage of superior division of right bundle branch that is located in the RVOT. Thus, VCG could easily clear the doubt confirming the real presence of RBBB when the characteristic RECD in 'glove finger' is present in the right anterior quadrant (complete RBBB) or in the right posterior quadrant (incomplete RBBB) in the horizontal plane (HP) and the RECD is located in the top right quadrant of the frontal plane (FP).

Electro-vectocardiographically, diagnosis is always a supposition, since the only constant element is the presence of RECD, located in the superior, middle, or inferior portions, which could be the consequence or not of a dromotropic disorder. In most cases, it corresponds to normal patients (normal variant) and its clinical interest lies in the fact that it causes electro-vectocardiography patterns that are easily confused with left fascicular blocks (LAFB and LPFB), besides, at times, causing morphologies that simulate electrically inactive areas or myocardial infarction (pseudo-electrically inactive areas) both in the anterior and the inferior walls:[85] here lies the importance and the need of a perfect individualization.

Table 7.3 shows the clinical diagnosis in 100 cases of divisional right bundle branch block (vectorcardiography diagnosis).

The incidence of RECD is still unknown; but it is surely more frequent than any other intraventricular conduction disorder. The scant reference in the literature is due to the fact that ECG is interpreted as a normal variant, incomplete RBBB morphology without clinical significance, or misinterpreted as LAFB (Type 1A), LPFB (Type B), or electrically inactive areas (inferior or antero-septal). Pastore *et al.*,[85]

Table 7.3 Clinical diagnosis in 100 cases of divisional right bundle branch block.

Etiology	Cases
Without disease (normal variant):	29
Systemic hypertension light or/light to moderate:	10
Mitral valve prolapse without significance:	6
Mitral valve prolapse with significance:	5
Systemic hypertension and Mitral valve prolapse in association:	5
Severe hypertension:	5
Coronary heart disease:	5
Systemic hypertension and coronary heart disease in association:	4
Cor pulmonale	4
Secundum atrial septal defect (fossa ovalis):	4
Mitral stenosis:	3
Chagas disease:	3
Aortic stenosis associated with mitral annular calcification:	2
Dilated cardiomyopathy:	2
Pectus excavatum:	2
Straight-back syndrome:	2
Transplanted heart:	2
Massive pulmonary embolism:	2
Ebstein's anomaly:	1
During cardiac catheterization (intermittent):	1
Beri-beri cardiomyopathy:	1
Brugada syndrome:	1
Arrhythmogenic right ventricular cardiomyopathy/dysplasia:	1

after VCG analysis, considered the existence of three types according to the location of RECD in the frontal plane:

1 superior right end conduction delay (SRECD), sub pulmonary, type I or right antero-superior divisional block (RASDB), corresponding to the set of fibers located in the RVOT — this variant was found in one of our cases of BS;

2 inferior right end conduction delay (IRECD), type II or right postero-inferior divisional block (RPIDB);

3 middle right end conduction delay (MRECD), type III or right middle divisional block (RMDB).

Figure 7.14 show the location of right end conduction delay (RECD) in peripheral divisional blocks of right bundle branch on frontal plane.

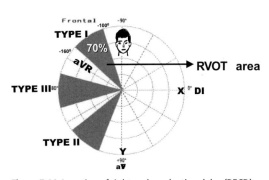

Figure 7.14 Location of right end conduction delay (RECD) in peripheral divisional blocks of right bundle branch on frontal plane.

Eight years later, Pérez Riera *et al.*,[86] on the basis of the analysis of 100 VCGs, subdivided type 1 into three varieties according to the rotation of the QRS loop and QRS axis on the frontal plane: type 1A; type 1B and type 1C. The clinical significance of this subdivision lies in the fact that the type 1A is easily confused with LAFB because both dromotropic disorders cause extreme deviation of the QRS axis to the left in the frontal plane and present a counterclockwise rotation of the QRS loop; nevertheless, in type 1A, RECD is observed and in LAFB there is a possible discrete LECD.

Figure 7.15 show the vectorcardiographic variants of superior right end conduction delay (SRECD), type 1 or right antero-superior divisional block (RASDB): types IA, IB and IC, in the frontal plane.

The Consensus on resting electrocardiography by the Brazilian Society of Cardiology published in 2003, admits the characterization of His right bundle branch fascicular blocks; on the other hand, it agrees that there are only two variants.

1 Superior right end conduction delay (SRECD), type 1 or right antero-superior divisional block (RASDB). The criteria for this are:
- extreme deviation of QRS axis on FP between −45° and +/−180°;
- QRS duration <120 ms;
- rS in DII, DIII and aVF;
- SII > SIII;
- presence of S wave in DI;
- qR in aVR with wide final R wave;

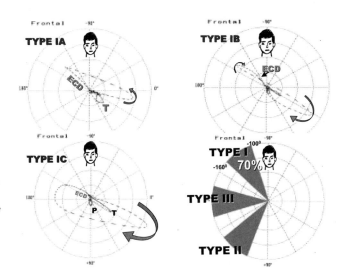

Figure 7.15 Vectorcardiographic variants of SRECD, type 1, or RASDB, types 1A, 1B and 1C, frontal plane. Only type 1A can be confused with LAFB because both have marked QRS axis deviation to the left and QRS frontal loop rotates counterclockwise.

- possible rSr' in V_1–V_2 or rS with wide and notched final S wave.

2 Inferior right end conduction delay (IRECD), type 2 or right postero-inferior divisional block (RPIDB). The criteria for this are:

- QRS axis on FP to the right of +90°;
- QRS duration <120 ms;
- R wave DII > R wave DIII with SII < 10 mm;
- qR in DII, DIII and aVF;
- DI and aVL rS;
- qR in aVR with R wave wide and prominent;
- possible rSr' in V_1–V_2 or rS with wide and notched final S wave.

In the case of true LAFB, VCG in most cases will show in the FP:

1 vector from onset 10 to 20 ms pointed downwards and to the right: qR in DI and aVL leads;

2 QRS loop with counterclockwise rotation;

3 possible discrete left end conduction delay (LECD) located in the top left quadrant.

Or, when there is right bundle branch block type 1A, we verify in the FP:

1 vector from onset 10 to 20 ms pointed downwards and to the left: R in DI and aVL;

2 counterclockwise rotation of QRS loop;

3 RECD in the area corresponding to the RVOT.

In the next examples, we show a typical Brugada syndrome ECG, plus type 1A block of superior division of right bundle branch. Figures 7.16 and 7.17 show a typical ECG of Brugada syndrome, Fig. 7.18 shows a VCG/ECG in the horizontal plane, and Fig. 7.19 gives the differential diagnosis on the frontal plane between BSDRBB and LAFB.

Figure 7.20 shows the 12 lead ECG for one patient. Figure 7.21 shows the ECG/VCG correlation in frontal plane and Fig. 7.22 shows the ECG/VCG correlation in horizontal plane.

Stress test

The stress test can induce repolarization change as a consequence of an increase of adrenergic tone and a concomitant decrease in vagal tone. This may be related to a decrease in phase 1 amplitude I_{to1} at faster rates, leading to a decrease in J point and ST segment elevation, and therefore a decrease in the incidence of ventricular arrhythmias.[87,88] Normalization of the ECG during exercise can also be due to a (relative) increase in Ca^{2+} current. The recording of changes in the width of J point and ST segment elevation, dependent on heart rate and autonomous

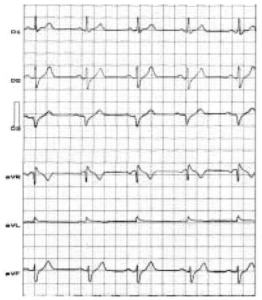

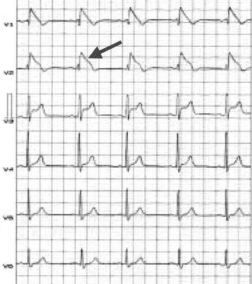

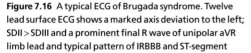

Figure 7.16 A typical ECG of Brugada syndrome. Twelve lead surface ECG shows a marked axis deviation to the left; SDII > SDIII and a prominent final R wave of unipolar aVR limb lead and typical pattern of IRBBB and ST-segment elevation of the 'coved-type' in leads V_1–V_2 (Type 1 Brugada pattern). Conclusions: 1. Block of superior division of right bundle-branch (BSDRBB); 2. Type 1 Brugada pattern.

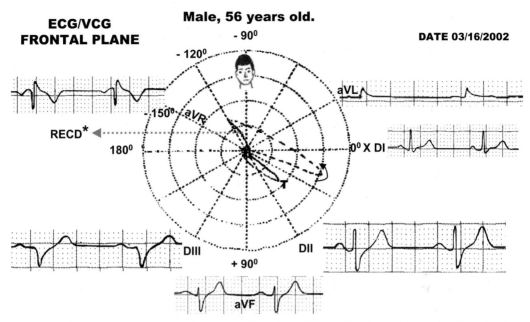

Figure 7.17 ECG/VCG, frontal plane. This is the first VCG of Brugada disease shown in medical literature. SDII > SDIII, there is a marked axis deviation to the left, QRS frontal loop rotates counterclockwise and right end conduction delay (RECD*) is located on the top right quadrant (−120°) on the territory of the superior division of RBB. This division is inside the free wall of the RVOT. Conclusion: block of superior division of right bundle branch type 1A.

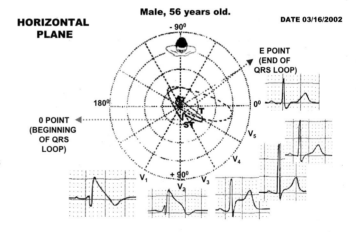

Figure 7.18 VCG/ECG, horizontal plane. The beginning of QRS loop (0 point) does not coincide with the end (E point) as seen in normal conditions, because the J point and the ST segment are upwardly unleveled.

tone, may be a useful marker for the detection of patients with high risk of SCD.[89]

Ambulatory electrocardiography or long-term electrocardiographic recording (Holter monitoring and looper)

Long-term ECG (Holter monitoring) or 15-day looper can:

1 record an increase of J point and ST segment elevation during sleep (nocturnal vagal worsening);[19]

2 record ventricular repolarization changes induced by rate increase;

3 detect and characterize tachyarrhythmic events and their relationship with the circadian pattern of the development of PVT/VF in patients with BS;

4 determine the coupling of the initial extrasystole.

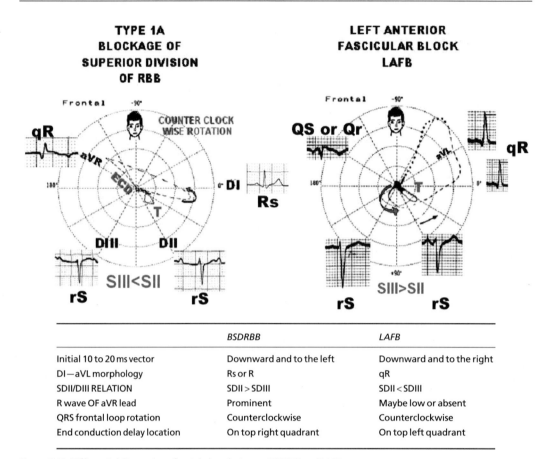

	BSDRBB	LAFB
Initial 10 to 20 ms vector	Downward and to the left	Downward and to the right
DI—aVL morphology	Rs or R	qR
SDII/DIII RELATION	SDII > SDIII	SDII < SDIII
R wave OF aVR lead	Prominent	Maybe low or absent
QRS frontal loop rotation	Counterclockwise	Counterclockwise
End conduction delay location	On top right quadrant	On top left quadrant

Figure 7.19 Differential diagnosis on frontal plane between BSDRBB and LAFB.

Signal-averaged ECG (SAECG) or high-resolution electrocardiography

Late potentials (LP) are low amplitude (microvolt: 1–25 µV level) and very high frequency potentials, which occur at the end of QRS (within the ST segment) and are related to delayed electric activity and fragmented conduction of the ventricles. Ikeda *et al.* proved that this method is a significant non-invasive marker in identifying patients with high risk of SCD in BS.[10,11] However, these studies do not provide prospective data on SCD risk. These authors verified that the SAECG displays 89% sensitivity, 50% specificity, 70% positive predictive value, and 77% negative predictive value for the presence of LP, but no correlation with ST segment elevation and HV interval duration. The SAECG is the only non-invasive significant marker for SCD, in contrast to TWA and QT dispersion. The main limitation of SAECG is its sensitivity in the presence of RBBB, which may mask

the test. There are no standardized criteria for LP diagnosis in the presence of RBBB or LBBB; however, the frequency domain analysis allows detecting LP14. Taking into account this limitation, the SAECG is a highly accurate method as a non-invasive marker for fatal ventricular arrhythmias in BS. Positive SAECG indicates the presence of abnormal LP to the end of the filtered QRS, and it is present in 0 to 6% among normal volunteers.[90] The presence of LP in SAECG and the body surface area correlate to inducibility in PES.[91]

The criteria for positivity in SAECG are:

1 root mean square (RMS): the mean amplitude of the terminal 40 ms of QRS complex, mean voltage of the final 40 ms of filtered QRS under 25 µV. (The normal value is >25 µV.)

2 low amplitude signal (LAS): the low amplitude terminal component of the complex with amplitude <40 mV exceeds 40 ms. Total duration of electric

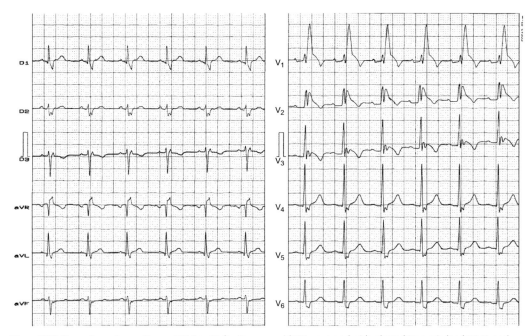

Figure 7.20 Brugada syndrome. Name: ALP. Sex: Male. Age: 32-year-old. Race: Caucasian. Weight: 76 kg. Height: 1.70 m. Date: 02/09/2003. Case number: 455. ECG diagnosis: 1. LAFB: marked QRS axis deviation to the left, SIII > SII, initial q wave is recorded in lead DI and an r wave in the inferior leads. 2. CRBBB: QRS duration > 120 ms, rsR' pattern in lead V_1 with wide R' wave, and wide, slurred S wave in leads DI, V_5 and V_6. 3. Bifascicular block (1 + 2): In frontal plane the first portions of QRS complex has the characteristics of and isolated LAFB, and the last portion have characteristics of a CRBBB. 4. Type 1 Brugada pattern.

Figure 7.21 ECG/VCG correlation in the frontal plane. Name: ALP. Sex: Male. Age: 32-year-old. Race: Caucasian. Weight: 76 kg. Height: 1.70 m. Date: 02/09/2003. Case number: 455. The QRS loop has the initial part, which resembles that seen in LAFB, and the terminal part, which resembles that seen in RBBB. The 10 to 20 ms vector is downward and to the right (initial r wave in inferior leads and qRs pattern in DI lead), SIII > SII. The QRS frontal loop rotates in a counterclockwise direction with extreme deviation of QRS axis: LAFB. There are RECD: RBBB.

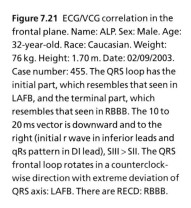

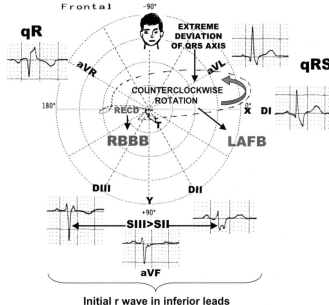

Initial r wave in inferior leads

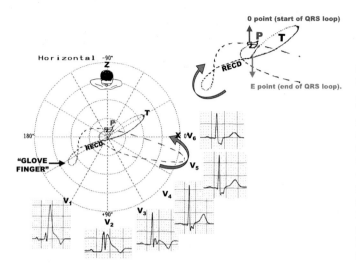

Figure 7.22 ECG/VCG correlation in horizontal plane. Name: ALP. Sex: Male. Age: 32-year-old. Race: Caucasian. Weight: 76 kg. Height: 1.70 m. Date: 02/09/2003. Case number: 455. VCG diagnosis: 1. CRBBB Kennedy Type 1 or Grishman Type (the afferent limb is located behind X line). Right end conduction delay (RECD) located on right anterior quadrant: finger like appendage or 'glove finger morphology'. E point (end of QRS loop) is not coincident with 0 point (start of QRS loop). 2. Brugada Type I of repolarization.

signals of low amplitude >40 μV to the end of the filtered QRS. (Normal value is <40 μV if 25 to 250 Hz filters are used and under 35 μV if 40 to 250 Hz filters are used.)

3 QRSD: total duration of the filtered QRS complex in absence of bundle branch block (QRSD) >114 ms (or 120 ms). (Normal value is <114 ms—some authors consider a 120 ms limit.[92])

The presence of two or more altered variables turns the SAECG into a positive one. The method is useful in risk stratification for the appearance of VT with lethal potential; low amplitude and very high frequency LP detected and recorded in the end of QRS and in the beginning of the ST segment, are non-invasive markers of an arrhythmogenic circuit. This special technique of averaging, filtering, and high gain results from the detection of the ECG sign and uses time as a variable (time domain) or the frequency response of the sign (frequency domain), with the results of the former better established. The presence of BBB harms the conclusions about LP with the SAECG.[93] LP in SAECG is present in 70% of cases of BS. The SAECG does not allow a differentiation between BS and arrhythmogenic right ventricular dysplasia: in both entities LP are frequently recorded.

QT-interval dispersion

QT dispersion is defined as the difference between maximal and minimal QT duration found in the classical 12 lead ECG. The ECG must be conducted

at a velocity of 50 mm/s and with the 12 leads vertically aligned, in order to analyze one beat simultaneously from the first deflection of the QRS complex until the point of return of the T wave to the baseline or in the lowest point between the T and U waves.[94] The normal value of QT dispersion is 32 ± 8 ms.[95] QT dispersion is higher in men than in women[12] and is a non-invasive marker of myocardial electrical stability and, consequently, a marker for the risk of SCD. Thus, the higher the dispersion, the higher the risk of severe VT. QT dispersion is a sensitive marker of spontaneous or induced VT: 88% sensitivity and 57% specificity; and an independent predictor of cardiovascular mortality.[13] QT dispersion shows daytime variations, higher in the first hours of the morning, and lower at night, and in carriers of coronary disease. It is not considered a significant marker for mortality in BS.[11–14]

Microvolt T wave alternans (TWA)

The alternans can be defined by amplitudes or alternating configurations, beat to beat of the P wave, QRS complex or T waves, isolated or combined. The most frequent type of alternans is the one that affects only QRS. Electrical alternans involving the P wave, QRS complex, ST segment (depolarization alternans), and the T wave (repolarization alternans) is a rare finding.[96] T wave alternans relates to alternating low and high voltage of the T wave in a 1:1, 2:1, or 3:1 sequence. The isolated alternans of the T-wave (phase 3 of the AP in the absence of changes in the

QRS complex (phase 0 of AP) or of the P wave, was described for the first time by Hering in 1909[97] and in the papillary muscle of cats by Taussing in 1928.[98]

The causes for isolated TWA are:

1 spontaneous tachycardia, or tachycardia induced by exercise, drugs or a pacemaker;

2 sudden changes in the extension of the HR cycle;[99]

3 hydro electrolytic disorders: severe hyperkalemia of uremia;

4 experimentally in hypocalcemia in puppies;[100]

5 hypothermia;

6 severe myocardial damage: cardiomyopathy;

7 acute myocardial ischemia, particularly in variant angina;

8 post-resuscitation;

9 acute pulmonary embolism;

10 following amiodarone treatment (rare);

11 family-inherited long QT syndromes of the Romano–Ward or Jervell–Lange-Nielsen types;[101–103]

12 BS[15] — intravenous administration of class IA and IC antiarrhythmic drugs induced TWA in a patient with BS,[13–16] class I antiarrhythmic drug and variant angina induced TWA and VT in a patient with BS and vasospastic angina,[17] while during febrile illness in a patient with BS, spontaneous TWA was described.[18]

Measurement of microvolt TWA is by:

1 special, multi-segmented electrodes with multi-contact sensors developed by the Cambridge Heart Inc. Company;

2 a special conductor gel;

3 a system for processing electric signs based in the method of spectral analysis with a patented system for noise reduction.

With this technology, it is possible to obtain a more accurate measurement with a volt millionth, and to remove artifacts during exercise and muscular noises.

Contraindications are:

1 acute phase of MI;

2 recent acute ischemia;

3 current severe arrhythmia;

4 endocarditis;

5 aortic stenosis;

6 pulmonary embolism;

7 neuromuscular disease or disabling osteomuscular disease;

8 severe ventricular dysfunction.

Limitations are that it is not valid:

1 if beta-blockers or drugs that lead to bradycardia are present;

2 for a carrier of atrial flutter;

3 for a carrier of chronic atrial fibrillation.

In conclusion, TWA is not considered a significant marker of mortality; however, class IA (procainamide) and class IC (pilsicainide) antiarrhythmic drugs can induce TWA in patients with BS.

Heart rate variability (HRV)

Heart rate variability is a useful tool for the detection of sympathetic–parasympathetic balance in the autonomous nervous system. A recent paper using linear methods of time domain or non-spectral and frequency domain HRV analysis (time-domain frequency) were performed at daytime and nighttime, showing that patients with BS had low HRV at night, which may predispose to the occurrence of PVT/VF episodes.[20]

Body surface potential mapping (BSM)

This a method developed to record simultaneous cardiac potentials in body surface, through isopotential lines, which can be reunited by a computer, generating the BSM. The method improves the capacity of identification of cardiac electric activity compared to 12 lead ECG and VCG. It uses 87 electrodes (59 anterior and 28 posterior ones, besides the 12 conventional leads of ECG and VCG: X, Y, Z in the surface of the chest with the aim of obtaining additional information. More than two decades ago, Mirvis made an evaluation of normal variation in ST segment patterns by BSM and ST segment elevation in the absence of heart disease.[104] Fontaine et al., in an editorial, drew attention for the first time to the importance of this method to understand the source of cardiac arrhythmias.[105]

Himatsu et al., using BSM, found differences in the characteristics and the area of ST segment elevation between asymptomatic and symptomatic carriers of BS.[106] Izumida et al. demonstrated the beneficial effect of isoproterenol on repolarization, and its worsening with fast Na^+ channel blockers.[107] Shimizu et al. studied 25 patients, carriers of BS, and compared them to 40 controls, finding the following facts about ST elevation.[21]

1 The maximum ST segment elevation measured 20 ms after the end of QRS (max ST 20) in the area

corresponding to RVOT was significantly higher in patients carriers of BS when compared to controls (0.37 ± 0.13 versus 0.12 ± 0.04 mV).

2 The maximum ST elevation was observed in the fourth intercostal space in 18 of the 25 patients.

3 In 7 patients, the maximum ST elevation was located in the second or third intercostal space.

The authors concluded that, by recording the leads from V_1 to V_3 in the second and third intercostal space ($V_{1H}–V_{2H}$), diagnostic sensitivity could be improved. Eckardt et al. showed the existence of a correlation between the size of the area of ST segment elevation assessed by BSM and the presence of LP in SAECG and inducibility in PES.[91] Finally, Bruns et al. using BSM demonstrated that in BS, the mirror or reciprocal image might be recorded in the left precordial leads.[108]

The authors thank Prof. Arthur Wilde head of the Department of Cardiology, Academic Medical Center, University of Amsterdam, The Netherlands and the staff at the Masonic Medical Research Laboratory, for their text corrections and helpful suggestions.

References

1 Alings M, Wilde A. 'Brugada' syndrome: Clinical data and suggested pathophysiologic mechanism. *Circulation* 1999; **99**: 666–673.

2 Farre J. The Brugada syndrome: do we need more than the 12-lead ECG? *Eur. Heart J.* 2000; **21**: 264–265.

3 Sangwatanaroj S, Prechawat S, Sunsaneewitayakul B, Sitthisook S, Tosukhowong P, Tungsanga K. Right ventricular electrocardiographic leads for detection of Brugada syndrome in sudden unexplained death syndrome survivors and their relatives. *Clin. Cardiol.* 2001; **24**: 776–781.

4 Sangwatanaroj S, Prechawat S, Sunsaneewitayakul B et al. New electrocardiographic leads and the procainamide test for the detection of the Brugada sign in sudden unexplained death syndrome survivors and their relatives. *Eur. Heart J.* 2001; **22**: 2290–2296.

5 Nagatomo T, Abe H, Oginosawa Y et al. Reproduction of typical electrocardiographic findings of the Brugada syndrome using modified precordial leads. J UOEH 2002; **24**: 383–389.

6 Nagase S, Kusano KF, Morita H et al. Epicardial electrogram of the right ventricular outflow tract in patients with the Brugada syndrome. Using the epicardial lead. *J. Am. Coll. Cardiol.* 2002; **39**: 1992–1995.

7 Takagi M, Toda I, Takeuchi K et al. Utility of right precordial leads at higher intercostal space positions to diagnose

Brugada syndrome. *Pacing Clin. Electrophysiol.* 2002; **25**: 241–242.

8 Cabezon Ruiz S, Errazquin Saenz De Tejada F, Pedrote Martinez A et al. Normal conventional electrocardiogram with negative pharmacological stress test does not rule out Brugada syndrome. *Rev. Esp. Cardiol.* 2003; **56**: 107–110.

9 Pérez Riera AR, Fortunato de Cano S, Cano MN, Schapachnik E. Significance of electrocardiogram in the Brugada Syndrome and in other arrthmogenic entities. Guidelines for prevention of sudden death. Virtual Symposium about the Brugada syndrome: ten years of history: 1992/2002) www.simposio-brugada.com.ar

10 Ikeda T, Sakata T, Sakabe K et al. Noninvasive risk stratification markers in the Brugada syndrome: comparison of late potentials, T-wave alternans and QT dispersion. *Pacing Clin. Electrophysiol.* 2000; **23**: 731.

11 Ikeda T, Sakurada H. and Sakabe K et al. Assessment of noninvasive markers in identifying patients at risk in the Brugada syndrome: insight into risk stratification. *J. Am. Coll. Cardiol.* 2001, 37: 1628–1634.

12 Battur MK, Aloseyed S, Oto A et al. Circadian variations of QTc dispersion: is it a clue to morning increase in sudden cardiac death? *Clin. Cardiol.* 1999; **22**: 103–106.

13 Chinushi M, Washizuka T, Okumura H, Aizawa Y. Intravenous administration of class I antiarrhytmic drugs induced T wave alternans in a patient with Brugada syndrome. *J. Cardiovasc. Electrophysiol.* 2001; **12**: 493–495.

14 Ruskin JN. Role of invasive electrophysiology testing in the evaluation and treatment of patients at high risk of sudden cardiac death. *Circulation* 1992; **85** (suppl I): 1152–1159.

15 Tada H, Nogami A, Shimizu W et al. ST segment and T wave alternans in a patient with Brugada syndrome. *Pacing Clin. Electrophysiol.* 2000; **23**: 413–415.

16 Takagi M, Doi A, Takeuchi K, Yoshikawa J. Pilsicanide-induced marked T wave alternans and ventricular fibrillation in a patient with Brugada syndrome. *J. Cardiovasc. Electrophysiol.* 2002; **13**: 837.

17 Chinushi Y, Chinushi M, Toida T, Aizawa Y. Class I antiarrhythmic drug and coronary vasospasm-induced T wave alternans and ventricular tachyarrhythmia in a patient with Brugada syndrome and vasospastic angina. *J. Cardiovasc. Electrophysiol.* 2002; **13**: 191–194.

18 Morita H, Nagase S, Kusano K, Ohe T. Spontaneous T wave alternans and premature ventricular contractions during febrile illness in a patient with Brugada syndrome. *J. Cardiovasc. Electrophysiol.* 2002; **13**: 816–818.

19 Maia IG, Soares MW, Boghossian SH, Sa R. The Brugada syndrome. Outcome of one case. *Arq. Bras. Cardiol.* 2000; **74**: 437–445.

20 Krittayaphong R, Veerakul G, Nademanee K, Kangkagate C. Heart rate variability in patients with Brugada syndrome in Thailand. *Eur. Heart J.* 2003; **24**: 1771–1778.

21 Shimizu W, Matsuo K and Takagi M *et al.* Body surface distribution and response to drugs of ST segment elevation in Brugada syndrome: clinical implication of eighty-seven-lead body surface potential mapping and its application to twelve-lead electrocardiograms. *J. Cardiovasc. Electrophysiol.* 2000; **11**: 396–404.

22 Pérez Riera AR, Fortunato de Cano S, Fleury de Padua Neto LA, Schapachnik E. Síndrome de Brugada: Nuevos conceptos y expectativas futuras. *Rev. Argent. Cardiol.* 2001; **69**: 652–662.

23 Pérez Riera AR, Schapachnik E, Ferreira C. Brugada disease: chronology of discovery and paternity. Preliminary observations and historical aspects. *Indian Pacing Electrophysiol. J.* 2003; **3**: 244.

24 Wilde AA, Antzelevitch C, Borggrefe M *et al.* Proposed diagnostic criteria for the Brugada syndrome *Eur. Heart J.* 2002; **23**: 1648–1654.

25 Balser JR. Sodium 'channelopathies' and sudden death: Must you be so sensitive? *Circ. Res.* 1999; **85**: 872–874.

26 Kirsch GE. Ion channel defects in primary electrical diseases of the heart. In F. Lehmann-Horn, ed., *Channelopathies.* 2000; 115–151. Elsevier Science.

27 Celesia GG. Disorders of membrane channels or channelopathies. *Clin. Neurophysiol.* 2001; **112**: 2–18.

28 Marbán E. Cardiac channelopathies. Virtual Symposium about the Brugada syndrome: ten years of history: 1992/2002) www.simposio-brugada.com.ar

29 Cau C. The Brugada syndrome. A predicted sudden juvenile death. *Minerva Med.* 1999; **90**: 359–364.

30 Tan HL, Bezzina CR, Smits JP, Verkerk AO, Wilde AA. Genetic control of sodium channel function. *Cardiovasc. Res.* 2003; **57**: 961–973.

31 Hari P, Chemiti GK, Joshi A. Brugada syndrome also linked to sudden cardiac death. *Postgrad. Med.* 2001; **109**: 18.

32 Futterman LG, Lemberg L. Brugada. *Am. J. Crit. Care* 2001; **10**: 360–364.

33 Matsuo K, Kurita T, Inagaki M *et al.* The circadian pattern of the development of ventricular fibrillation in patients with Brugada syndrome. *Eur. Heart J.* 1999; **20**: 465–470.

34 Di Diego JM, Cordeiro JM, Goodrow RJ *et al.* Ionic and cellular basis for the predominance of the Brugada syndrome phenotype in males. *Circulation* 2002; **106**: 2004–2011.

35 Antzelevitch C. Androgens and male predominance of the Brugada syndrome phenotype. *Pacing Clin. Electrophysiol.* 2003; **26**: 1429–1431.

36 Matsuo K, Akahoshi M, Seto S, Yano K. Disappearance of the Brugada-type electrocardiogram after surgical castration. *Pacing Clin. Electrophysiol.* 2003; **26**: 1551–1553.

37 Antzelevitch C, Brugada P, Brugada J *et al.* Brugada syndrome a decade of progress *Circ. Res.* 2002; **91**: 1114–1118.

38 Remme CA, Wever EF, Wilde AA *et al.* Diagnosis and long-term follow-up of the Brugada syndrome in patients with idiopathic ventricular fibrillation. *Eur. Heart J.* 2001; **22**: 400–409.

39 Nademanee K, Veerakul G, Nimmannit S *et al.* Arrhythmogenic marker for the sudden unexplained death syndrome in Thai men. *Circulation* 1997; **96**: 2595–2600.

40 Nademanee K. Sudden unexplained death syndrome in Southeast Asia. *Am. J. Cardiol.* 1997; **79**: 10–11.

41 MacKenzie R. The Brugada syndrome – an electrocardiogram with important mortality implications. *J. Insur. Med.* 2001; **33**: 106–109.

42 Takenaka S, Kusano KF, Hisamatsu K *et al.* Relatively benign clinical course in asymptomatic patients with Brugada-type electrocardiogram without family history of sudden death. *J. Cardiovasc. Electrophysiol.* 2001; **12**: 2–6.

43 Brugada P, Brugada J. Right bundle branch block, persistent ST segment elevation and sudden cardiac death: a distinct clinical and electrocardiographic syndrome. *J. Am. Coll. Cardiol.* 1992; **20**: 1391–1396.

44 Villacorta H, Faig Torres RA, Simões de Castro IR, Lambert H. de Araujo Gonzáles, Alonso R. Morte súbita em paciente com bloqueio de ramo direito e elevação persistente do segmento ST. *Arq. Bras. Cardiol.* 1996; **66**: 229–231.

45 Itoh H, Shimizu M, Ino H, Okeie K, Yamaguchi M, Fujino N, Mabuchi H. Hokuriku Brugada Study Group. Arrhythmias in patients with Brugada-type electrocardiograph findings. *Jpn. Circ. J.* 2001; **65**: 483–486.

46 Eckardt L, Kirchhof P, Loh P *et al.* Brugada syndrome and supraventricular tachyarrhythmias: a novel association? *J. Cardiovasc. Electrophysiol.* 2001; **12**: 680–685.

47 Eckardt L, Kirchhof P, Johna R, Haverkamp W, Breithardt G, Borggrefe M. Wolff–Parkinson–White syndrome associated with Brugada syndrome. *Pacing Clin. Electrophysiol.* 2001; **24**: 1423–1424.

48 Smits JP, Eckardt L, Probst V *et al.* Genotype–phenotype relationship in Brugada syndrome: electrocardiographic features differentiate *SCN5A*-related patients from non-*SCN5A*-related patients. *J. Am. Coll. Cardiol.* 2002; **40**: 350–356.

49 Kobayashi T, Shintani U, Yamamoto T *et al.* Familial occurrence of electrocardiographic abnormalities of the Brugada-type. *Intern. Med.* 1996; **35**: 637–640.

50 Atarashi H, Ogawa S, Harumi K *et al.* Idiopathic ventricular fibrillation investigators. Three-year follow-up of patients with right bundle branch block and ST segment elevation in the right precordial leads: Japanese Registry

of Brugada Syndrome. Idiopathic Ventricular Fibrillation Investigators. *J. Am. Coll. Cardiol.* 2001; **37**: 1916–1920.

51 Bianco M, Bria S, Gianfelici A, *et al.* Does early repolarization in the athlete have analogies with the Brugada syndrome? *Eur. Heart J.* 2001; **22**: 504–510.

52 Gussak I, Antzelevitch C. Early repolarization syndrome: clinical characteristics and possible cellular and ionic mechanisms. *J. Electrocardiol.* 2000; **33**: 299–309.

53 Chinushi M, Kuroe Y, Ito E, *et al.* Vasospastic angina accompanied by Brugada-type electrocardiographic abnormalities. *J. Cardiovasc. Electrophysiol.* 2001; **12**: 108–111.

54 Nakamura W, Segawa K, Ito H *et al.* Class IC antiarrhytmic drugs: flecainide and pilsicainide, produce ST segment elevation simulating inferior myocardial ischemia. *J. Cardiovasc. Electrophysiol.* 1998; **9**: 855–858.

55 Ortega-Carnicer J, Bertos-Polo J, Gutierrez-Tirado C. Aborted sudden death, transient Brugada pattern, and wide QRS dysrrhythmias after massive cocaine ingestion. *J. Electrocardiol.* 2001; **34**: 345–349.

56 Kataoka H. Electrocardiographic patterns of the Brugada syndrome in 2 young patients with pectus excavatum. *J. Electrocardiol.* 2002; **35**: 169–171.

57 Kalla H, Yan GX, Marinchak R. Ventricular fibrillation in a patient with prominent J (Osborn) waves and ST segment elevation in the inferior electrocardiographic leads: a Brugada syndrome variant? *J. Cardiovasc. Electrophysiol.* 2000; **11**: 95–1198.

58 Gonzalez Rebollo JM, Hernandez Madrid A *et al.* Recurrent ventricular fibrillation during a febrile illness in a patient with the Brugada syndrome. *Rev. Esp. Cardiol.* 2000; **53**: 755–775.

59 Scheinman MM. Is the Brugada syndrome a distinct clinical entity? *J. Cardiovasc. Electrophysiol.* 1997; **8**: 332–336.

60 Fischer S, Reinhold S, Kettner W. Kardiologische Abteilung der Medizinischen Klinik, Stadtisches Klinikum Magdeburg, Krankenhaus. *Altstadt Med. Klin.* 2001; **96**: 485–488.

61 Fujiki A, Usui M, Nagasawa H *et al.* ST segment elevation in the right precordial leads induced with class IC antiarrhytmic drugs: insight into the mechanism of Brugada syndrome. *J. Cardiovasc. Electrophysiol.* 1999; **10**: 214–218.

62 Shimizu W, Antzelevitch C, Suyama K *et al.* Effect of sodium channel blockers on ST segment, QRS duration, and corrected QT interval in patients with Brugada syndrome. *J. Cardiovasc. Electrophysiol.* 2000; **11**: 1320–1329.

63 Brugada R, Brugada J, Antzelevitch C. *et al.* Sodium channel blockers identify risk for sudden death in-patients with ST-segment elevation and right bundle branch block but structurally normal hearts. *Circulation* 2000; **101**: 510–515.

64 Brugada R. Use of intravenous antiarrhythmics to identify concealed Brugada syndrome. *Curr. Control Trials Cardiovasc. Med.* 2000; **1**: 45–47.

65 Brugada J, Brugada P, Brugada R. Ajmaline unmasks right bundle branch block-like and ST segment elevation in V1-V3 in-patients with idiopathic ventricular fibrillation. *Pacing Clin. Electrophysiol.* 1996; **19**: 599 (Abstract).

66 Nishizaki M, Sakurada H, Ashikaga T *et al.* Effects of glucose-induced insulin secretion on ST segment elevation in the Brugada syndrome. *J. Cardiovasc. Electrophysiol.* 2003; **14**: 243–249.

67 Nogami A, Nakao M, Kubota S *et al.* Enhancement of J-ST-segment elevation by the glucose and insulin test in Brugada syndrome. *Pacing Clin. Electrophysiol.* 2003; **26**: 332–337.

68 Shimizu W, Kamakura S. Catecholamines in children with congenital long QT syndrome and Brugada syndrome. *J. Electrocardiol.* 2001; **34**: 173–175.

69 Asenjo R, Madariaga R, Morris R *et al.* Sudden death due to recuperated ventricular fibrillation: Brugada syndrome? *Rev. Med. Chil.* 1998; **126**: 814–821.

70 Tanaka H, Kinoshita O, Uchikawa S *et al.* Successful prevention of recurrent ventricular fibrillation by intravenous isoproterenol in a patient with Brugada syndrome. *Pacing Clin. Electrophysiol.* 2001; **24**: 1293–1294.

71 Ayerza MR, de Zutter M, Goethals M, Wellens F, Geelen P, Brugada P. Heart transplantation as last resort against Brugada syndrome. *J. Cardiovasc. Electrophysiol.* 2002; **13**: 943–944.

72 Chalvidan T, Deharo JC, Dieuzaide P *et al.* Near fatal electrical storm in a patient equipped with an implantable cardioverter defibrillator for Brugada syndrome. *Pacing Clin. Electrophysiol.* 2000; **23**: 410–412.

73 Araújo N, Godinho F, Maciel W *et al.* Pesquisa de Portadores Assintomáticos da Síndrome de Brugada Através do Teste da Ajmalina e Dobutamina. LIV Congresso Brasileiro de Cardiologia Tema Livre 084 Hospital Universitário Clementino Fraga Filho UFRJ; Clínica São Vicente Rio de Janeiro-RJ Brasil.

74 Bjerregaard P, Gussak I, Antzelevitch C. The enigmatic ECG of the Brugada syndrome. Letter to the Editor. *J. Cardiovasc. Electrophysiol.* 1998; **9**: 109–111.

75 Kakishita M, Kurita T, Matsuo K *et al.* Mode of onset of ventricular fibrillation in patients with Brugada syndrome detected by implantable cardioverter defibrillator therapy. *J. Am. Coll. Cardiol.* 2000; **36**: 1646–1653.

76 Sastry BK, Narasimhan C, Soma Raju B. Brugada syndrome with monomorphic ventricular tachycardia in a one-year-old child. *Indian Heart J.* 2001; **53**: 203–205.

77 Boersma LV, Jaarsma W, Jessurun ER, Van Hemel NH,

Wever EF. Brugada syndrome: a case report of monomorphic ventricular tachycardia. *Pacing Clin. Electrophysiol.* 2001; **24**: 112–115.

78 Ogawa M. Sustained monomorphic ventricular tachycardia originating from right ventricular outflow tract in Brugada syndrome. Virtual Symposium about the Brugada syndrome: ten years of history: 1992/2002) www.simposio-brugada.com.ar

79 Pinar Bermudez E, Garcia-Alberola A, Martinez Sanchez J, *et al.* Spontaneous sustained monomorphic ventricular tachycardia after administration of ajmaline in a patient with Brugada syndrome. *Pacing Clin. Electrophysiol.* 2000; **23**: 407–409.

80 Shimada M, Miyazaki T, Miyoshi S *et al.* Sustained monomorphic ventricular tachycardia in a patient with Brugada syndrome. *Jpn. Circ. J.* 1996; **60**: 364–370.

81 Ogawa M, Kumagai K, Saku K. Spontaneous right ventricular outflow tract tachycardia in a patient with Brugada syndrome. *J. Cardiovasc. Electrophysiol.* 2001; **12**: 838–840.

82 Martinez Sanchez J, Garcia Alberola A, Jose Sanchez Munoz J *et al.* Concurrent long QT and Brugada syndrome in a single patient. *Rev. Esp. Cardiol.* 2001; **54**: 645–648.

83 Maarten P, van den Berg MD, Arthur AM. *et al.* Possible bradycardic mode of death and successful pacemaker treatment in a large family with features of long QT syndrome Type 3 and Brugada syndrome *J. Cardiovasc. Electrophysiol.* 2001; **12**: 630–636.

84 Pastore CA *et al.* Diretrizes do ECG de repouso. Diretriz Normatização da interpretação do eletrocardiograma de repouso. *Arq. Bras. Cardiol.* 2003; **80** supl I: 1–17.

85 Pastore CA, Moffa PJ, Tobias MO *et al*: Bloqueios divisionais do ramo direito e áreas eletricamente inativas. Diagnóstico diferencial eletro-vetorcardiográfico. *Arq. Bras. Cardiol.* 1985; **45**: 309–317.

86 Pérez Riera AR. 'Right end conduction delay (RECD). Electorcardiographic criteria: proposal for classification and clinical significance.' Presented at the XLIX Congress of the Brazilian Society of Cardiology. Belo Horizonte — MG (August/1993).

87 Guevara-Valdivia ME, Iturralde Torres P, de Micheli A *et al.* Exercise test unmask apparent right bundle branch and ST segment elevation in the Brugada syndrome. *Arch. Cardiol. Mex.* 2001; **71**: 66–72.

88 Lee KL, Lau CP, Tse HF *et al.* Prevention of ventricular fibrillation by pacing in a man with Brugada syndrome. *J. Cardiovasc. Electrophysiol.* 2000; **1**: 935–937.

89 Miyazaki T, Mitamura H, Miyoshi S *et al.* Autonomic and antiarrhythmic drug modulation of ST segment elevation in patients with Brugada syndrome. *J. Am. Coll. Cardiol.* 1996; **27**: 1061–1070.

90 Zipes DP. Genesis of cardiac arrhytmias electrophysiological considerations. In: Braunwald E. *Heart Disease.* Philadelphia: W.B. Saunders, 1997.

91 Eckardt L, Bruns HJ, Paul M *et al.* Body surface area of ST elevation and the presence of late potentials correlate to the inducibility of ventricular tachyarrhythmias in Brugada syndrome. *J. Cardiovasc. Electrophysiol.* 2002; **13**: 742–749.

92 Simsom MB, MacFarlane PW. In: *Comprehensive Electrocardiology. Theory and Practice in Heath and Disease*, Vol. 2. *The Signal-Averaged Electrocardiogram.* Chapter 33, 1204. Pergamon Press, 1989.

93 Buckingham TA, Thessen CC, Stevens LL *et al.* Effect of conduction defects on the signal-averaged electrocardiographic determination of late potentials. *Am. J. Cardiol.* 1988; **61**: 1265–1271.

94 Lepesckin E, Surawicz B. The measurement of the Q-T interval of the electrocardiogram, *Circulation* 1952; **6**: 378–388.

95 Fei L, Statters DJ, Camm AJ. QT-interval dispersion on 12-lead electrocardiogram in normal subjects: its reproducibility and relation to the T wave. *Am. Heart J.* 1994; **127**: 1654–1655.

96 Schulze-Bahr E, Zoelch KA, Eckardt L, Haverkamp W, Breithardt G, Borggrefe M. Electrical alternans in long QT syndrome resembling a Brugada syndrome pattern. *Pacing Clin. Electrophysiol.* 2003; **26**: 2033–2035.

97 Hering HE. Experientell studien na saugetieren uber das elektrocardiogramm. *Exp. Med.* 1909; **7**: 363.

98 Taussig HB. Electrograms taken from isolated strips of mammalian ventricle cardiac muscle. *Bull. Johns Hopkins Hosp.* 1928; **43**: 81.

99 Fisch C, Edmands RE. Greenpan K. T wave alternans: Na association with abrupt rate change. *Am. Heart J.* 1971; **81**: 817.

100 Navarro-Lopez F, Cinca J, Sanz G *et al.* Isolated T wave alternans elicited by hypocalcemia in dogs. *J. Electrocardiol.* 1978; **11**: 103–108.

101 Hiejima K, Sano T. Electrical alternans of TU wave in Romano-Ward syndrome. *Br. Heart J.* 1976; **38**: 767–770.

102 Schwartz PJ, Malliani A. Electrical alternations of the T-wave: clinical and experimental evidence of its relationship with the sympathetic nervous system and with the QT long syndrome. *Am. Heart J.* 1975; **89**: 45–50.

103 Zareba W, Modd SJ, Le Cessie S *et al.* T-wave alternans in idiopathic long QT syndrome. *J. Am. Coll. Cardiol.* 1994; **23**: 1541–1546.

104 Mirvis DM. Evaluation of normal variation in ST segment patterns by body surface isopotential mapping: S-T segment elevation in absence of heart disease. *Am. J. Cardiol.* 1982; **50**: 122–128.

105 Fontaine G, Aouate P, Fontaliran F. Repolarization and the genesis of cardiac arrhytmias: role of body surface

mapping [editorial comment]. *Circulation* 1997; **95**: 2600–2602.

106 Hismatsu K, Kusano KF, Morita H *et al.* ST elevation characteristics in asymptomatic patients with Brugada ECG evaluated by body surface mapping: comparison with symptomatic Brugada syndrome. *Circulation* 2000; **102**: 584.

107 Izumida N, Asano Y, Doi S *et al.* Changes in body surface maps by isoproterenol and Na channel blocker in patients with Brugada syndrome. *Circulation* 2000; **102**: 583.

108 Bruns HJ, Eckardt L, Vahlhaus C *et al.* Body surface potential mapping in patients with Brugada syndrome: right precordial ST segment variations and reverse changes in left precordial leads. *Cardiovasc. Res.* 2002; **54**: 58–66.

CHAPTER 8

Brugada syndrome: relationship to other arrhythmogenic syndromes

D. Corrado, MD, PhD, *C. Basso,* MD, PhD, *G. Buja,* MD, *A. Nava,* MD, *G. Thiene,* MD

Introduction

In 1992 Brugada and Brugada reported a distinct subgroup of patients with episodes of 'idiopathic' ventricular tachycardia or ventricular fibrillation, characterized by a unique ECG pattern consisting of right bundle branch block (RBBB) and high take-off ST segment elevation from V_1 to V_2/V_3 (Brugada syndrome).[1] As in patients with long QT syndrome, the ECG changes and the ventricular electrical instability of Brugada syndrome are not explainable by structural heart disease, myocardial ischemia, or electrolyte disturbances. This 'primary electrical heart disease' selectively affects the right ventricle, as suggested by the ECG abnormalities, which are confined to right precordial leads. Distinctive clinical manifestations consist of dynamic changes of the ECG over time, polymorphic ventricular tachycardia, and exercise-unrelated sudden death.[2,3] A genetically induced cardiac sodium channel dysfunction due to a mutation in the gene *SCN5A* has been discovered in some patients with Brugada syndrome.[4]

Limits between Brugada syndrome and other arrhythmogenic conditions remain to be defined. Clinical conditions strongly related to Brugada syndrome are the 'sudden unexpected death syndrome (SUDS)' of young Southern Asians[5] and the 'vagally induced idiopathic ventricular fibrillation'.[6] Both conditions exhibit a Brugada-like ECG pattern and predispose to ventricular fibrillation in the absence of clinically demonstrable organic heart disease.

On the other hand, the high take-off ST segment elevation in right precordial leads, with or without the associated risk of sudden arrhythmic death, may

also be observed in patients with other diseases/ abnormalities or in individuals with early repolarization syndrome (mostly young competitive athletes).[7] Table 8.1 lists the causes which have been demonstrated to lead to a Brugada-like ECG pattern. It is mandatory for the clinician to carefully exclude each of these conditions before coming to the diagnosis of Brugada syndrome. Differential diagnosis between Brugada syndrome and ARVC/D (arrhythmogenic right ventricular cardiomyopathy/dysplasia) may be particularly difficult because this condition may mimic Brugada syndrome and structural abnormalities may be found only at postmortem investigation.[8–10]

Differential diagnosis between Brugada syndrome and ARVC/D

ARVC/D is a well-recognized cause of sudden arrhythmic death, mostly in young people and athletes.[11–16] This disease is an inherited heart muscle disease, which is characterized by loss of right ventricular myocardium, typically progressing from the epicardium to the endocardium and fibrofatty substitution.[12,14,15,17] Common clinical features of ARVC/D include structural and functional abnormalities of the right ventricle, ECG depolarization/repolarization changes such as prolongation of QRS interval and inversion of T waves in right precordial leads, presentation with ventricular arrhythmias of right ventricular origin, and exercise-related sudden death.[13,16,18–20]

Table 8.2 reports the main characteristics of Brugada syndrome and ARVC/D that may be useful in making a differential diagnosis. Both Brugada

Table 8.1 Conditions that can lead to ST segment elevation in the right precordial leads.

Right or left bundle branch block, left ventricular hypertrophy

Acute myocardial ischemia or infarction

Acute myocarditis

Right ventricular ischemia or infarction

Dissecting aortic aneurysm

Acute pulmonary thromboemboli

Various central and autonomic nervous system abnormalities

Heterocyclic antidepressant overdose

Duchenne muscular dystrophy

Friedreich's ataxia

Thiamine deficiency

Hypercalcemia

Hyperkalemia

Cocaine intoxication

Mediastinal tumor compressing right ventricular outflow tract

Arrhythmogenic right ventricular cardiomyopathy/dysplasia

Long QT syndrome, type 3

Other conditions that can lead to ST segment elevation in the right precordial leads

Early repolarization syndrome

Other normal variants (particularly in men)

Modified from Wilde *et al.*[7]

syndrome and ARVC/D are genetic disorders with an autosomal dominant pattern of inheritance, in which young adults present clinically with right precordial ECG abnormalities, late potentials, and life-threatening ventricular arrhythmias leading to syncope or sudden death.[19–24] The two conditions, however, demonstrate important differences with respect to involved genes, underlying cardiomyopathic changes, autonomic and antiarrhythmic drug modulation of ECG abnormalities, and mechanisms of arrhythmias.

Brugada syndrome and ARVC/D show a different genetic background. The only gene thus far linked to the Brugada syndrome is the cardiac sodium channel gene which is the same gene implicated in the LQT3 form of the long QT syndrome.[4,25,26] Instead, ARVC/D has been linked to nine different chromosomal loci and three putative genes,[24] which are unrelated to those discovered for Brugada syndrome.

Patients with Brugada syndrome have no evidence of significant structural heart disease at different imaging techniques such as echocardiography, angiography, magnetic resonance imaging, and radionuclide scintigraphy, whereas ARVC/D patients characteristically show overt right ventricular

morpho-functional changes such as global dilatation, bulgings/aneurysms, and wall motion abnormalities.[1,3,19,20,27] The most important mechanism of ventricular tachycardia with a left bundle branch block morphology in patients with ARVC/D is thought to be a 'scar-related' reentry, similarly to ventricular tachycardia observed in post-myocardial infarction.[28] In contrast, the electrogenesis of ventricular arrhythmias in patients with Brugada syndrome is consistent with a 'phase-2 reentry' (or 'local re-excitation') inducing rapid polymorphic ventricular tachycardia, which can degenerate into ventricular fibrillation.[27,29] Ventricular arrhythmias in patients with ARVC/D are facilitated by catecholamines and exercise, thus accounting for sudden death of young competitive athletes during sport; instead, ST segment elevation and arrhythmias are characteristically enhanced by vagotonic agents or beta-adrenergic blockers in Brugada patients, and cardiac arrest has been documented to occur usually at rest or during sleep.[27,29–31] Unlike ARVC/D, the ECG abnormalities in patients with Brugada syndrome can vary considerably from time to time, until complete transient normalization, mostly because of variable influences of autonomic

Table 8.2 Differential diagnosis between ARVC and Brugada syndrome.

Clinical characteristics	ARVC	Brugada syndrome
Age	25–35	35–40
Sex (male/female)	M > F (3 : 1)	M > F (8 : 1)
Distribution	Worldwide (Italy)	Worldwide (Southeast Asia)
Inheritance	AD (AR)	AD
Chromosomes	1, 2, 3, 6, 10, 14 (17)	3
Gene	hRYR2, plakobin, desmoplakin	SCN5A
Symptoms	Palpitations, syncope, cardiac arrest	Syncope, cardiac arrest
Circumstances	Effort	Rest
Imaging	Morpho-functional RV (and LV) abnormalities	Normal
Pathology	Fibrofatty replacement	Normal
ECG repolarization	Inverted T waves in right precordial leads	High take-off, ST segment V_1–V_3
ECG depolarization	Epsilon waves, QRS-prolongation, late potentials	RBBB/LAD, late potentials
AV conduction	Normal	50% abnormal PR/HV intervals
Atrial arrhythmias	Late (secondary)	Early (primary 10–25%)
ECG changes	Fixed (mostly)	Variable
Ventricular arrhythmias	Monomorphic VT/VF	Polymorphic VT/VF
Mechanism of arrhythmias	Scar-related reentry	Phase 2 reentry
Drug effect class I	↓	↑
Drug effect class II	↓	↑
Drug effect class III	↓	–/↑
Drug effect class IV	–/↓	–
Beta-stimulation	↑	↓
Natural history	Sudden death, heart failure	Sudden death

Arrows denote changes in ST segment elevation (↑, increased; ↓, decreased; –/, small change, if any). Modified from Wilde et al.[7]

nervous system over the time.[2,30] Finally, administration of sodium channel blockers such as flecainide, ajmaline, and procainamide can accentuate or unmask ST segment elevation in Brugada patients, whereas it does not affect ventricular repolarization in patients with ARVC/D or other arrhythmic conditions.[32]

'Phenotype overlapping' between Brugada syndrome and ARVC/D

Although Brugada syndrome and ARVC/D are two separate entities, there is a subset of ARVC/D patients displaying the ECG pattern of right precordial high take-off ST segment elevation that shares some clinical features and electrogenetic mechanisms with Brugada patients.

Previous reports from our group clearly established the relationship between the ECG pattern of RBBB and right precordial ST segment elevation to a

right ventricular cardiomyopathy. In 1986, Martini et al.[8] described six patients with 'apparent' idiopathic ventricular fibrillation, three of whom had the ECG pattern of early repolarization in right precordial leads. In these patients, underlying structural abnormalities of the right ventricle were clinically documented.

Familial cardiomyopathy underlying the syndrome of RBBB, ST segment elevation, and sudden death

Corrado et al.[9] studied 16 members of an affected family and provided definitive evidence that a structural abnormality of both the right ventricular myocardium and the specialized conduction system may present clinically as 'RBBB, right precordial ST segment elevation and sudden death'. The proband had been resuscitated from sudden cardiac arrest due to ventricular fibrillation 5 years before sudden death. Serial ECGs showed sinus rhythm, first degree AV block (PR interval of 220 ms), RBBB with left axis deviation, and high take-off ST segment elevation with inverted T waves in right precordial leads, in the absence of *clinical* heart disease. Postmortem investigation disclosed right ventricular dilation and myocardial atrophy with fibrofatty replacement of the right ventricular free wall as well as sclerotic interruption of the right bundle branch. A variable degree of RBBB, left axis deviation, and ST segment elevation was observed in seven family members; four of them had structural right ventricular abnormalities on echocardiography and late potential on signal-averaged ECG. A sib of the proband also had a prolonged HV interval, inducible ventricular tachycardia, and fibrofatty replacement on endomyocardial biopsy. These findings suggest that a 'double' right ventricular conduction defect, both 'septal' (due to the conduction system disease) and 'parietal' (due to the fibrofatty replacement of ventricular myocardium), may underlie the syndrome.

Right precordial ST segment elevation and sudden death in young people

More recently, we addressed prevalence, substrates, and clinical profile of young sudden death victims with the ECG pattern of right precordial ST segment elevation.[33] Among a series of 273 young (≤35 years) victims of cardiovascular sudden death who were prospectively studied according to a specific clinical and morphological protocol from 1979 to 1998 in the Veneto Region of Italy, 12 lead ECG was available in 96 cases (36%). Thirteen (14%; 12 males, 1 female, aged 24 ± 8 years) showed ST segment elevation in leads V_1 to V_2/V_3, either isolated (9 cases) or associated with RBBB (4 cases). At autopsy, all these patients had ARVC/D (92%) except one, who had no evidence of structural heart disease. Compared with the 19 young sudden death victims with ARVC/D and no ST segment abnormalities from the same series, those with ARVC/D and right precordial ST segment elevation included fewer competitive athletes (17% versus 58%; $p = 0.03$), more died suddenly at rest or during sleep (83% versus 26%, $p = 0.003$), and showed serial ECG changes over time (83% versus 0, $p = 0.015$), polymorphic ventricular tachycardia (33% versus 0, $p = 0.016$), and predominant fatty replacement of the right ventricular anterior wall (58% versus 21%; $p = 0.05$). Therefore, the right precordial ST segment elevation, which was found in 14% of young sudden death victims with available ECG, reflected an underlying ARVC/D (with predominant right ventricular anterior wall involvement) and characterized a subgroup of patients who share with Brugada patients the propensity to die from non-exercise-related cardiac arrest and to exhibit dynamic ECG changes and polymorphic ventricular tachycardia, all clinical and ECG features typically observed in Brugada syndrome.

ECG abnormalities

Most of the patients with the syndrome of RBBB and right precordial ST segment elevation described in the literature were of South Asian origin. Nademanee *et al.* reported that the syndrome was the commonest cause of natural sudden death in South Asian males below 50 years of age, with a prevalence of one sudden death per 2500 inhabitants per year in Thailand and as high as one sudden death per 1000 inhabitants per year in Laos.[5] Our data provided a prevalence of 14% of the pattern of RBBB and/or right precordial ST segment among the ECG recordings obtained from a homogeneous series of young sudden death victims (≤35 years) from the Veneto Region of Italy, suggesting that this ECG abnormality is not so rare even in the Western countries and should be considered as a worldwide marker of arrhythmic sudden death.

A widened S wave in left lateral leads, which is typical for RBBB, was observed in only four of our sudden death victims with right precordial ST segment elevation (28%). This indicates that though the ST segment elevation in V_1-V_2/V_3 mimics a RBBB, the pattern is rarely consistent with a *true* RBBB. When two or more ECGs were available, serial changes over the time of the ST segment elevation, up to transient normalization of the tracing, were noted in over 80% of cases. Therefore, the previous concept that dynamic ECG changes are the proof against an underlying structural substrate[3,27–30] is not in keeping with our findings showing that ECG variations over time occur even in patients with organic heart disease, namely ARVC/D proven at autopsy. The variability of the autonomic nervous system activity modulating a conduction defect or a repolarization abnormality in the setting of a structural right ventricular myocardial disease is the most likely explanation for these ECG changes.[15,29]

Morphologic studies

Morphologic studies in sudden death victims with the ECG pattern of RBBB and right precordial ST segment elevation are rare and limited to case reports.[8–10,33–35] However, when available, autopsy findings consistently showed fibrofatty replacement of right ventricular myocardium, frequently associated with a conduction system pathology.[8,9,33] We definitely showed that a structural heart disease, namely ARVC/D, was the most prevalent substrate underlying the above ECG abnormalities in a homogeneous series of young sudden death victims. A functional electrical disease (like Brugada syndrome) could have accounted for ECG abnormalities and arrhythmic cardiac arrest in the only heart that did not exhibit any structural abnormality.

In patients with transient right precordial ST segment elevation and vagal-induced ventricular fibrillation, Kansanuki *et al.*, by using body-surface mapping, demonstrated conduction abnormalities which were predominantly localized between the anterior RV wall and the outflow tract, and advanced the hypothesis that this clinical condition may reflect an early subclinical stage of ARVC/D, characterized by a very localized lesion in the right ventricular outflow tract.[6] Our data do not support Kansanuki's theory. The pathologic findings in sudden death victims with right precordial ST segment elevation were all consistent with a widespread form of ARVC/D, which did not differ in terms of cardiomegaly and extent of myocardial atrophy with fibrofatty replacement from that without ST segment abnormalities. The peculiar arrangement of fibrofatty tissue across the right ventricular free wall, with predominant involvement of epicardial and mediomural layers, rather than the extent of right ventricular involvement, may have played a role in the genesis of the ECG abnormalities and arrhythmias. Kirschner *et al.*[36] performed autopsy studies in south Asian victims of SUDS in 1986, when the morphologic features of ARVC/D were still incompletely known and found structural changes in the specialized conduction system in 14 out of 18 hearts. Similarly, we found an involvement of the branching bundle and proximal right bundle branch, ranging from mild fibrous atrophy to interruption, in 3 of 4 patients with the ECG pattern of true RBBB. These findings confirm that a structural His–Purkinje system disease may underlie the electrophysiologic

finding of prolonged HV interval in a subset of patients with the RBBB and right precordial ST segment.[1,9]

Mechanisms of ST segment elevation and ventricular arrhythmias

The ventricular arrhythmogenicity of ARVC/D is traditionally explained by the existence of islands of surviving myocardium surrounded by replacing fibrofatty tissue that act as a substrate for an inhomogeneous intraventricular conduction predisposing to reentrant ventricular arrhythmias.[12–15] These depolarization abnormalities are mediated by a sympathetic mechanism that distinctively predispose to sudden death during enhanced adrenergic drive, such as sports activity.[12,13,16]

Instead, in the majority of patients with Brugada and related syndromes, the malignant ventricular arrhythmias occur at rest and in many cases during night time;[1–3,5,6,37] a sudden rise of vagal activity has been reported to occur just before ventricular fibrillation episodes.[6,31] Our data suggest that an increased vagal activity and/or withdrawal of sympathetic activity may play a significant arrhythmogenic role even in the subset of ARVC/D patients with right precordial ST segment elevation, who show a propensity to die suddenly at rest or during sleep. Like patients with Brugada syndrome, the presumed arrhythmogenic mechanisms in this group of patients is a vagal-induced ventricular fibrillation originating in the setting of a dispersion of right ventricular repolarization.

Right ventricular transmural dispersion of repolarization

Antzelevicth *et al.*[38–40] provided experimental evidence that a heterogeneous distribution of action potentials duration across the right ventricular wall may be the basis for both a right precordial ST segment elevation and rapid ventricular arrhythmias (polymorphic ventricular tachycardia or ventricular fibrillation), which may be precipitated by enhanced parasympathetic activity. In contrast to endocardial myocytes, right ventricular epicardial myocytes distinctively exhibit a 'spike and dome configuration' of action potential, due to a pronounced 'phase 1' that coincides with the J wave in the surface ECG. A series of pathologic conditions or pharmacologic interventions such as sodium channel blockade may cause the loss of action potential dome in the epicardium (but not in the endocardium) and provoke a transmural current flow from epicardium to endocardium, which accounts for ST segment elevation. Moreover, propagation of action potential dome from sites at which it is maintained to sites at which it is abolished may result in local re-excitation ('phase 2 reentry') and may induce very rapid ventricular arrhythmias of the form of polymorphic ventricular tachycardia or ventricular fibrillation. The ionic basis for the loss of action potential dome in right ventricular epicardium is an outward shift in the balance of currents active at the end of phase 1 of the action potential, mostly enhancement of the 'transient outward current (I_{to})' and reduction of the 'inward calcium current (I_{Ca})'. Litovsky and Antzelevitch demonstrated that acetylcholine facilitates the loss of the action potential dome and accentuates both ST segment elevation and dishomogeneity of ventricular repolarization by suppressing the calcium current and/or augmenting the potassium current.[41]

Etiopathogenesis

Loss of the action potential plateau in the epicardium but not the endocardium by any causes, either functional or structural, would be expected to induce elevation of the ST segment and ventricular arrhythmias elicited by 'phase 2 reentry'.[42–44] In Brugada syndrome, a genetically induced sodium channel dysfunction with current inhibition is the most likely mechanism of the loss of the epicardial action potential dome with transmural dispersion of repolarization, which in turn may predispose to the development of ventricular fibrillation.[29,38] In our sudden death victims, the ARVC/D lesions predominantly involved the epicardial and midmural layers and created a transmural gradient of myocyte degeneration and death in the setting of the fibrofatty replacement. This pathologic substrate potentially accounted for a 'structural' epicardial–endocardial heterogeneity of repolarization in the right ventricular wall, predisposing to 'phase 2 reentry'. Accordingly, experimental damage of canine ventricular epicardium secondary to metabolic inhibition and simulated ischemia have been demonstrated to provoke electrical inhomogeneity and local reexcitation.[38,40] In addition, Krishan and Antzelevitch showed a synergism between heterogeneous repolarization and delayed conduction in giving rise to arrhythmic activity in canine ventricular epicardium.[44] In our sudden death victims, therefore, a delayed intraventricular conduction caused by the disarrangement of surviving myocardium in islands interspersed with fibrofatty tissue, may have contributed importantly to the induction and maintenance of reentrant activity, in association with the dispersion of repolarization.

There are other explanations for the 'phenotype overlapping' between Brugada syndrome and ARVC/D. A double genetic defect may account for the coexistence of both Brugada and ARVC/D phenotypes. Alternatively, right ventricular structural changes can be a consequence of a genetically defective cardiac sodium channel, which with time can induce myocyte death. In this regard, familial Lenègre disease (also known as 'progressive cardiac conduction disease'), which is a progressive disease of the specialized conduction tissue and characterized by fibrofatty atrophy of the His–Purkinje system, has been recently linked to mutations in SCN5A,[45,46] the same gene involved in 'primary electrical diseases' such as Brugada syndrome and the LQT3 variant of long QT syndrome.

Conclusions and clinical implications

There is clinical and pathologic evidence of an overlap in clinical manifestation and mechanisms of ventricular arrhythmias between patients with ARVC/D and Brugada syndrome. This suggests caution in using 'class IC' antiarrhythmic agents that may enhance ST segment elevation and precipitate arrhythmic events in ARVC/D patients with Brugada-like ECG abnormalities.[2,29,44] Follow-up studies in Brugada syndrome demonstrated a highly malignant outcome of both untreated or pharmacologic treated patients, the implantable defibrillator being the only effective measure for prevention of sudden death.[47,48] Whether an aggressive antiarrhythmic approach with implantable defibrillator represents a more appropriate strategy in the subset of patients with ARVC/D and right precordial ST segment elevation, needs to be assessed by future prospective studies.

Since patients with ARVC/D may present clinically with the same ECG pattern and clinical features, the diagnosis of Brugada syndrome should be based on the definitive exclusion of demonstrable structural right ventricular abnormalities by extensive non-invasive and invasive cardiac evaluation.

Further studies aimed to identify all genes involved in Brugada syndrome and ARVC/D, to screen for *SCN5A* mutations in family members of sudden death victims with ARVC/D, and to investigate heart morphologic findings of Brugada sudden death victims, may provide in the near future important insights in understanding the relationship of Brugada syndrome to ARVC/D.

This study was supported by the Veneto Region, Italy.

References

1 Brugada J, Brugada P. Right bundle branch block, persistent ST segment elevation and sudden cardiac death: a distinct clinical and electrocardiographic syndrome. A multicenter report. *J. Am. Coll. Cardiol.* 1992; **20**: 1391–1396.

2 Brugada J, Brugada P. Further characterization of the syndrome of right bundle branch block, ST segment elevation, and sudden cardiac death. *J. Cardiovasc. Electrophysiol.* 1997; **8**: 325–331.

3 Brugada J, Brugada R, Brugada P. Right bundle branch block and ST-segment elevation in leads V1 through V3. A marker for sudden death in patients without demonstrable structural heart disease. *Circulation* 1998; **97**: 457–460.

4 Chen Q, Kirsch GE, Zhang D *et al.* Genetic basis and molecular mechanism for idiopathic ventricular fibrillation. *Nature* 1998; **392**: 293–296.

5 Nademanee K, Veerakul G, Nimmannit S *et al.* Arrhythmogenic marker for the sudden unexplained death syndrome in Thai men. *Circulation* 1997; **96**: 2595–2600.

6 Kasanuki H, Ohinishi S, Ohtuka M *et al.* Idiopathic ventricular fibrillation induced with vagal activity in patients without obvious heart disease. *Circulation* 1997; **95**: 2277–2285.

7 Wilde AA, Antzelevitch C, Borggrefe M *et al.* Proposed diagnostic criteria for the Brugada syndrome: consensus report. *Circulation* 2002; **106**: 2514–2519.

8 Martini B, Nava A, Thiene G *et al.* Ventricular fibrillation without apparent heart disease: description of 6 cases. *Am. Heart J.* 1989; **118**: 1203–1209.

9 Corrado D, Nava A, Buja GF *et al.* Familial cardiomyopathy underlies syndrome of right bundle branch block, ST segment elevation and sudden death. *J. Am. Coll. Cardiol.* 1996; **27**: 443–448.

10 Tada H, Aihara N, Ohe T *et al.* Arrhythmogenic right ventricular cardiomyopathy underlies syndrome of right

bundle branch block, ST segment elevation, and sudden death. *Am. J. Cardiol.* 1998; **81**: 519–522.

11 Marcus FI, Fontaine G, Guiraudon G *et al.* Right ventricular dysplasia. A report of 24 adult cases. *Circulation* 1982; **65**: 384–398.

12 Thiene G, Nava A, Corrado D, Rossi L, Pennelli N. Right ventricular cardiomyopathy and sudden death in young people. *N. Engl. J. Med.* 1988; **318**: 129–133.

13 Corrado D, Thiene G, Nava A, Rossi L, Pennelli N. Sudden death in young competitive athletes: clinicopathologic correlation in 22 cases. *Am. J. Med.* 1990; **89**: 588–596.

14 Basso C, Thiene G, Corrado D *et al.* Arrhythmogenic right ventricular cardiomyopathy. Dysplasia, dystrophy, or myocarditis? *Circulation* 1996; **94**: 983–991.

15 Corrado D, Basso C, Thiene G *et al.* Spectrum of clinicopathologic manifestations of arrhythmogenic right ventricular cardiomyopathy/dysplasia: a multicenter study. *J. Am. Coll. Cardiol.* 1997; **30**: 1512–1520.

16 Corrado D, Basso C, Schiavon M, Thiene G. Screening for hypertrophic cardiomyopathy in young athletes. *N. Engl. J. Med.* 1998; **339**: 364–369.

17 Nava A, Thiene G, Canciani B *et al.* Familial occurrence of right ventricular dysplasia: a study involving nine families. *J. Am. Coll. Cardiol.* 1988; **12**: 1222–1228.

18 Rampazzo A, Nava A, Danieli GA *et al.* The gene for arrhythmogenic right ventricular cardiomyopathy maps to chromosome 14q23-q24. *Hum. Mol. Genet.* 1994; **3**: 959–962.

19 Corrado D, Fontaine G, Marcus FI *et al.* Arrhythmogenic right ventricular dysplasia/cardiomyopathy. Need for an international registry. *Circulation* 2000; **101**: e101–e106.

20 Corrado D, Basso C, Thiene G. Arrhythmogenic right ventricular cardiomyopathy: diagnosis, prognosis, and treatment. *Heart* 2000; **83**: 588–595.

21 Alings M, Wilde A. Brugada syndrome: clinical data and suggested pathophysiological mechanism. *Circulation* 1999; **99**: 666–673.

22 Corrado D, Buja G, Nava A, Basso C, Thiene G. What is Brugada syndrome? *Cardiol. Rev.* 1999; **7**: 191–195.

23 Corrado D, Buja G, Basso C, Thiene G. Clinical diagnosis and management strategies in arrhythmogenic right ventricular cardiomyopathy. *J. Electrocardiol.* 2000; **33** Suppl: 49–55.

24 Corrado D, Basso C, Nava A, Thiene G. Arrhythmogenic right ventricular cardiomyopathy: current diagnostic and management strategies. *Cardiol. Rev.* 2001; **9**: 259–265.

25 Priori SG, Napolitano C, Gasparini M *et al.* Clinical and genetic heterogeneity of right bundle branch block and ST-segment elevation syndrome: a prospective evaluation of 52 families. *Circulation* 2000; **102**: 2509–2515.

26 Priori SG, Napolitano C, Gasparini M *et al.* Natural history of Brugada syndrome: insights for risk stratification and management. *Circulation.* 2002; **105**: 1342–1347.

27 Gussak I, Antzelevitch C, Bjerregaard P, Towbin JA, Chaitman BR. The Brugada syndrome: clinical, electrophysiological and genetic aspects. *J. Am. Coll. Cardiol.* 1999; **33**: 5–15.

28 Fontaine G, Frank R, Tonet JL *et al.* Arrhythmogenic right ventricular dysplasia: a clinical model for the study of chronic ventricular tachicardia. *Jpn. Circ.* 1984; **48**: 515–538.

29 Antzelevitch C The Brugada syndrome: ionic basis and arrhythmia mechanisms. *J. Cardiovasc. Electrophysiol.* 2001; **12**: 268–272.

30 Miyazaki T, Mitamura H, Miyoshi S *et al.* Autonomic and antiarrhythmic drug modulation of ST segment elevation in patients with Brugada syndrome. *J. Am. Coll. Cardiol.* 1996; **27**: 1061–1070.

31 Matsuo K, Kurita T, Inagaki M *et al.* The circadian pattern of the development of ventricular fibrillation in patients with Brugada syndrome. *Eur. Heart J.* 1999; **20**: 465–470.

32 Brugada R, Brugada J,. Antzelevitch C *et al.* Sodium channel blockers identify risk for sudden death in patients with ST-segment elevation and right bundle branch block but structurally normal hearts. *Circulation* 2000; **101**: 510–515.

33 Corrado D, Basso C, Buja G *et al.* Right bundle branch block, right precordial ST-segment elevation, and sudden death in young people. *Circulation* 2001; **103**: 710–717.

34 Morgera T, Sinagra GF, Viel E *et al.* The syndrome of right bundle branch block, persistent ST segment elevation, and sudden cardiac death. Which is the histological substrate? *Eur. Heart J.* 1997; 1190–1191.

35 Fontaine G, Piot O, Sohal PS *et al.* Sus-decalage du segment ST en derivations precordiales droites et mort subite: relation avec la dysplasie ventriculaire droite arythmogene. *Arch. Mal Coeur* 1996; **89**: 1323–1329.

36 Kirschner RH, Echner FAO, Baron RC. The cardiac pathology of sudden unexplained nocturnal death in Southeast Asian refugees. *JAMA* 1986; **256**: 2700–2075.

37 Atarashi H, Ogawa S, Harumi K *et al.* Characteristics of patients with right bundle branch block and ST-segment elevation in right precordial leads. *Am. J. Cardiol.* 1996; **78**: 581–583.

38 Yan GX, Antzelevitch C. Cellular basis for the electrocardiographic J wave. *Circulation* 1996; **93**: 372–379.

39 Antzelevitch C. The Brugada syndrome. *J. Cardiovasc. Electrophysiol.* 1998; **9**: 513–516.

40 Xan G-X, Antzelevitch C. Cellular basis for the Brugada syndrome and other mechanisms of arrhythmogenesis associated with ST-segment elevation. *Circulation* 1999; **100**: 1660–1666.

41 Litovsky SH, Antzelevitch C. Differences in the electrophysiological response of canine ventricular subendocardium and subepicardium to acetylcholine and isoproterenol. A direct effect of acetylcholine in ventricular myocardium. *Circ. Res.* 1990; **67**: 615–627.

42 Antzelevitch C, Sicouri S, Lucas A *et al.* Clinical implications of electrical heterogeneity in the heart: the electrophysiology and pharmacology of epicardial, M and endocardial cells. In: Podrid PJ, Kowey PR eds. *Cardiac Arrhythmias: Mechanisms, Diagnosis and Management.* Baltimore, MD: Williams & Wilkins, 1994: 88–107.

43 Lucas A, Antzelevitch C. Differences in the electrophysiological response of canine ventricular epicardium and endocardium to ischemia. Role of the transient outward current. *Circulation* 1993; **88**: 2903–2915.

44 Krishnan SC, Antzelevitch C. Flecainide-induced arrhythmias in canine ventricular epicardium. Phase 2 reentry? *Circulation* 1993; **87**: 562–572.

45 Lenegre J, Moreau PH. Le bloc auriculo–ventriculaire chronique, Etude anatomique, clinique et histologique. *Arch Mal Coeur* 1963; **56**: 867–888.

46 Schott JJ, Alshinawi C, Kyndt F *et al.* Cardiac conduction defects associate with mutations in *SCN5A*. *Nature Genet.* 1999; **23**: 20–21.

47 Brugada J, Brugada R, Brugada P. Pharmacological and device approach to therapy of inherited cardiac diseases associated with cardiac arrhythmias and sudden death. *J. Electrocardiol.* 2000; **33** (Suppl): 41–47.

48 Brugada J, Brugada R, Antzelevitch C *et al.* Long-term follow-up of individuals with the electrocardiographic pattern of right bundle-branch block and ST-segment elevation in precordial leads V1 to V3. *Circulation* 2002; **105**: 73–78.

CHAPTER 9

ST segment elevation and sudden death in the athlete

D. Corrado, MD, PhD, *A. Pelliccia*, MD, *C. Antzelevitch*, PhD, *L. Leoni*, MD,
M. Schiavon, MD, *G. Buja*, MD, *B. Maron*, MD, *G. Thiene*, MD,
C. Basso, MD, PhD

Sudden death in young people and athletes with apparently normal hearts

A structural cardiac abnormality is found at autopsy in most cases of sudden death.[1–10] Fatal events in adults usually occur as an arrhythmic complication of atherosclerotic coronary artery disease, in the setting of either acute coronary syndromes or previous myocardial infarction.[1–6] Other cardiovascular disorders implicated in sudden death, predominantly in younger people and athletes, include cardiomyopathy, valve heart disease, congenital anomaly of coronary arteries, conduction system disease, and congenital heart disease.[7–10] Sudden death may occur in patients with 'apparently' normal hearts.[11–14] The mechanism is usually arrhythmic, namely a rapid ventricular tachycardia or fibrillation leading to cardiac arrest with no demonstrable structural heart disease. Failure to detect structural abnormalities may depend on the unknown or concealed nature of the underlying pathologic substrates, along with the low sensitivity of currently available clinical tests. Subtle structural heart conditions potentially at risk of sudden arrhythmic cardiac arrest include coronary artery spasm superimposed on a non-obstructive coronary artery plaque, focal myocarditis, segmental cardiomyopathy, and abnormalities of the conduction system.[12,13] The ultimate diagnosis of these structural lesions which remain clinically concealed may require histologic examination by endomyocardial biopsy or at postmortem. On the other hand, life-threatening ventricular arrhythmias may be the result of primary electrical heart diseases ('idiopathic

ventricular fibrillation') in the absence of structural heart disease.[14]

Corrado *et al.*[15] recently assessed the relative prevalence of both subtle morphologic substrates and truly structurally normal heart in a series of 273 consecutive cases of sudden cardiac death in young people and athletes (≤35 years) which occurred in the Veneto Region of Italy from 1979 to 1998. Following exclusion of extracardiac causes of sudden death, the heart was examined according to a detailed morphologic protocol consisting of macroscopic and histologic examination, including study of the specialized conduction system by serial sections. At macroscopic examination, 197 SCD victims (72%) had an overt underlying structural heart disease such as cardiomyopathy, obstructive coronary atherosclerosis, valve disease, non-atherosclerotic coronary artery disease, aortic rupture, postoperative congenital heart disease, and other. The remaining 76 cases (28%) had a macroscopically normal heart. In 79% of them, histologic examination disclosed concealed pathologic substrates consisting of focal myocarditis, regional arrhythmogenic right ventricular cardiomyopathy/dysplasia, and conduction system abnormalities (leading to either ventricular preexcitation or heart block). In 16 hearts (6%) there was no evidence of structural heart disease even after detailed histologic examination of both ordinary ventricular myocardium and specialized conduction system, and the cause of sudden death remained unexplained. These findings are very similar to those recently reported by Chug *et al.*[16] showing a 5% prevalence of structurally normal hearts (without any evidence of either macroscopic and histologic structural abnormalities) in a large autopsy series of sudden death victims aged 42 ± 14 years from Minneapolis-St. Paul. In conclusion, macroscopic heart features are normal in nearly one-third of sudden deaths in young people and athletes. In the majority of them, however, histologic study unmasks concealed pathologic substrates such as focal myocarditis or cardiomyopathy and conduction system diseases. Six per cent of sudden death victims have no evidence of structural heart disease and the cause of their sudden death is in all likelihood related to a primary electrical heart disease such as inherited cardiac ion channels defects (channelopathies) including long QT syndrome,[17] catecholaminergic polymorphic ventricular tachycardia,[18] and Brugada syndrome.[19]

No data exist that directly relate Brugada syndrome to the risk of participating in sports. There is only an anecdotal report of a previously asymptomatic Brugada patients who experienced cardiac arrest during a competitive athletic activity (J. A. Camm, personal communication). This chapter will address the potential relationship between arrhythmogenic mechanisms of Brugada syndrome and the risk of sudden death during sports, with particular reference on the effects of autonomic nervous system modulation and genetics. Moreover, the need for a differential diagnosis between Brugada syndrome and early repolarization abnormalities associated with 'athlete's heart' will be discussed.

Mechanisms underlying ST segment elevation and arrhythmogenesis

Brugada syndrome is an inherited ion channel disease characterized by a distinctive ECG pattern of right bundle branch block and ST segment elevation in right precordial leads (V_1 to V_2–V_3) (Fig. 9.1).[19,20] This ECG pattern and the electrical ventricular instability have been explained by dispersion of repolarization within the right ventricular wall which predisposes to local re-excitation of myocytes with different action potential durations.[20,21] A mutant cardiac sodium channel gene SCN5A has been discovered in up to 25% of patients with Brugada syndrome.[22] Experimental studies by Antzelevitch et al.[21,23] elucidated the ionic basis for ST segment elevation in the Brugada syndrome: an outward shift in the balance of currents active at the end of phase 1,

namely enhancement of the transient outward current (I_{to}) and reduction of the L type inward calcium current (I_{Ca}). Such an outward shift of currents further shifts the end of phase 1 of the action potential in the right ventricular epicardium to a more negative potential at which the L type calcium current is overwhelmed by the outward repolarizing currents (mainly I_{to}) and the action potential dome fails to develop, leading to marked shortening of action potential. The loss of the action potential dome occurs in the right ventricular epicardium, but not in the endocardium. Marked accentuation of the right ventricular action potential notch or loss of action potential dome leads to a 'coved type' ST segment elevation (i.e., 'high take-off' and 'down-sloping') and inversion of the T wave on the ECG (Fig. 9.1), and is associated with the propensity to develop rapid polymorphic ventricular tachycardia or ventricular fibrillation.[21,23] A lesser accentuation of the action potential notch is associated with a smaller prolongation of the right ventricular epicardial action potential, leading to a 'saddleback' configuration of ST segment elevation, i.e., a J wave followed by a positive T wave, that is generally thought not to be arrhythmogenic.[24] In Brugada patients, transition from 'saddleback type' to 'coved type' ST segment elevation may occur either spontaneously as a consequence of autonomic changes or can be induced by sodium channel blockers.[25–27] Patients may remain asymptomatic if such a transition does not occur. It is noteworthy that pharmacologic interventions or pathophysiologic alterations may facilitate this transition and lead to development of ventricular arrhythmias.[28–34] Arrhythmogenesis has been related to a marked dispersion of repolarization on the epicardial surface, as a result of a non-uniform loss of the epicardial action potential dome (i.e., complete loss of the dome at some sites but not others), probably due to intrinsic differences of I_{to} in epicardium. Propagation of the action potential dome from sites at which is maintained to sites at which it is abolished may lead to local re-excitation (so called 'phase 2 reentry') and the development of a closely coupled extrasystole ('R on T' phenomenon).[21,23,35] An increase in epicardial–endocardial heterogeneity of repolarization, also present under these conditions, may facilitate transmural propagation of phase 2 reentry, providing further substrate for malignant ventricular arrhythmias.

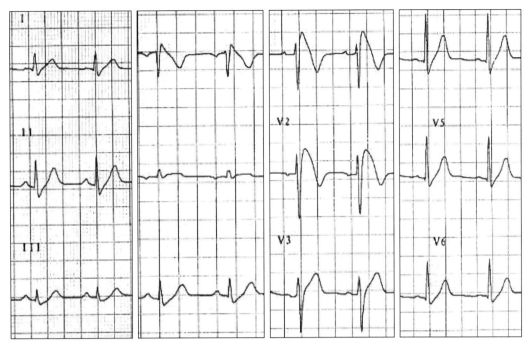

Figure 9.1 Basal 12 lead ECG showing the distinctive features of Brugada syndrome. Note the diagnostic 'coved type' configuration of ST-T in V_1 and V_2 due to a high take-off J point giving rise to a downsloping ST segment which is followed by a negative T wave.

A *partial* depression of epicardial action potential dome is likely to underlie another type of early repolarization pattern which is characterized by an 'up-sloping' ST segment elevation. A typical clinical example is the early repolarization pattern in the leads exploring the left ventricle,[36,37] where epicardial action potential 'notch' and I_{to} are relatively smaller. Another condition is the right precordial ST segment elevation seen in highly trained athletes.[38,39] The mechanisms underlying this latter condition are most likely related to hypervagotonia associated with the adaptation to athletic training. In the wedge, acetylcholine depresses the action potential plateau in right ventricular epicardium but not endocardium, by suppressing the calcium current and/or augmenting the potassium current, and leads to an 'up-sloping' and 'concave' ST segment elevation, that is readily reversed with atropine (Fig. 9.2).[23] Although acetylcholine *alone* is capable of causing loss of the action potential dome in isolated right ventricular epicardial tissues,[40] acetylcholine or vagotonia alone are unlikely to lead to loss of the action potential dome *in vivo* or to provoke phase 2 reentry. This may explain why the right precordial early repolarization pattern in the normal athlete does not evolve to a coved type and 'in itself' is not associated with the risk of sudden arrhythmic death.[38] In theory, an athlete with the Brugada syndrome may be at greater arrhythmic risk due to associated hypervagotonia (see below).

Sudden death during sports: role of autonomic imbalance

In patients with structural heart diseases, such as idiopathic or ischemic cardiomyopathy, the ventricular arrhythmogenicity is explained by the electrical heterogeneity of ventricular myocardium which acts as a substrate for inhomogeneous intraventricular conduction predisposing to ventricular arrhythmias.[6,41] These depolarization abnormalities are mediated by a sympathetic mechanism that distinctively predispose to sudden death during enhanced adrenergic activity, such as that during physical exercise or mental stress.[42] In contrast, in the majority of patients with Brugada syndrome the

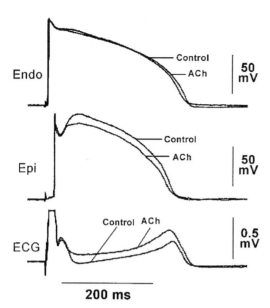

Figure 9.2 Acetylcoline-induced ST segment elevation in arterially perfused right ventricular wedge preparation. Transmembrane action potentials from epicardium and endocardium and an ECG are recorded simultaneously. Superimposed traces are recorded under control conditions and after addition of 3 μmol/L acetylcholine (ACh). Acetylcholine depresses action potential plateau in epicardium but not endocardium. BCL = 2000 ms. Modified from Yan et al.[23]

malignant ventricular arrhythmias occur at rest and, in many cases, at night.[43–46] The circadian pattern of ventricular fibrillation, established by the analysis of implantable cardioverter–defibrillator storage data, suggests that an increase in nocturnal vagal activity and/or withdrawal of sympathetic activity may play an important role in precipitating sudden death.[43]

Miyazaki et al. showed the effects of autonomic receptor stimulation on ST segment elevation in Brugada syndrome. During β-adrenoceptor stimulation by isoproterenol, the ST segment elevation was eliminated, whereas it was augmented by muscarinic stimulation with intravenous edrophonium.[47] Accentuation of ST segment elevation in patients with the Brugada syndrome following vagal maneuvers and normalization of the ST segment during exercise are consistent with these findings. Moreover, sympathetic agonists have an inhibitory effect on ventricular arrhythmias.[48] These findings

have been explained by the opposite effects of acetylcholine and isoproterenol, which respectively depresses and restore the epicardial action potential dome.[23]

Sudden cardiac death is usually the result of an interaction between transient acute abnormalities ('triggers') and underlying heart disease ('substrate'). Acute triggers of sudden death during sports include emotional stress, myocardial ischemia, sympathovagal imbalance, and hemodynamic changes, potentially leading to life-threatening ventricular arrhythmias. On the other hand, intensive and systematic athletic training in itself increases the risk of sudden death in the presence of heart diseases, by promoting over time disease progression or worsening the arrhythmogenic substrate (either structural or primary electrical). In patients with hypertrophic cardiomyopathy, recurrent episodes of exercise-induced myocardial ischemia during intensive training, may result in progressive further increase of left ventricular hypertrophy and post-necrotic myocardial fibrosis which enhances ventricular electrical instability.[49] Likewise, in patients with arrhythmogenic right ventricular cardiomyopathy/dysplasia, regular physical training may provoke a right ventricular volume overload and cavity enlargement, which in turn, may accelerate fibrofatty atrophy by stretching the 'genetically diseased' right ventricular myocardium.[50] According to distinctive ion and cellular pathophysiological mechanisms,[20,21,23] 'acute' sympathetic stimulation and catecholamine exposure such as that during sports activity has an inhibitory effect on the arrhythmogenic mechanisms of Brugada syndrome and may be expected to reduce the risk of sudden death. However, in the risk assessment it should be taken into account that systematic conditioning in athletes with Brugada syndrome may enhance the resting vagal tone and exaggerate the vagal reaction during the post-exercise recovery period, thus facilitating the occurrence of syncope or sudden death at rest or immediately after sports. Neurohumoral factors are considered important in governing the cardiovascular responses to training. It is well known that systematic athletic conditioning induces resting sinus bradycardia. The mechanism involved is thought to be mainly mediated by an adaptation of the cardiac autonomic nervous system to athletic training and consists of increased cardiac parasympathetic modulation and decreased cardiac sympathetic activity.[51–55] The enhanced vagal drive has been inferred from the finding of raised levels of acetylcholine in the myocardium of trained rats,[56] as well as a greater gain of baroreceptive mechanisms in physically conditioned men[57] and animals.[58] Determinants of plasma catecholamines have suggested that sympathetic activity at rest is reduced in both trained men[59] and animals.[60] A reduction of both the parasympathetic and sympathetic tone with the major reduction being the sympathetic tone has also been advanced. Other possible mechanisms involved include an intrinsic slowing of the sinus node rate[61] and alterations in β-adrenoreceptor density[62] produced by training. Moreover, the endurance training influences the cardiac autonom-

ic control during the post-exercise recovery period. During exercise, heart rate increases through a combined effect of sympathetic activation and parasympathetic withdrawal. Immediately after exercise, heart rate recovery is mainly attributed to vagal reaction. Trained athletes characteristically exhibit more rapid heart rate recovery after exercise than their untrained counterparts at similar relative work-loads, as an expression of an enhanced vagal rebound.[63] Therefore, there is a possibility that an adaptation of the cardiac autonomic nervous system to training, which results in increased vagal activity and/or withdrawal of sympathetic activity, may enhance the propensity of athletes with Brugada syndrome to die suddenly at rest, during sleep, or immediately after exercise (Fig. 9.3).

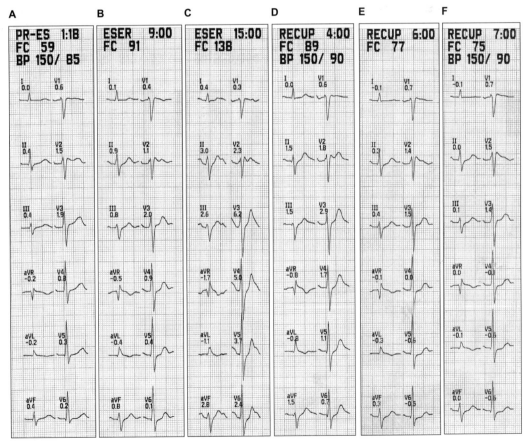

Figure 9.3 ECG recorded at pre-exercise (**A**), exercise (**B, C**), and post-exercise (**D–F**) steps in a 31-year-old athlete with Brugada syndrome. Note the distinctive increase of the ST segment elevation (up to 3.5 mm at the J point in lead V_2) during post-exercise as a consequence of enhanced vagal rebound. Sympathetic stimulation aggravates the concomitant intraventricular conduction defect as shown by QRS prolongation from 90 to 130 ms and deeper S waves in infero-lateral leads during exercise.

Sudden death during sports: predisposing genetic defects

Specific mutations of the *SCN5A* gene may result in clinical variants of Brugada syndrome characterized by an enhanced risk of SD during sports performance. A single C terminal aspartic acid insertion (1795insD) has been described to lead to the electrocardiographic manifestations of both long QT and Brugada syndromes: QT interval prolongation and distinctive right precordial ST segment elevations.[64] The molecular mechanism have been recently elucidated.[65] The mutation affects the fast inactivation component of the sodium channel, causing a plateau of persistent I_{Na} which prolongs the QT interval at slow heart rates. At the same time, 1795insD induces depolarized sodium channels to undergo excessive slow inactivation which reduces sodium channel availability primarily at rapid heart rates. This channel dysfunction accounts for a variant of Brugada syndrome in which the ST segment elevation atypically occurs during β-adrenergic stimulation. The 1795insD carriers are expected to exhibit right precordial ST segment elevation and to increase their arrhythmic risk during an enhanced sympathetic drive such as that during sports exercise.

The threonine at position 1620 in the coding sequence of *SCN5A* is an important determinant of the temperature sensitivity of the human cardiac sodium channel. This missense mutation (Thr1620Met) causes a temperature-dependent speeding up of the inactivation of I_{Na}, which results in the preponderance of the 'outward' early repolarization current, ST segment elevation, and dispersion of repolarization predisposing to ventricular fibrillation.[66] The dysfunction of the mutant channel is exaggerated at higher temperatures with the decay of the Thr1620Met current being 2.4, 3, and 3.4 times faster than wild type at 37°C, 39°C, and 40°C, respectively. This increased temperature sensitivity of the Thr1620Met current decay may predispose some Brugada patients to life-threatening arrhythmias either during a febrile state[67] or during a body temperature increase due to intensive physical exercise, mostly if performed in concomitance with an increased environmental temperature and humidity.

Differential diagnosis between Brugada syndrome and athlete's heart

'Athlete's heart' is a condition characterized by reversible structural and electrical heart remodeling due to long-term athletic training.[68] Typical features include an increase in left ventricular mass, left ventricular diastolic cavity dimension, and wall thickness[69] as well as ECG abnormalities such as increased QRS voltages suggestive of left ventricular hypertrophy, and repolarization abnormalities.[70,71] The most common repolarization change is the so-called 'early repolarization' most often characterized as upward displacement of ST segment in inferior and precordial leads.[36,37] A prominent ST segment elevation in right precordial leads ('right precordial early repolarization') is characteristically observed in a small subgroup of trained athletes in whom it has been considered a benign consequence of the intensive athletic conditioning and deprived of any clinical significance.[38,39]

The boundaries between right precordial early repolarization due to 'athlete's heart' and Brugada syndrome are still undefined Therefore, the finding of right precordial ST segment elevation in a young trained athlete may raise clinical suspicion of Brugada syndrome and the need for a differential diagnosis. In a professional and elite athlete, this differential diagnosis has relevant clinical, ethical, and economic implications, due to potential adverse clinical outcome implicit with diagnosis of Brugada syndrome.

We recently compared the ECG pattern of right precordial early repolarization pattern in trained athletes and in patients with Brugada syndrome in order to identify possible criteria for differential diagnosis.[39] Amplitude of maximum ST segment was measured at J point (ST_J) and after 80 ms (ST_{80}), and a ST_J/ST_{80} ratio was calculated (Fig. 9.4). A right precordial ST segment elevation was found in 4% of athletes. Despite similar degree of maximum amplitude of ST_J (3.1 ± 0.9 mm versus 3.2 ± 0.6 mm), athletes had a ST_J/ST_{80} ratio of 0.7 ± 0.13 compared to 1.6 ± 0.3 in Brugada patients ($p < 0.001$). A ST_J/ST_{80} ratio ≤1 had a sensitivity of 87% and a specificity of 100% in identifying athletes. Compared with athletes, Brugada patients had a significantly higher heart rate (75 ± 9 bpm versus 50 ± 8 bpm; $p < 0.001$), a shorter QT_c interval (0.35 ± 0.04 s versus 0.39 ± 0.02 s; $p < 0.001$) and longer QRS duration (0.11 ± 0.02 s versus 0.09 ± 0.01 s; $p < 0.001$) as well as exhibiting more often a 'S1S2S3 pattern' (53% versus 27%; $p = 0.04$). In conclusion, right precordial early repolarization was not an uncommon ECG pattern (4% prevalence) in a large population of highly trained competitive athletes and it was characterized by distinctive features allowing an accurate differential diagnosis from the ECG abnormalities of patients with Brugada syndrome. ST_J/ST_{80} ratio and QRS interval duration accurately differentiated the ECG pattern of early repolarization in athletes from that of patients with Brugada syndrome, thus implying different electrogenetic mechanisms (Fig. 9.5).

Sports recommendations for patients with Brugada syndrome

Patients with Brugada syndrome, i.e., with distintive ECG abnormalities *plus* cardiac arrest, syncope, or inducibility at programmed ventricular stimulation, are currently treated with implantable cardioverter–defibrillator therapy with the inherent limitations in sports practice.

No data exist that directly relate asymptomatic Brugada syndrome, i.e., individuals with just a Brugada-like ECG pattern, asymptomatic Brugada gene carriers with or without ECG abnormalities, or asymptomatic family members—family history of BS or SD due to proven or strongly suspected BS — with ECG abnormalities, to the risk of participating

A

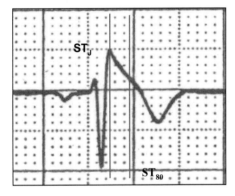

B

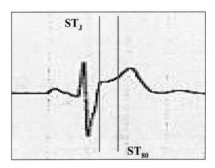

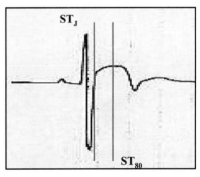

Figure 9.4 Morphologic patterns and methods of measurement of ST segment elevation in (**A**) representative right precordial ECG complex from a Brugada patients and (**B**) two trained athletes. Vertical lines marks the J point (ST_J) and the point 80 ms after the J point (ST_{80}) where the amplitudes of ST segment elevation are calculated. 'Coved' type ST segment elevation in the patient with Brugada syndrome is characterized by a ST_J/ST_{80} ratio of 1.9. The right precordial early repolarization pattern show a ST_J/ST_{80} ratio <1 in both athletes: 0.7 for the 'concave' toward the top (**B**, top) and 0.68 for the 'convex' toward the top (**B**, bottom) ST segment elevation. See text for more details.

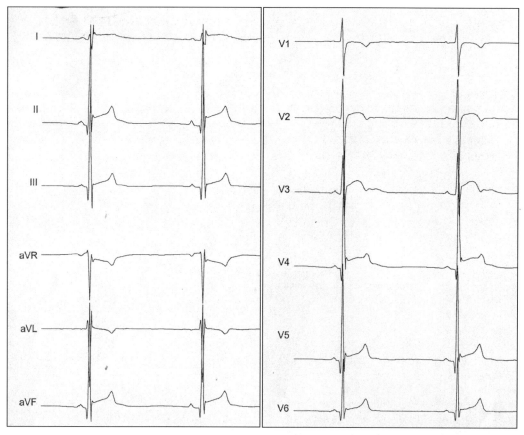

Figure 9.5 Twelve lead ECG of a 23-year-old highly trained cyclist showing right precordial repolarization abnormalities which may simulate Brugada syndrome. In the leads V_2 and V_3, the J point is displaced upward (up to 3 mm) and gives rise to a more elevated ST segment (up to 5 mm), which is followed by a negative T wave. The 'up-sloping' shape of the elevated ST segment allows differential diagnosis with Brugada syndrome which is characterized by a 'high take-off and down-sloping' ST segment elevation. Also note the early repolarization pattern in the leads exploring the inferolateral wall of the left ventricle and the increased QRS voltages.

in sports. Therefore, this subgroup of 'patients' can engage in all recreational and competitive sports, with the exceptions of sports which involve the potential for traumatic injury and water related-activity because of the specific risk of impaired consciousness.

Patients should be made aware of the danger of practicing intensive sports activity at high temperature and/or humidity due to the specific arrhythmic risk associated with an exaggerated increase of the body temperature. Also electrolytes alteration, mainly hypokalemia, associated with strenuous physical activity may facilitate the development of malignant ventricular arrhythmia.

This study was supported by the 'Sudden death in the athlete' Research Project, Rome, Italy.

References

1 Spain DM, Brodness VA, Moh C. Coronary atherosclerosis as a cause of unexpected and unexplained death: autopsy study from 1949–1959. *J. Am. Med. Assoc.* 1950; **174**: 384–389.

2 Kuller L. Sudden death in arteriosclerotic heart disease. *Am. J. Cardiol.* 1969; **24**: 617–624.

3 Friedman M, Manwaring JH, Rosenmann RH *et al.* Instantaneous and sudden death: clinical and pathological differentiation in coronary artery disease. *J. Am. Med. Assoc.* 1973; **225**: 1319–1328.

4 Liberthson RR, Nagel EL, Hirshman JC *et al.* Pathophysiologic observations in pre-hospital ventricular fibrillation and sudden cardiac death. *Circulation* 1974; **49**: 790–798.

5 Roberts WC. Sudden cardiac death: definitions and causes. *Am J Cardiol* 1986; **57**: 1410–1413.

6 Myerburg RJ, Castellanos A. Cardiac arrest and sudden cardiac death. In: E. Braunwald, ed. *Heart Disease: A Textbook of Cardiovascular Medicine* (4th edn), Philadelphia, PA: W.B. Saunders, 1992: 756–789.

7 Thiene G, Nava A, Corrado D *et al.* Right ventricular cardiomyopathy and sudden death in young people. *N. Engl. J. Med.* 1988; **318**: 129–133.

8 Corrado D, Thiene G, Nava A *et al.* Sudden death in young competitive athletes: clinicopathologic correlation in 22 cases. *Am. J. Med.* 1990; **89**: 588–596.

9 Corrado D, Basso C, Poletti A *et al.* Sudden death in the young: is coronary thrombosis the major precipitating factor? *Circulation* 1994; **90**: 2315–2323.

10 Myerburg RJ, Conde CA, Sung RJ *et al.* A clinical, electrophysiologic and hemodynamic profile of patients resuscitated from pre-hospital cardiac arrest. *Am. J. Med.* 1980; **68**: 568–576.

11 Wellens HJJ., Lemery R, Smeets JL *et al.* Sudden arrhythmic death without overt heart disease. *Circulation* 1992; **85** Suppl 1: 92–97.

12 Myerburg RJ. Sudden cardiac death in persons with normal (or near normal) hearts. *Am. J. Cardiol.* 1997; **79**: 3–9.

13 Consensus Statement of the Joint Steering Committees of the Unexplained Cardiac Arrest Registry of Europe and of the Idiopathic Ventricular Fibrillation Registry of the United States, Survivors of out-of-hospital cardiac arrest with apparently normal hearts. Need for definition and standardized clinical evaluation. *Circulation* 1997; **95**: 265–272.

14 Viskin S, Belhassen B. Idiopathic ventricular fibrillation. *Am. Heart J.* 1990; **120**: 661–671.

15 Corrado D, Basso C, Thiene G. Sudden cardiac death in young people with apparently normal heart. *Cardiovasc. Res.* 2001; **50**: 399–408.

16 Chug SS, Kelly KL, Titus JL. Sudden cardiac death with apparently normal heart. *Circulation* 2000; **102**: 649–654.

17 Schwartz PJ, Priori SG, Spazzolini C *et al.* Genotype-phenotype correlation in the long QT syndrome. Gene-specific triggers for life-threatening arrhythmias. *Circulation* 2001; **103**: 89–95.

18 Priori SG, Napolitano C, Memmi M *et al.* Clinical and molecular characterization of patients with cathecolaminergic polymorphic ventricular tachycardia. *Circulation* 2002; **106**: 69–74.

19 Brugada P, Brugada J. Right bundle branch block, persistent ST-segment elevation and sudden cardiac death: a multicenter report. *J. Am. Coll. Cardiol.* 1992; **20**: 1391–1396.

20 Yan GX, Antzelevitch C. Cellular basis for the electrocardiographic J-wave. *Circulation* 1996; **93**: 372–379.

21 Antzelevitch C. The Brugada syndrome: ionic basis and arrhythmia mechanisms. *J. Cardiovasc. Electrophysiol.* 2001; **12**: 268–272.

22 Chen Q, Kirsch GE, Zhang D *et al.* Genetic basis and molecular mechanisms for idiopathic ventricular fibrillation. *Nature* 1998; **392**: 293–296.

23 Yan GX, Antzelevitch C. Cellular basis for the Brugada syndrome and other mechanisms of arrhythmogenesis associated with ST-segment elevation. *Circulation* 1999; **100**: 1660–1666.

24 Wilde AA, Antzelevitch C, Borggrefe M *et al.* Proposed diagnostic criteria for the Brugada syndrome: consensus report. *Circulation* 2002; **106**: 2514–2519.

25 Antzelevitch C, Brugada P, Brugada J *et al.* Brugada syndrome: a decade of progress. *Circ. Res.* 2002; **91**: 1114–1118.

26 Brugada R, Brugada J, Antzelevitch C *et al.* Sodium channel blockers identify risk for sudden death in patients with ST-segment elevation and right bundle branch block but structurally normal hearts. *Circulation* 2000; **101**: 510–515.

27 Shimizu W, Antzelevitch C, Suyama K *et al.* Effect of sodium channel blockers on ST-segment, QRS duration, and corrected QT interval in patients with Brugada syndrome. *J. Cardiovasc. Electrophysiol.* 2000; **11**: 1320–1329.

28 Brugada P, Brugada J, Brugada R. Arrhythmia induction by antiarrhythmic drugs. *Pacing Clin. Electrophysiol.* 2000; **23**: 291–292.

29 Babaliaros VC, Hurst JW. Tricyclic antidepressants and the Brugada syndrome: an example of Brugada waves appearing after the administration of desipramine. *Clin. Cardiol.* 2002; **25**: 395–398.

30 Goldgran-Toledano D, Sideris G, Kevorkian JP. Overdose of cyclic antidepressants and the Brugada syndrome. *N. Engl. J. Med.* 2002; **346**: 1591–1592.

31 Rouleau F, Asfar P, Boulet S *et al.* Transient ST-segment elevation in right precordial leads induced by psychotropic drugs: relationship to the Brugada syndrome. *J. Cardiovasc. Electrophysiol.* 2001; **12**: 61–65.

32 Tada H, Sticherling C, Oral H *et al.* Brugada syndrome mimicked by tricyclic antidepressant overdose. *J. Cardiovasc. Electrophysiol.* 2001; **12**: 275.

33 Pastor A, Nunez A, Cantale C *et al.* Asymptomatic Brugada syndrome case unmasked during dimenhydrinate infusion. *J. Cardiovasc. Electrophysiol.* 2001; **12**: 1192–1194.

34 Ortega-Carnicer J, Bertos-Polo J, Gutierrez-Tirado C. Aborted sudden death, transient Brugada pattern, and wide QRS dysarrhythmias after massive cocaine ingestion. *J. Electrocardiol.* 2001; **34**: 345–349.

35 Kanda M, Shimizu W, Matsuo K *et al.* Electrophysiologic characteristics and implications of induced ventricular

fibrillation in symptomatic patients with Brugada syndrome. *J. Am. Coll. Cardiol.* 2002; **39**: 1799–1805.

36 Wassemburg RM, Alt WJ, Lloyd C. The normal RS-T segment elevation variant. *Am. J. Cardiol.* 1961; **8**: 184–189.

37 Kambara H, Phillips J. Long term evaluation of early repolarization syndrome (normal variant RS-T elevation) *Am. J. Cardiol.* 1976; **38**: 157–161.

38 Bianco M, Bria S, Gianfelici A *et al.* Does early repolarization in the athlete have analogies with the Brugada syndrome? *Eur. Heart J.* 2001; **22**: 504–510.

39 Corrado D, Leoni L, Pelliccia A *et al.* Need for a differential diagnosis between trained athletes with right precordial early repolarization and Brugada patients. *Pacing Clin. Electrophysiol.* 2003; **26**: 449 (Abstract).

40 Litovsky SH, Antzelevitch C. Differences in the electrophysiological response of canine ventricular subendocardium and subepicardium to acetylcholine and isoproterenol. A direct effect of acetylcholine in ventricular myocardium. *Circ. Res.* 1990; **67**: 615–627.

41 Thiene G, Basso C, Corrado D. Cardiovascular causes of sudden death. In: Silver MD, Gotlieg AI, Schoen FJ, eds. *Cardiovascular Pathology.* Philadelphia, PA: Churchill Livingstone, 2001: 326–374.

42 Lampert R, Jusk T, Bury M *et al.* Emotional and physical precipitants of ventricular arrhythmias. *Circulation* 2002; **106**: 1800–1805.

43 Matsuo K, Kurita T, Inagaki M *et al.* The circadian pattern of the development of ventricular fibrillation in patients with Brugada syndrome. *Eur. Heart J.* 1999; **20**: 465–470.

44 Nademanee K, Veerakul G, Nimmannit S *et al.* Arrhythmogenic marker for the sudden unexplained death syndrome in Thai men. *Circulation* 1997; **96**: 2595–2600.

45 Kasanuki H, Ohnishi S, Ohtuka M *et al.* Idiopathic ventricular fibrillation induced with vagal activity in patients without obvious heart disease. *Circulation* 1997; **95**: 277–285.

46 Corrado D, Basso C, Buja G *et al.* Right bundle branch block, right precordial ST segment elevation, and sudden death in young people. *Circulation* 2001; **103**: 710–717.

47 Miyazaki T, Mitamura H, Miyoshi S *et al.* Autonomic and antiarrhythmic drug modulation of ST-segment elevation in patients with Brugada syndrome. *Am. Coll. Cardiol.* 1996; **27**: 1061–1070.

48 Tanaka H, Kinoshita O, Uchikawa S *et al.* Successful prevention of recurrent ventricular fibrillation by intravenous isoproterenol in a patient with Brugada syndrome. *Pacing Clin. Electrophysiol.* 2001; **24**: 1293–1294.

49 Basso C, Thiene G, Corrado D *et al.* Hypertrophic cardiomyopathy and sudden death in the young: pathologic evidence of myocardial ischemia. *Hum. Pathol.* 2000; **31**: 988–998.

50 Corrado D, Thiene G, Nava A *et al.* Sudden death in young competitive athletes: clinicopathologic correlation in 22 cases. *Am. J. Med.* 1990; **89**: 588–596.

51 Scheuer J, Tipton CM. Cardiovascular adaptations to physical training. *Annu. Rev. Physiol.* 1977; **39**: 221–251.

52 Ekblom B, Kilborn A, Soltysiak J. Physical training, bradycardia and autonomic nervous system. *Scand. J. Clin. Lab. Invest.* 1973; **32**: 251–256.

53 Smith ML, Hudson DL, Graitzer HM *et al.* Exercise training bradycardia: the role of autonomic balance. *Med. Sci. Sports Exerc.* 1989; **21**: 40–44.

54 Goldsmith RL, Bigger JT Jr, Bloomfield DM *et al.* Physical fitness as a determinant of vagal modulation. *Med. Sci. Sports Exerc.* 1997; **29**: 812–817.

55 Svendenhag J, Wallin BG, Sundloff G *et al.* Skeletal muscle sympathetic activity at rest in trained and untrained subjects. *Acta Physiol. Scand.* 1984; **120**: 499–504.

56 De Schryver C, Mertens-Strythagen J. Heart tissue acetylcholine in chronically exercised rats. *Experientia* 1975; **31**: 316–318.

57 Stegemann J, Busert A, Brock D. Influence of fitness on blood pressure control system in man. *Aerospace Med.* 1974; **45**: 45–48.

58 Bedford TG, Tipton CM. Exercise training and the arterial baroreflex. *J. Appl. Physiol.* 1987; **63**: 1926–1932.

59 Cousineau D, Ferguson RJ, de Champlain J *et al.* Catecholamines in coronary sinus during exercise in man before and after training. *J. Appl. Physiol.* 1977; **43**: 801–806.

60 De Schryver C, Mertens-Strythagen J, Istvan B *et al.* Effects of training on heart rate and skeletal muscle catecholamine concentration in rats. *Am. J. Physiol.* 1969; **217**: 1589–1592.

61 Katona PG, McLean M, Dighton DH *et al.* Sympathetic and parasympathetic cardiac control in athletes and non-athletes at rest. *J. Appl. Physiol.* 1982; **52**: 1652–1657.

62 Butler J, O'Brien M, O'Malley K *et al.* Relationship of beta-adrenoreceptor density to fitness in athletes. *Nature* 1982; **298**: 60–62.

63 Aral Y, Saul JP, Albrecht P *et al.* Modulation of cardiac autonomic activity during and immediately after exercise. *Am. J. Physiol.* 1989; **256**: H132–H141.

64 Bezzina C, Veldkamp MW, van den Berg MP *et al.* A single Na^+ channel mutation causing both long-QT and Brugada syndromes. *Circ. Res.* 1999; **85**: 1206–1213.

65 Veldkamp MW, Viswanathan PC, Bezzina C *et al.* Two distinct congenital arrhythmias evoked by a multidysfunctional Na^+ channel. *Circ. Res.* 2000; **86**: e91–e97.

66 Dumaine R, Towbin JA, Brugada P *et al.* Ionic mechanisms responsible for the electrocardiographic phenotype of the Brugada syndrome are temperature dependent. *Circ. Res.* 1999; **85**: 803–809.

67 Antzelevitch C, Brugada R. Fever and the Brugada syndrome. *Pacing Clin. Electrophysiol.* 2002; **25**: 1537–1539.

68 Huston P, Puffer JC, MacMillan RW. The athletic heart syndrome. *N. Engl. J. Med.* 1985; **315**: 24–32.

69 Maron BJ, Pelliccia A, Spirito P. Cardiac disease in young trained athletes: insights into methods for distinguishing athlete's heart from structural heart disease, with particu-lar emphasis on hypertrophic cardiomyopathy. *Circulation* 1995; **91**: 1596–1601.

70 Oakley DG, Oakley CM. Significance of abnormal electro-cardiograms in highly trained athletes. *Am. J. Cardiol.* 1982; **50**: 985–989.

71 Pelliccia A, Maron BJ, Culasso F *et al.* Clinical significance of abnormal electrocardiographic patterns in trained ath-letes. *Circulation* 2000, **102**: 278–84.

CHAPTER 10

Brugada syndrome: role of genetics in clinical practice

R. Brugada, MD

Introduction

Since its initial description in the early 1990s,[1] Brugada syndrome has been progressively attracting more and more attention in the cardiology community. There are several reasons for it becoming such a focal point of attention. First, the disease takes the lives, in many instances as a first symptom, of previously healthy individuals in their forties, during their most productive years.[2] This has created a very important concern, for the diagnosis and treatment implications in the affected persons, and especially for the identification of mutation carriers in their offspring, usually very young children. Second, once thought to be very rare, the Brugada syndrome is now recognized worldwide and has a relatively high prevalence in certain parts of the world, particularly Southeast Asia. Third, the identification of the disease has coincided with a burst of activity in the molecular biology of cardiology. Brugada syndrome has benefited tremendously from the experience gained in the field of molecular cardiology and genetics in other arrhythmogenic diseases. Fourth, in few diseases have we seen the link between clinical application and basic sciences as well connected and interacting as in Brugada syndrome. Research findings are continuously applied to the clinical field and vice versa. This can only be possible in a disease where there is a good understanding of both the basic mechanisms of disease, and of the limitations of the different diagnostic and clinical tools available to the physician. Lastly, there still remain many important challenges regarding clinical, cellular, and genetic mechanisms. The ECG pattern may be concealed and even transiently normalize. It may also appear under the influence of some external factors like tricyclic overdose, fever, cocaine, anesthetics, etc.[3] We do not know yet whether these patients are at higher or lower risk of sudden death. But the biggest challenge by far is the limited therapeutic options available for the disease. Brugada syndrome is a very malignant disease with a high rate of recurrence of events, which kills young individuals, and with the only possible treatment at this point being the implantable defibrillator, unaffordable where the disease is most prevalent. It becomes then a pressing issue to be able to provide some form of treatment to these individuals. All these factors continue to drive both clinical and basic research in many centers.

Basic research into the mechanisms underlying the Brugada syndrome is in its infancy and the next 10 years will probably provide still better understanding of this lethal disease. What started as an electrocardiographic curiosity has become a great challenge for electrophysiologists, cardiologists, biophysicists, geneticists, and molecular biologists. We have several diagnostic tools available, the latest one being genetic testing. This chapter deals with the use of genetic testing in the diagnosis of Brugada syndrome and its possible role in clinical decision making and especially in the risk stratification of the patient. We will focus on the reality of this diagnostic modality, indicating the present limitations and future advances that can be provided. Genetics as a diagnostic tool is extremely new, and better technology and better analysis will certainly improve all aspects of this test to provide better understanding of the risk that patients have of dying suddenly.

Genetic terminology

There are some genetic terms that require a clear understanding if one wants to draw any conclusions from the genetic data and apply it to the clinical arena.

Genetic locus versus genetic mutation

There exists a very important difference between knowing the genetic locus and knowing an exact mutation. A genetic locus refers to the position where the gene causing the disease can be statistically expected in a chromosome. However, a genetic locus does not tell us anything about the gene that is affected, the type of problem in the gene, and the pathophysiologic consequences of the defect. A locus is an area within a chromosome. For instance, a genetic locus for familial atrial fibrillation has been localized to chromosome 10; but the exact gene and the mutation causing the arrhythmia are not yet known.[4] Thus, the exact pathophysiologic mechanisms leading to the arrhythmia remain unknown. On the contrary, several mutations have been described in the long QT syndrome which affect the genes encoding for the K^+ channel (HERG, minK, KVLQT1) or the human cardiac Na^+ channel *SCN5A*. Expression of these mutations in different preparations has shown why the cardiac repolarization is prolonged with these mutations: loss of function for the mutations affecting the K^+ channel, gain of function for the mutations affecting the Na^+ channel.[5] Because the specific mutations and the definitive mechanisms responsible for the disease are known, the approach to therapy is more rational. Theoretically, there may be the possibility to genetically manipulate and correct these defects in the future. From a practical point of view, when only a genetic locus is known we can only identify individuals at risk for the disease if the family is linked to the same locus.

When the gene causing the disease is known, families and sporadic cases of the disease can be tested for the gene by using the 'candidate gene' approach. That means that the investigation is concentrated in a certain known gene which is expected to have a relation with the disease. This approach was successfully used for the identification of mutations causing the Brugada syndrome. In order to conclude that the mutation is causing the disease, the mutation cannot be present in any of the 100 control patients of the same ethnic background, the mutation is required to cause a biophysical alteration in the electrophysiological analysis, and it has to be present in all the affected individuals in the family.

Mutation versus polymorphism

Our genome is 99.9% similar to the one from somebody not related to us. 0.1% is different, and this variability allows individuals to be distinguished by means of genetic testing. It also allows the tracking of chromosomes across generations in a family, and is the basis of genetic linkage analysis. These changes, present every 1000 bases, usually fall into the non-codifying region and have no functional role that we know of yet. Those that fall in the areas codifying for proteins, exons, may have some function and play a role in the modulation of the gene where they lay. When these changes occur in more than 1% of the general population they are called polymorphisms. Research in polymorphisms is ongoing, and some of them have been linked to different electrocardiographic parameters, and even to a higher risk of sudden death. The question is whether there is a casual relationship or whether they are markers closer to a genetic determinant of the disease. The answer is probably both. Unfortunately, there are very few cases where the data is robust enough to draw meaningful conclusions. Polymorphisms have been used recently for the association studies, and many of them have been linked to a disease, even though further data in some of them have not reproduced the same association. So this is an open field of research, and great caution has to be taken when considering results.

A mutation is a change in the reading of the DNA molecule that will bring a change in the amino acid sequence and/or conformation of the protein. Different mutations have been described, from a missense mutation which causes a change in one amino acid, to a nonsense mutation or a splicing mutation that cause a truncation or alteration of the protein. To make the diagnosis of a mutation, it should not be present in 200 unrelated control chromosomes of the same genetic background. The mutation has to change the protein conformation, the mutation has to have a functional effect, and it has to track with the affected individuals in the family. These factors, which appear to be common sense, are not trivial issues, especially when dealing with the disease in a single individual.

Penetrance

Penetrance is the probability that the disease will ap-

A   B

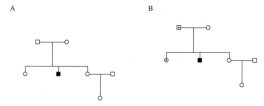

Figure 10.1 In this family one individual is affected by Brugada syndrome (**A**) but three carry a mutation in *SCN5A* (**B**). The penetrance is 33%.

pear when the individual is carrying the genetic defect.

Figure 10.1A shows a pedigree with one individual affected by Brugada syndrome. The genetic testing in Fig. 10.1B shows that three family members were carriers of a mutation in the gene *SCN5A*, but the other two individuals did not have an abnormal pattern on the electrocardiogram. The penetrance in this family is therefore 33%.

Expressivity

Variable expressivity means the different degrees of severity in the phenotypes in individuals with the same mutation. Individuals in the same family, who therefore carry the same *SCN5A* mutation, can show different electrocardiographic abnormalities, from Brugada syndrome to conduction disease.

Genetic testing as a diagnostic tool

Recently acquired knowledge on the genetic basis of arrhythmias is having a major impact on how we approach patients with a family history of a disease. It is understandable that when confronted with a hereditary disease, patients, physicians, and family members want information about who is and who is not a carrier of the mutation. Genetics have become the gold standard test for inherited diseases. Either you have the familial mutation or you do not, and therefore you have inherited the disease or you have not. This, except in very rare situations, is a central dogma of clinical genetic testing. And this is continuously being used in population screening for many diseases, from tests on newborns to the identification of carriers of cystic fibrosis genes. For some diseases, analysis of the gene provides an accurate estimate of the likelihood of the person being a carrier of the disease. This is the case for mutations in β-globin and sickle cell disease. If there is no mutation, the patients are spared from the disease. In other diseases, like cystic fibrosis, it is possible to identify around 85% of the mutation carriers in the population. A negative result indicates that there still a small likelihood that the patient is a carrier of an unknown mutation, albeit a very small likelihood. These justify without a doubt the use of genetic testing in these diseases as a diagnostic tool.

The use of genetic testing in the diagnosis of arrhythmogenic diseases is much more controversial. As is the case for several inherited cardiac diseases, inherited arrhythmias are highly heterogeneous, indicating that more than one gene can cause the disease, and we are still not able to genotype a large portion of the affected individuals. In long QT syndrome, with seven genes identified, we are able to genotype 60–70% of the patients. In Brugada syndrome, with one gene identified, we are able to find the mutation in 20% of the affected individuals. In these cases, genetics can help in the understanding of the basic mechanisms of the disease, and in familial screening we are able to identify the mutation if we are fortunate.

But the big question remains for the clinician. Can genetics be used to help in the diagnosis of the patient, especially in those cases where the diagnosis is not clear? Can genetics be used to diagnose a long QT in a patient with a QTc of 440 ms and a history of sudden death in the family? Or can genetics diagnose Brugada syndrome in a patient with aborted sudden death? While identification of the mutation can have important implications for the individual and the family members, the likelihood of having a positive test in individuals with no clear diagnosis is low.

Genetics in Brugada syndrome

Despite linkage data not being robust in Brugada syndrome, a more than definitive link between the sodium currents and Brugada syndrome has been provided by research in genetics. This has been achieved through the candidate gene approach. Linkage data is lacking mainly for a few reasons:
- Brugada syndrome causes sudden death in young individuals, making families rather small for a powerful linkage analysis
- penetrance of the disease is very low, usually less

than 30%, and we have to rely on diagnostic tools which probably carry their own limitations
- diagnostic identification of affected individuals is becoming a tremendous challenge, not just because of penetrance, but because mutations in *SCN5A* cause a variable expressivity.

SCN5A mutations can cause events from ST elevation in precordial leads to alterations in the electrocardiogram, such as conduction disease, which are very prevalent in the general population. These are parameters that have to be taken into account before linkage analysis is run, and have limited our ability to find the statistical power to a positive result.

However, it would be unfair to ignore the largest body of evidence provided in genetics of Brugada syndrome, even with the lack of a positive LOD score, and this is the fact that dozens of centers have identified mutations in *SCN5A* which are linked to individuals with the disease and that the biophysical data have also linked the disease to a basic mechanism. So it is assumed in the medical community that *SCN5A* is responsible for part of the disease.

The relationship between *SCN5A* and Brugada syndrome was identified in 1998.[6] *SCN5A*, the α-subunit of the cardiac sodium channel gene, is responsible for phase 0 of the cardiac action potential. The identification of disease-causing mutations and the decrease in availability of sodium currents, suggest that a shift in the ionic balance in favor of I_{to} current during phase 1 of the action potential may be the determinant of the disease. To date, this is the only gene linked to Brugada syndrome. *SCN5A* has been identified in approximately 20% of patients with Brugada syndrome, indicating that there is at least one other gene responsible for the disease. In 2002, a second locus, on chromosome 3, was identified, although the gene responsible has not been found as yet.[7] Close to 80 different mutations in *SCN5A* have been reported to date and approximately half of them have been biophysically characterized. The common denominator in the analysis of the mutations is the decrease in Na current availability by two main mechanisms: (1) lack of expression of the mutant channel or (2) acceleration of inactivation of the channel.

Steps in genetic testing in Brugada syndrome

Collection of patients
Patient identification
Identification of the individuals is the first basic step in research in genetics. There are many inherited diseases which follow some classic patterns of transmission of the disease. In Brugada syndrome, the pattern so far described is autosomal dominant disease, in which there is vertical transmission of the disease (each generation has affected individuals), both males and females can inherit and transmit the disease, and each child has a 50% chance of inheriting the abnormal gene from the affected parent.

Several questions are important in the pre-genetic screening for the disease.

Is there a family history of sudden death?
This is the question that usually triggers research in genetics of sudden death. Having several members in the family with sudden death is the wake-up call to an inherited disease. The challenge though is to ascertain that the sudden death was caused by the disease. Could a car accident, drowning, or seizure be caused by cardiac arrest? It certainly could, but it is difficult to prove. One has to take into account all possible variables. When performing an analysis of sudden death in families with Brugada syndrome, we concluded that up to 50% of the cases of sudden death were not related to the disease. This has very important implications in research using genetic linkage, as one of the parents of somebody who had sudden death would be wrongly presumed to have carrier status.

Is the disease genetic?
In Brugada syndrome there is a tremendous variability of the electrocardiographic pattern. Individuals with the disease with the typical coved-type ECG may come a few days later to the office with a completely normal electrocardiogram. We assume at this point that, if there once was a positive ECG, the diagnosis is made. The problem arises especially in patients in whom the electrocardiographic pattern has been found under the influence of certain external factors; for example a very low pH, high fever, cocaine abuse, tricyclic overdose, and many other factors that can cause the electrocardio-

graphic pattern. The issue is whether these patients are individuals that have a hidden Brugada syndrome, with some form of genetic predisposition, or are individuals with a different response to those stimuli that then creates a pattern resembling the disease.

Is a single individual enough?

When the diagnosis is made in a single patient, with no family history, it is difficult to prove causality. Electrophysiological data can help confirm the hypothesis that the mutation is causing the disease.

Confirming the diagnosis

There are a few tools to confirm the diagnosis of Brugada syndrome, usually based on the identification of the electrocardiographic pattern before or after the infusion of sodium blockers. Unfortunately different countries have different medications to test for the disease. For example, pilsicainide is available and used in Japan, ajmaline and flecainide in Europe, and procainamide is the only one available in the US. Procainamide is the weakest one, and many cases of false negative diagnosis have been reported to date. The electrocardiographic pattern, ST segment elevation in leads V_1 to V_3, is required to have a certain elevation and morphology. There is, as previously explained, an important variability in expressivity. Patients with mutations can have a completely normal electrocardiogram or can have conduction abnormalities.[8] Diagnosis of these alterations, especially if linkage analysis is considered, has to be taken into account.

Laboratory qualifications
Research versus clinical laboratory

Clinical laboratories performing DNA-based tests for genetic diseases must meet certain quality control requirements. In the USA, these are regulations established under the Clinical Laboratory Improvement Amendments of 1988 (CLIA). CLIA certification indicates that the laboratory has a qualified laboratory director, an approved laboratory facility with especial configuration to avoid contamination, and a standardized and approved test, with both positive and negative controls to make the test error proof. These are requirements that have to be met in order to perform the test on a clinical basis and which have to be verified during onsite inspections.

On the other hand, research laboratories collect patients and samples for research on the disease. Usually driven by universities and academic centers, these laboratories do not have the possibility of performing the tests on a clinical or diagnostic basis. Most, if not all, of the advances in genetics to date have come from research labs.

There are very important differences between the two kinds of laboratories, especially in the use of genetic data in Brugada syndrome.

- In very few instances is the result given back to the patient from research labs. The information is used to advance the understanding of the disease, but the data, despite the fact that is probably very accurate, has not met the rigorous controls to make it error proof.
- Cost. The cost of running the samples is probably the same, but not to the patient. Research labs do it for free, as it is for research purposes. Clinical labs do it on a fee-for-service basis.
- Timing. Because of the cost issue, research labs can not guarantee the speed for screening as they have to combine the screening service with the research projects. The screening service is provided at no cost to ensure a good number of samples for the research projects. CLIA approved labs guarantee a timing for screening.
- Knowledge about the disease. Research labs are usually more knowledgeable regarding the clinical aspects of the disease as the individuals in the laboratory are working to improve the understanding of the disease. Usually these are the investigators that are most up-to-date regarding therapeutic options. On the other hand, the CLIA laboratories are performing the genetic screening and provide results to the patient or to the provider, but this does not mean that the interpretation of the results will be completely accurate as to the clinical implications.
- Further phenotypic analysis. If a mutation is found the research laboratory will perform biophysical analysis to prove that the mutation is causing an electrophysiological abnormality that can explain the phenotype. This is becoming a very important issue in Brugada syndrome, and especially in families which are small. A CLIA-approved laboratory will provide the genetic information but not the electrophysiological data caused by the mutation. This will have to be done by other research labora-

tories. At present there are very few laboratories that are CLIA approved to screen for mutations in arrhythmias; they are very expensive and insurance companies do not cover it.

If the majority of advances come from research labs, if the individuals are more knowledgeable, and the test is cheaper, why is CLIA certification important? CLIA-approved laboratory status is becoming an indispensable requirement to provide feedback to the patient or to the physician regarding the results. This can lead to an important ethical dilemma, especially if the disease studied is causing sudden death in the family.

Techniques for screening

Several techniques are used to screen for a gene causing the disease. All of them require the amplification of the DNA of the region of interest in the gene with the use of polymerase chain reaction (PCR). Until a few years ago, single strand conformation polymorphism (SSCP) was the most commonly used technique for screening for mutations in known genes.[9] This technique has around 75% sensitivity. It is based on the different mobility pattern that the mutated and wild type molecules of DNA will have once they anneal to each other. This pattern of migration in a gel will be different than the control DNA or the DNA from a non-affected individual. This technique has been lately automated with the use of automated denaturing high-performance liquid chromatography (DHPLC), and the sensitivity to screen for mutations has increased probably to 85%. The main advantages are the speed and the cost. One of the main limitations is the lower sensitivity, significant in diseases such as Brugada syndrome, in which a priori there is the limitation that only 20% of the cases are caused by *SCN5A*.

Direct sequencing has been improved tremendously in the last 5 years, with much better reagents. Automation makes it a fast service and most importantly reliable for the task. It is unclear what the sensitivity is but it probably reaches the high 90s percentage wise. However, the most important limitation is the cost when compared to SSCP or DHPLC.

Possible screening scenarios
Screening for the single patient
SCN5A mutations are responsible for around 20%

of the cases of Brugada syndrome. All families with Brugada syndrome are first screened for this gene. If the disease in the family is not caused by *SCN5A*, then the proband is added to a pool of samples to be screened for other genes playing a role in cardiac electrical activity to identify another gene. But this is a fishing expedition at this point, and it can take many years before the new gene is identified. Screening for *SCN5A* in a patient can take less than 1 week. Unfortunately, laboratories had been collecting patients for many years before technology was available, and the backlog of samples in the main laboratories is considerable and screening usually takes much longer.

Screening for the family member of a family with a known mutation
This is certainly the easiest screening scenario to carry out. To find out whether an individual has inherited a known mutation from his parents does not require anything else than a few days.

Screening for a whole family
Once *SCN5A* is excluded, if the family has enough statistical power for genetic linkage, a full genome scan can be undertaken. This is performed to identify a new chromosomal locus or region, where the new gene will be localized. Different parameters will need to be taken into consideration before the genome analysis is started. Penetrance is the first one to consider as not all carriers of the mutation will show the phenotype. It is also possible that a patient in a family, despite having an electrocardiogram of Brugada syndrome, does not have the mutation. Therefore, the possibility of genetic heterogeneity or phenocopy variables (having a pattern resembling Brugada syndrome without having the mutation) have to be contemplated.

When applying these concepts to Brugada syndrome we can understand the limitations that we are facing. Penetrance with baseline ECG in Brugada syndrome is very low, and when using the diagnostic tools, especially ajmaline, the penetrance can actually improve. Unfortunately, we lack information on the sensitivity and specificity of this clinical test.

The variable expressivity in *SCN5A* mutations becomes clear in the paper by Kyndt *et al.*[8] In that paper they presented a family with the same sodium channel mutation, proven to be malignant for some of their members, which can actually present itself in different forms, from a normal ECG to a pattern of Brugada syndrome, to a pattern of conduction disease. The genetic mutation is the same, but the phenotype is completely different and it will require more research to understand what the true value of carrying this mutation will be.

Screening for the asymptomatic patient with a family history of sudden death

This is right now one of the most common reasons for a consultation about the genetics of sudden death: the possibility of performing genetic analysis on an individual that had a family member who died suddenly, of unknown causes. The main limitation is the lack of a positive diagnosis. If the patient, the family, or the deceased individual did not have a clear cause for sudden death, the probability of finding a positive result during the screening process becomes much lower.

Providing results
Genetic counseling

As genetics advance, so does the need for a better understanding of what the results mean. When studying a monogenic disease like Brugada syndrome, it can be understood that the mutation does not always cause the disease, but it may. When analyzing polygenic diseases (i.e., diseases caused by the interaction of many genes, such as hypertension and coronary artery disease), then the role that each gene plays in the final phenotype is not easy to ascertain. Genetic counseling becomes a necessity to unravel the many doubts that genetic data will put into the families. Genetics determines our makeup and our ability to respond to the different environmental exposures, be it to exercise, to smoking, or to stress. Genetics will continuously interact with the environment and will shape our response to it, in the form of a defensive mechanism or in the form of a disease. The situation in Brugada syndrome is not different. Not everybody that has the genetic defect will die of sudden death and not even everybody will show the ECG pattern. There are many other unknown factors that may shape us and protect us from the cardiac arrest, and there are other factors that may cause us to have a cardiac arrest. However, it is a popular belief in the general population that

genetics determines everything, and most people expect the worse from a positive diagnosis. Genetic counseling becomes in this issue the most important tool to return a family to a normal lifestyle.

When genetic diagnosis is negative

Consider the following. The screening of the exons of the sodium channel *SCN5A* has not provided any positive results as far as identification of mutations is concerned. The patient does not fall in the 20% of the cases of Brugada syndrome with a mutation in *SCN5A*. What can we say? The possibilities are:
- the patient has a mutation in another gene;
- the mutation affects an area of the gene that is not presently being screened, for example introns;
- the electrocardiographic pattern in the patient does not have a genetic basis; or
- we do not have the technical capability or enough sensitivity in the test to identify the mutation.

Does that mean that the patient does not have Brugada syndrome? Certainly not.

When genetic diagnosis is positive

When the genetic diagnosis is positive, it means that:
- a mutation has been identified;
- that the mutation is present in all affected individuals in the family;
- that it may be present in some individuals who are not phenotypically affected (do not show the disease but are carriers);
- that the mutation is not present in 200 control chromosomes from the same ethnic background; and
- that the biophysical analysis of the mutation indicates that it causes alterations in the electrical currents.

Having a positive result means that the patient has inherited a mutation that may be causing Brugada syndrome. He is probably at higher risk for the disease, and needs to be followed closely. However, inheriting the mutation does not mean that he will present symptoms of the disease.

Screening of exons indicates that the patient has some polymorphisms

Polymorphisms are very common, 1 in 1000 bases, and they will be found when screening for exons of the genes. The identification of the variations is like simply making a description of the genetic pattern of the individual. They are considered normal variants. However, as research progresses, we are realizing that some of these normal variations may determine gene modulation, or have a possible effect in the final phenotype. It is therefore possible that in the future, some of these polymorphisms may be linked to the disease, by causing a worse or better phenotype.

Limitations in the screening

When performing genetic analysis of a gene like *SCN5A*, we are actually looking at the exons of the gene — these are the segments of the DNA in the gene that codify for the amino acids and ultimately for the protein. We also look at the splice junctions, the areas where the exons and introns meet, for possible splicing mutations, mutations that do not allow the normal separation of exons and introns. We do not know at this point whether there are any mutations that cause the disease in the introns, or in the regulatory regions of the gene, like the promoter. It would be technically very demanding and financially very expensive to perform screening in the full gene.

Genetic background

Genetic background is not always easy to ascertain. A Hispanic is an individual from the Latin American countries, but the genetic background can be completely different if we compare a native Mexican from an individual from Argentina with a European descent. There are a few cases of polymorphisms and mutations identified in some genetic backgrounds and not present in others.

Functional effect

The mutation has to have a functional effect. In this case we are actually looking at our ability to identify a functional difference between the wild type and the mutant one, and if the difference is subtle, it is not always easy. All techniques have limitations, which become apparent when the functional effect is minimal.

In summary then, there are a few requirements that are important to verify whether a mutation is a true mutation and which are relevant to the diagnosis of the individual with Brugada syndrome, especially if this is a single patient in the family and is asymptomatic.

Limitations in the screening process
Single patient genetics

It is not easy to come to the conclusion that the mutation is causing the disease, especially if we are screening a single individual. In order to make the positive diagnosis we rely on the fact that the mutation changes the protein, that the mutation is not present in 200 control chromosomes, and that the biophysical data indicates an alteration in the ionic currents. These are the data that we have available, but we are missing the most important one in research in genetics and that is the tracking of the mutation with several affected individuals in the family. Unfortunately, research in genetics of sudden death, especially if it causes death in the young, carries the added difficulty of small families.

Negative genetic result in a family with an identified mutation

One of the great achievements in genetics was the possibility of making a negative diagnosis. We were certain that individuals without the familial mutation were spared of the familial disease. Centers have been providing a fee-for-service to screen individuals in families with identified mutations. While nobody can argue that the lack of the familial mutation is a better perspective than the presence of the mutation, research in genetics is emerging at this point with important challenges, especially as more and more families are identified. To illustrate this point we identified a family with Brugada syndrome and a mutation in 18 of their members, all of them carrying a mutation that disrupts the activity of the sodium channel and makes it non-functional.[10] It is clear from the data that those patients that do not have the mutation should be spared from the disease, but this is not the case. Two patients have a positive response to ajmaline, despite the fact that they do not carry the mutation. Several explanations arise from this observation: (1) the gene is not causing the disease because not everybody carries the mutation, (2) the ajmaline test is providing a false positive result, not described, but possible in any stimulation challenge, and (3) the patients have a different genetic mutation. These are all possibilities.

From the data shown it is understandable that we are faced with an important dilemma to reach the right conclusion. We are never able to provide evidence that the test is a false positive, because, with 35 000 genes in the genome, there always will be a possibility of a second mutation. Moreover, the identification of the mutation in these very few out-liners will always carry doubt of whether there is enough evidence that the second mutation is caus-ing the disease. This indicates the importance of genetic counseling that outlines all the possible re-sults and explanations.

Despite this limitation, the likelihood of a family inheriting two mutations is low, and a member with-out the familial mutation is very likely to be spared from the familial disease.

Bringing basic science into clinical arena

Data in genetics research is available on a daily basis. Findings in the most important journals are embar-goed and press-released to every single magazine and newspaper. Research is not a simple task, it does require hard work, and most of the big findings will have important implications in patient care in the future. Unfortunately, to the lay public, especially if affected with a devastating disease, the future needs to be as soon as possible. It is difficult for them to understand that a novel compound that shrinks tumors in mice is part of a research project that will take years to be fully developed and applied to patients. But genetics, molecular biology, and espe-cially all the information that is available from the Human Genome Project, have increased awareness of the advances is such a way that it seems that the so-lution to the diseases will be available in no time. It is granted that we advance more now in one day than we could in a decade 100 years ago. But genetics are just at the beginning. We are still at the descrip-tive phase of the genome and there is much still to learn.

Genetics and risk stratification

Genetics in Brugada syndrome are not ready to help in risk stratification. There has been no correlation yet between the kind of mutation and the risk of dying. This has been attempted in other diseases, such as hypertrophic cardiomyopa-thy, and despite that it appeared possible to predict, the reality has been that each family carries its own mutation and that the malignancy of the mutation probably depends on several other genetic factors.

What is the patient and health care provider expecting from genetics in Brugada syndrome and what should be expected?

To the single patient, genetics can only provide in-formation regarding whether he carries a mutation in *SCN5A* or not. But it does not provide informa-tion on the clinical status, on the risk of sudden death, or on being spared from the disease. Only 20% of the cases of Brugada syndrome carry a muta-tion in *SCN5A*. That means that the negative result does not provide relief to the patient, as it is very pos-sible that he carries a mutation in another, not yet identified, gene. To the member of a family with a known mutation, genetics can provide the positive diagnosis (indicating that he needs closer follow-up) or the negative diagnosis, which keeping in mind the rare possibility of a second gene, does at least provide the relief that they have not inherited the affected gene from the family so they are at less risk of having the disease.

Genetic testing as a gold standard for the other diagnostic tests

Genetics allows the validation of the different diag-nostic tools, especially the electrocardiographic parameters and the assessment of the response to class I blockers. We can use genetics as the best gold standard in the families with an identified mutation to assess whether we are using the right parameters to make the diagnosis. This is the genotype–pheno-type correlation and is explained at length in chapter 11 of this book.

The long-term benefit of genetics research for the patient

The most important benefit that the patient can ob-tain from research in genetics of Brugada syndrome is the possibility of gaining a better understanding of the disease, which will then make us able to provide better tools to diagnose and treat the disease. Despite that this is a long term goal, it is certainly an impor-tant one for families with inherited diseases, trans-mitted through the generations.

Placing all data into the patient perspective to provide the best care possible

The past decade has witnessed the identification of a

new clinical entity responsible for sudden death in the young and the evolution of a strategy to diagnose, risk stratify, and treat patients with this syndrome. This has been possible thanks to the efforts of many centers around the world and to the collaboration of hundreds of physicians. This is still a very new disease, with a high social impact due to the fact that it involves the death of young individuals. Through research and continued collaboration among the basic and clinical groups involved, we look forward to advances that will enable us to better identify those at risk and provide the means to treat them more effectively, so as to reduce the burden of this disease on the affected families.

Genetics are providing a link between the basic and clinical science. Advances in genetics will probably have an impact on future diagnosis, prevention, and risk stratification. In large families, genetics can provide very important information on who is carrying the familial mutation. In the single patient the issue is much more complicated, as the lack of segregation of the mutation with several members makes the conclusions regarding the mutation less robust. However, we are just at the beginning of the era of molecular genetics and we have already understood that genetics have a tremendous potential in the diagnosis and identification of possible affected individuals. It is likely that in the near future, it will also impact risk stratification parameters, and that in the long term it will provide, by gaining knowledge and understanding of the disease, better forms of treatment. The physicians and patients are the most important link to the achievement of these goals, and are encouraged to participate in this endeavor by providing genetic and clinical data to the investigators. It is only thanks to them that we have achieved so much in such a short time.

Final thought

Genetics are moving extremely fast, sometimes faster than printing of a book can handle. This chapter was finished in April 2004. It is possible that the knowledge, understanding, and information provided in this chapter will become obsolete as soon as the book is published. In this digital era, we recommend validation of the present data, intended for general information, with the most up-to-date knowledge in Brugada syndrome. This can be found at www.brugada.org.

References

1 Brugada P, Brugada J. Right bundle branch block, persistent ST segment elevation and sudden cardiac death: a distinct clinical and electrocardiographic syndrome: a multicenter report. *J. Am. Coll. Cardiol.* 1992; **20**: 1391–1396.

2 Brugada J, Brugada R, Brugada P. Right bundle-branch block and ST-segment elevation in leads V_1 through V_3. A marker for sudden death in patients without demonstrable structural heart disease. *Circulation* 1998; **97**: 457–460.

3 Wilde AA, Antzelevitch C, Borggrefe M *et al.* Proposed diagnostic criteria for the Brugada syndrome: Consensus Report. *Eur. Heart J.* 2002; **23**: 1648–1654.

4 Brugada R, Tapscott T, Czernuszewicz GZ *et al.* Identification of a genetic locus for familial atrial fibrillation [see comments]. *N. Engl. J. Med.* 1997; **336**: 905–911.

5 Roden DM, George AL, Jr., Bennett PB. Recent advances in understanding the molecular mechanisms of the long QT syndrome. *J. Cardiovasc. Electrophysiol.* 1995; **6**: 1023–1031.

6 Chen Q, Kirsch GE, Zhang D *et al.* Genetic basis and molecular mechanisms for idiopathic ventricular fibrillation. *Nature* 1998; **392**: 293–296.

7 Weiss R, Barmada MM, Nguyen T *et al.* Clinical and molecular heterogeneity in the Brugada syndrome. A novel gene locus on chromosome 3. *Circulation* 2002; **105**: 707–713.

8 Kyndt F, Probst V, Potet F *et al.* Novel *SCN5A* mutation leading either to isolated cardiac conduction defect or Brugada syndrome in a large French family. *Circulation* 2001; **104**: 3081–3086.

9 Gross E, Arnold N, Goette J *et al.* A comparison of BRCA1 mutation analysis by direct sequencing, SSCP and DHPLC. *Hum. Genet.* 1999; **105**: 72–78.

10 Hong K, Berruezo-Sanchez A, Poungvarin N *et al.* Phenotypic characterization of a large European family with Brugada syndrome displaying a sudden unexpected death syndrome mutation in *SCN5A. J. Cardiovasc. Electrophysiol.* 2004; **15**: 64–69.

CHAPTER 11

Genotype–phenotype relationship in the Brugada syndrome

J. P. P. Smits, MD, *A. A. M. Wilde,* MD, PhD

Introduction

In their initial report in 1992 on the disease that is now known as the Brugada syndrome, Pedro and Josep Brugada mentioned concerning its etiology that 'a hereditary factor could be suspected from the occurrence of the syndrome in two siblings and the family history of unexplained sudden death in two other patients'.[1]

Since then, the inherited nature of the Brugada syndrome has been convincingly established and was proven in 1998 by linking the syndrome to mutations in the *SCN5A* gene on chromosome 3p21 (Table 11.1).[2] However, in only 15–30% of Brugada syndrome cases and families a mutation in the *SCN5A* gene has been found.[3] In one family, the syndrome has been linked to a locus on chromosome 3, 3p22–25; however, the affected gene awaits identification (Table 11.2).[4] In the remaining cases of Brugada syndrome, although many of them are familial, no responsible gene or chromosome has been identified yet.[3]

Because the *SCN5A* gene encodes the pore forming α-subunit of the cardiac sodium channel (hH1), and the fact that the resulting reduction in depolarizing sodium current theoretically explains the Brugada syndrome phenotype, the syndrome is considered to be an ion channel disease.[2,5] Whether this is true for all Brugada syndrome cases remains to be established, but it is our current working hypothesis.

Knowing that other genes have to be involved, we may wonder if a genotype–phenotype relationship in the Brugada syndrome exists, as in the inherited long QT syndrome.[6,7] If such a relationship exists, knowledge of it may speed up a clinical and genetic diagnosis. Additionally, it may have consequences for mutation-specific prognosis and treatment, and possibly of identification of pro-arrhythmic effects of drugs and/or environmental triggers.

However, before such possibilities might become available, we will first have to identify those other genes. Isolation of those genes may be possible if we carefully look at Brugada syndrome patients and families and search for what may be minute phenotypic differences between them. What these phenotypic differences may be, considering the theoretical basis for the Brugada syndrome, the involved genes and proteins, will be discussed in the following sections.

Factors that are theoretically involved in the Brugada syndrome

Ion currents

The cardiac action potential is shaped by balanced and strictly regulated depolarizing and repolarizing ion currents traversing through and controlled by ion selective transmembrane channels. In general, ion channels consist of a transmembrane, pore forming, α-subunit which may co-express with one or more modulator β-subunit(s).[8]

The action potential (AP) shape in different regions of the heart and myocardium depends on the ion currents that are present and reflects differences in functional requirements.[8] Changes in ion cur-

Table 11.1 Clinical data from Brugada syndrome mutations that have been studied in heterologous expression systems predicting a reduction in sodium current.

Mutation	Index event proband	Family history*	ECG	Conduction disease	Flecainide challenge	EPS arrhythmia inducible?	HV (ms)	Reference
L567Q	SCD	+	ST↑	?	nd.	nd.	nd.	22, 23
G752R	none	+	ST↑ atypical	PR↑	+	nd.	nd.	23
G1406R (ICCD + Brugada)	palp. dizziness	+	'typical'	PR↑ RBBB, LAHB	PR↑↑ QRS↑↑	PVT	↑	25
R1432G	syncope	?	RBBB pattern ST↑	PR 240 ms RBBB pattern	ST↑	nd.	nd.	26, 27
R1512W	syncope	−	RBBB pattern ST↑ c	PR 220 ms RBBB pattern	ST↑	no	55	28
S1710L (ICCD/ IVF/BS)	syncope VF	−	+	1st degree AV block QRS↑ non-typical ST↑ at increased HR	1st degree AV block QRS↑ non-typical ST↑ at increased HR	VF	↑	29, 30
1795InsD (LQT3 + Brugada)	SCD	+	RBBB ST↑ QT↑	PR↑ QRS↑	ST↑	no	↑	31–33
Y1795H	none	−	(i)RBBB pattern ST↑ c/s	RBBB pattern	ST↑ c	non-sustained VT	↑	34
A1924T	none	−	'typical' RBBB pattern	no	no	nd.	?	28

SCD, sudden cardiac death; palp., palpitations; ICCD, inherited cardiac conduction disease; (c)RBBB, (complete) right bundle branch block; LAHB, left anterior hemi block; c, coved; VT, ventricular tachycardia; PVT, polymorphic ventricular tachycardia. *Family history positive or negative for sudden cardiac death.

rents and AP shape underlie changes of the ECG and abnormalities in cardiac conduction and rhythm. The proposed pathophysiologic basis for the Brugada syndrome is a rebalancing of the currents that contribute to phase 1, leading to an accentuation of the action potential notch in right ventricular epicardium.[5] The presence of a prominent I_{to} in this tissue makes it more sensitive to a reduction in depolarizing currents, such as I_{Na} during phase 0 (the rapid upstroke) or I_{Ca-L} during phase 2 (the plateau phase). Thus, a reduction of depolarizing ion currents, I_{Na} and I_{Ca-L}, or an increase in early repolarizing ion current, I_{to}, during the early phase of the cardiac action potential due to abnormal expression

Table 11.2 The only non *SCN5A* related Brugada syndrome mutation. Clinical characteristics.

Mutation	Index event proband	Family history	ECG	Conduction disease	INa challenge	EPS arrhythmias inducible?	HV (ms)	Reference
3p22-25	syncope	+	RBBB left axis ST↑ V_1–V_3 c	1st degree AV block	ST↑↑	VF	60	4

RBBB, right bundle branch block; c, coved; VF, ventricular fibrillation.

or function, may give rise to the Brugada syndrome phenotype. Table 11.3 summarizes the genes and the chromosomal locations of the α- and β-subunits of depolarizing and repolarizing ion channel currents involved in rapid depolarization, early repolarization, and the plateau phase of the cardiac action potential.

Presently, all *SCN5A* mutations in Brugada syndrome have been found to encode non-expressing or totally or partially dysfunctional sodium channels, resulting in a reduction in I_{Na}.

Table 11.3 Ion currents, their subunits, encoding genes and chromosome location.

Current	Gene	Chromosome
I_{Na}	SCN5A	3p21
α-subunit	$β_1$ (SCN1B)	19q13.1-q13.2
β-subunit	$β_2$ (SCN2B)	11q23
I_{Ca-L}	$α_1C$ (CACNL1A1)	12pter-p13.2
α-subunit	$β_1$ (CACNB1)	17q21-q22
β-subunit	$β_2$ (CACNB2)	10q12
	$α_2β$ (CACNA2D1)	7q21–22
I_{to}	Kv4.3 (KCND3)	1p13.2
α-subunit	kChip2 (KCNIP2)	10q24
β-subunit		

Modulatory subunits

Modulatory subunits of cardiac ion channels may significantly affect the function of the pore-forming subunit of the ion channel (Table 11.3). The presence of modulatory subunits may be needed for channel assembly, trafficking, and membrane expression.[8] Finally, β-subunits may associate with the pore forming α-subunit in the cell membrane and modulate its function. In the Brugada syndrome, no mutations have been found in genes that encode β-subunits.

A potential role for the Na$^+$ channel β-subunit is, however, shown by the fact that the $β_1$-subunit of the cardiac sodium channel modifies the effects of mutations in the α-subunit, and it possibly has a role as a chaperone protein for the Na$^+$ channel α-subunit.[9,10]

Ion channel expression

Expression of hH1 in the surface membrane of the myocyte is not a random process, but is guided by intracellular proteins.[10] The C terminus of Na$^+$ channels from several different tissues interacts with the PDZ domain of syntrophin, a protein in the dys-

trophin-associated protein complex, directing Na$^+$ channels to specific sites on the membrane.[11] Mutations in PDZ domains may therefore be expected to disrupt this interaction and proper channel expression. The recently resolved mechanism of the long QT syndrome type 4 illustrates the role of the cytoskeleton in ion channel expression. In a family suffering from LQT4, a loss of function mutation in the gene encoding ankyrin B was found.[12] Through ankyrin, the spectrin–actin cytoskeleton of cells connects with ion channels, and other ion transporting proteins, anchoring it to the cell membrane.

In a heterozygous mouse model of this mutation, several cardiac ion pumps were affected, due to abnormal protein localization and reduced expression levels.[13] Mutations in proteins regulating ion channel expression, which may be a role for β-subunits, would therefore be a possible cause for reduced expression of Na$^+$ channels, and other ion channels in Brugada syndrome.

Ion channel modification

While in the ER, and when expressed in the cell membrane, ion channel function will be affected by processes such as (de)glycolysation[14] and (de)phosphorylation.[14,15] These processes may affect sodium channel expression, and also channel gating properties.[16]

Direct modification of ion channel function by protein–protein interaction has recently been shown for hH1, by binding of calmodulin (CaM)[16] to it in a Ca^{2+} dependent manner.[17] Due to the binding of CaM, the gating properties of hH1 changed, enhancing slow inactivation. Because CaM is an intracellular Ca^{2+}-sensing protein, the intracellular Ca^{2+} concentration therefore affects sodium channel function.[17] This and similar mechanisms may be very well involved in Brugada syndrome.

Potential parameters that may reflect a genotype–phenotype relationship in Brugada syndrome

Parameters that may reflect a genotype–phenotype relationship may be similar to those in the long QT syndrome. In the long QT syndrome, these parameters are: the presenting symptoms, the age at which the first symptoms occur, the triggering event, and the ECG morphology.[6,7] All these parameters are easily available.

Presently, the only known parameters, discriminating two genotypically different groups in Brugada syndrome, are those related to cardiac conduction.[18]

Demographic characteristics

Although Brugada syndrome is an autosomal inherited disease, it affects males 8–10 times more than females.[3] The male predominance probably reflects the gender differences in expression of I_{to} and I_{Ca-L}.[19,20] An increase in I_{to} or a reduction in I_{Ca-L} may theoretically alter the normal AP, similarly to a reduction in I_{Na}. When such alterations occur, for example due to mutations in the genes encoding I_{to} and I_{Ca-L}, this must have a different effect on male or female carriers. The observation that surgical castration in males alleviates ST segment elevation suggests that male hormones also play a role.[21]

In the long QT syndrome, age-related, genotypical differences have been well established.[6,7] The mean age for a first arrhythmic event to occur in the Brugada syndrome is approximately 40 years (range: 1 to 77 years).[3] Presently, neither gender nor age at the moment of the first arrhythmic event have been identified to be specific for a subgroup of Brugada patients.

Clinical characteristics

Triggering events

Similarly to the congenital long QT syndrome, differences in the genes underlying the disease may theoretically result in different arrhythmia triggers.

Presently, two triggers are known to unmask the typical ECG and induce arrhythmias: these are sleep and fever. Whether the rise in body temperature, the changes in the (humoral) immune system, or both, trigger symptoms, is not known. Until now, no remarkable differences in triggers between Brugada syndrome patients or families have been established.

ECG characteristics

In the inherited long QT syndrome, the morphology of the T wave and QTc duration are genotype-specific.[6,7] A similar relationship for the Brugada syndrome is possible, because the shape of the ST segment is critically dependent on the magnitude and timing of the balance of ion currents.[8] Two different shapes of the ST segment are recognized, the coved and the saddleback types. The magnitude and shape of the ST segment shows considerable intra- and inter-individual variation. Patients may show spontaneous ST segment changes in time, the abnormalities may become aggravated, or may normalize. Inter-individual variation in the ST segment abnormalities can frequently be observed between family members who carry the same *SCN5A* mutation. Both the intra- and inter-individual ST segment variation may reflect normal and abnormal modification of ion channels. These spontaneous variations will make the establishment of a genotype-specific ST segment unlikely. In a recent report, the magnitude of the spontaneous ST segment elevation was not found to be different between carriers of *SCN5A* mutations as compared to non-mutation carriers.[18]

Abnormalities in ion channel function or expression will not only affect the morphology of the ST segment, but also other electrical properties of the heart, for example conduction.

Loss of function mutations in the *SCN5A* gene, as

in the Brugada syndrome (Table 11.1),[23–34] have been identified in patients suffering from inherited cardiac conduction disease (ICCD) (Table 11.4).[25,29,30,35–39] SCN5A mutations in ICCD reduce the sodium current due to trafficking or gating defects of the channel. The functional differences between sodium channel dysfunction in Brugada syndrome and ICCD is often not easy to understand. Two SCN5A mutations, G1406R[25] and S1710L,[29,30] have been reported to result in both an ICCD and a Brugada syndrome phenotype. The phenotype of carriers of the G1406R mutation was gender-dependent. All Brugada syndrome patients were male, and all but one (6 out of 7) ICCD patients were female.[25] In addition to these two mutations, conduction abnormalities are often reported in Brugada syndrome patients.

The first report on a phenotype–genotype relationship in the Brugada syndrome stems from this observation. In this report, 23 Brugada syndrome patients, with 19 different SCN5A mutations, were compared to 54 Brugada syndrome patients in whom an SCN5A mutation had been excluded. The SCN5A mutation carriers were found to have significantly longer PQ intervals on their 12 lead ECG and longer His-to-ventricle (HV) intervals during EPS (Fig. 11.1). Therefore, it was concluded that the presence of impaired conduction in a Brugada syndrome patient points to an underlying SCN5A mutation and is genotype-specific.[18] Other ECG parameters, such as the QRS interval, the QTc interval, and the magnitude of ST segment elevations, were not found to be different.

Flecainide challenge

An important test in the diagnosis of the Brugada syndrome is a pharmacologic challenge with class I antiarrhythmic drugs, preferably flecainide or ajmaline.[40,41,43] Class I sodium channel blocking drugs will reduce the sodium current during phase 0 of the cardiac action potential, thereby, theoretically, disturbing the balance between depolarizing ion currents and repolarizing I_{to}. If this balance is already disturbed, because of a loss of function SCN5A mutation, the ST segment may become elevated or its shape may change.[5] Hence the effect of flecainide challenge might be expected to be ion channel-specific and probably mutation-specific. However, the change in ST segment shape or elevation, due to

flecainide challenge, was not found to be different between carriers of an SCN5A mutation and Brugada syndrome patients without a mutation.[18] Ion channel, or I_{Na}, specific effects have been shown in the greater QRS prolongation in carriers of an SCN5A mutation as compared to non-carriers (Fig. 11.1).[18] Another interesting finding is that flecainide testing preferentially puts Brugada syndrome patients who carry an SCN5A mutation at risk to develop ventricular tachyarrhythmias.[44]

Mechanistic proof for this ion channel specific effect, and for the effects on the ST segment in Brugada syndrome, comes from a study of the effects of flecainide on the 1795InsD.[45] The 1795InsD mutant channels were found to be more sensitive to the blocking effects of flecainide compared to wild-type channels. Thus, when cardiac conduction is already compromised by a reduction in I_{Na} due to an SCN5A mutation, flecainide may be expected to further aggravate this. Mutation-specific effects of the flecainide challenge may result from the fact that, depending on the amino acid substitution in the cardiac sodium channel, the effect of flecainide may be different.[18]

Synopsis

Brugada syndrome is a genetically heterogeneous inherited disease. Therefore genotype-specific differences may be present in Brugada syndrome patients and families. The variable penetrance of the disease complicates the establishment of a phenotype–genotype relationship. Without knowledge of possibly the majority of involved genes and proteins, and without full understanding of its pathophysiology, this search is even more complicated. A first step has been made by recognizing that there is one patient group carrying an SCN5A mutation, and another very large one that does not, and that these groups are indeed phenotypically different.

Additionally, we know that there is one family with a non-malignant disease course, in which the disease has been linked to an as yet unidentified gene on chromosome 3p22–25.[4]

Brugada syndrome SCN5A mutations, identified and investigated in cellular expression models, have consistently shown that I_{Na} is reduced.[42] This finding is consistent with the proposed pathophysiologic mechanism for the disease.[5] Between the Brugada syndrome and two other sodium channel

Table 11.4 Cardiac conduction disease mutations that have been studied in heterogeneous expression systems predicting a reduction in sodium current I_{Na}. Clinical characteristics.

Mutation	Index event proband	Family history* +/−	ECG	Conduction disease	EPS arrhythmia inducible?	HV (ms)	Reference
W156X + R225W†	broad complex tachycardia	+	–	progressive conduction disease in both atrium and ventricle	nd.	nd.	35
G298S	?/2nd degree AV block at age 6 years	?	2nd degree AV block progressive to 3rd degree	2nd degree AV block progressive to 3rd degree	?	?	36
T512I + H558R‡	irr. heart beat	–	2nd degree AV block	–	nd.	nd.	37
G514C	bradycardia	+	broad P wave PR↑, QRS↑	broad P wave PR↑, QRS↑	?	?	38
IVS22 + 2	syncope	+	RBBB complete AV block LBBB, LAHB, LPHB	–	nd.	?	29
G1406R (ICCD + Brugada)	palp. dizziness	+	'typical' PR↑ RBBB, LAHB	PR↑↑ QRS↑↑	PVT	↑	25
D1595N	2nd degree AV block	+	PR↑	PR↑ RBBB	AH 70 ms	210	36
S1710L (ICCD, IVF, BS)	syncope VF	+	1st degree AV block QRS↑ non-typical ST↑ at increased HR	1st degree AV block QRS↑ non-typical ST↑ at increased HR	VF	↑	29, 30
S1710 + 75X	1st degree AV block	+	1st degree AV block RBBB	–	nd.	nd.	39

†, compound heterozygosity; ‡, T512I mutation; H558R, polymorphism; SCD, sudden cardiac death; palp., palpitations; ICCD, inherited cardiac conduction disease; (c)RBBB, (complete) right bundle branch block; LAHB, left anterior hemi block; LPHB, left posterior hemi block; c, coved; VT, ventricular tachycardia; PVT, polymorphic ventricular tachycardia.
*Family history positive or negative for sudden cardiac death.

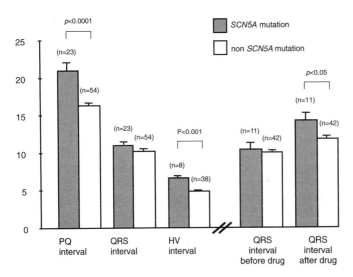

Figure 11.1 Conduction abnormalities are a discriminating phenotypical parameter, as evidenced by prolonged PQ and HV intervals, between Brugada syndrome patients with and without an *SCN5A* mutation. After administration of class I sodium channel blocking drugs, the QRS interval prolonged significantly more in Brugada syndrome patients carrying an *SCN5A* mutation.

associated arrhythmia syndromes, the long QT syndrome type 3 and cardiac conduction disease, phenotypic overlap exists.[25,29–33,42] There are several reports of loss of function *SCN5A* mutations that are causally related to both Brugada syndrome and cardiac conduction disease.[25,29,30] In Brugada syndrome patients with an *SCN5A* mutation, compromised conduction is therefore not surprising. Indeed, these differences in cardiac conduction are presently the only known differences that can discern between the group of *SCN5A*-related, and non-related Brugada syndrome patients.[18] Matters, however, are complicated already by the fact that the Brugada syndrome patients, in whom the disease was linked to a site on chromosome 3 (3p22–25), also have conduction abnormalities.[4] A possible explanation in this case, and others, may be that mutations in other proteins, also affecting the sodium current, may be involved.

ent types. Like in the long QT syndrome, this may lead to finding Brugada syndrome types. These different types may each have a different epidemiology and different clinical characteristics and require different, preferably pharmacologic, treatment.[6,7]

At present, only conduction parameters seem to discriminate between Brugada syndrome patients with and without a mutation in the *SCN5A* gene.[18]

Further phenotype–genotype relations may be established, if we are able to identify Brugada syndrome patients, or preferably families, who are phenotypically different from other Brugada syndrome patients. In such patients, an educated guess, for example based on some remarkable ECG recording, might lead to the identification of the causally involved gene.

This work was supported by a grant from NWO (the Netherlands Organisation for Scientific Research) grant no. 902–16–193.

Conclusion

Establishment of a phenotype–genotype relationship in the Brugada syndrome is important for understanding the pathophysiology of the disease. When we understand the basis of the disease, we may be able to develop an ion channel-, or protein mechanism-specific pharmacologic treatment. When indeed Brugada syndrome is caused by mutations in different genes, this could mean that in the future we can divide Brugada syndrome into differ-

References

1 Brugada P, Brugada J. Right bundle branch block, persistent ST segment elevation and sudden cardiac death: a distinct clinical and electrocardiographic syndrome. *J. Am. Coll. Cardiol.* 1992; **20**: 1391–1396.

2 Chen Q, Kirsch GE, Zhang D *et al.* Genetic basis and molecular mechanism for idiopathic ventricular fibrillation. *Nature.* 1998; **392**: 293–296.

3 Alings M, Wilde A. 'Brugada' syndrome: clinical data and suggested pathophysiological mechanism. *Circulation* 1999; **99**: 666–673.

4 Weiss R, Barmada M, Nguyen T *et al.* Clinical and molecular heterogeneity in the Brugada syndrome. A novel gene locus on chromosome 3. *Circulation* 2002; **105**: 707–713.

5 Antzelevitch C. The Brugada syndrome: ionic basis and arrhythmia mechanisms. *J. Cardiovasc. Electrophysiol.* 2001; **12**: 268–272.

6 Wilde AAM, Roden DM. Predicting the long-QT genotype from clinical data. From sense to science. *Circulation* 2000; **102**: 2796–2798.

7 Van Langen IM, Birnie E, Alders M *et al.* The use of genotype–phenotype correlations in mutation analysis for the long QT syndrome. *J. Med. Genet.* 2003; **40**: 141–145.

8 Roden DM, Balser JR, George AL Jr. *et al.* Cardiac ion channels. *Annu. Rev. Physiol.* 2002; **64**: 431–475.

9 Makita N, Shirai N, Wang DW *et al.* Cardiac Na+ channel dysfunction in Brugada syndrome is aggravated by β1-subunit. *Circulation* 2000; **101**: 54–60.

10 Zimmer T, Biskup C, Bollensdorff C *et al.* The beta1 subunit but not the beta2 subunit colocalizes with the human heart Na+ channel (hH1) already within the endoplasmic reticulum. *J. Membr. Biol.* 2002; **186**: 13–21.

11 Fanning AS, Anderson JM. PDZ domains: fundamental building blocks in the organization of protein complexes at the plasma membrane. *J. Clin. Invest.* 1999; **103**: 767–772.

12 Mohler PJ, Schott JJ, Gramolini AO *et al.* Ankyrin-B mutation causes type 4 long-QT cardiac arrhythmia and sudden cardiac death. *Nature* 2003; **421**: 634–639.

13 Chauhan VS, Tuvia S, Buhusi M *et al.* Abnormal cardiac Na(+) channel properties and QT heart rate adaptation in neonatal ankyrin(B) knockout mice. *Circ. Res.* 2000; **86**: 441–447.

14 Bennett ES. Isoform-specific effects of sialic acid on voltage-dependent Na+ channel gating: functional sialic acids are localized to the S5-S6 loop of domain I. *J. Physiol.* 2002; **538**: 675–690.

15 Ufret-Vincenty CA, Baro DJ, Lederer WJ *et al.* Role of sodium channel deglycosylation in the genesis of cardiac arrhythmias in heart failure. *J. Biol. Chem.* 2001; **276**: 28 197–28 203.

16 Zhang Y, Hartmann HA, Satin J. Glycosylation influences voltage-dependent gating of cardiac and skeletal muscle sodium channels. *J. Membr. Biol.* 1999; **171**: 195–207.

17 Tan HL, Kupershmidt S, Zhang R *et al.* A calcium sensor in the sodium channel modulates cardiac excitability. *Nature* 2002; **415**: 442–447.

18 Smits JPP, Eckardt L, Probst V *et al.* Genotype-phenotype relationship in Brugada syndrome: Electrocardiographic features differentiate *SCN5A*-related patients from non *SCN5A*-related patients. *J. Am. Coll. Cardiol.* 2002; **40**: 350–356.

19 Pham TV, Rosen MR. Sex, hormones and repolarization. *Cardiovasc. Res.* 2002; **53**: 740–751.

20 Di Diego JM, Cordeiro JM, Goodrow RJ *et al.* Ionic and cellular basis for the predominance of the Brugada syndrome phenotype in males. *Circulation.* 2002; **106**: 2004–2011.

21 Matsuo K, Akahoshi M, Seto S *et al.* Disappearance of the Brugada-type electrocardiogram after surgical castration. *Pacing Clin. Electrophysiol.* 2003; **26**: 1551–1553.

22 Priori SG, Napolitano C, Giordano U *et al.* Brugada syndrome and sudden cardiac death in children. *Lancet* 2000; **335**: 808–809.

23 Wan X, Chen S, Sadeghpour A *et al.* Accelerated inactivation in a mutant Na+ channel associated with idiopathic ventricular fibrillation. *Am. J. Physiol.* 2001; **280**: H354–H360.

24 Potet F, Mabo P, Le Coq G *et al.* Novel Brugada *SCN5A* mutation leading to ST segment elevation in the inferior or the right precordial leads. *J. Cardiovasc. Electrophysiol.* 2003; **14**: 200–203.

25 Kyndt F, Probst V, Potet F *et al.* Novel *SCN5A* mutation leading either to isolated cardiac conduction defect or Brugada syndrome in a large French family. *Circulation* 2001; **18**: 3081–3086.

26 Baroudi G, Pouliot V, Denjoy I *et al.* Novel mechanism for Brugada syndrome: defective surface localization of an *SCN5A* mutant (R1432G). *Circ. Res.* 2001; **88**: E78–E83.

27 Deschênes I, Baroudi G, Berthet M *et al.* Electrophysiological characterization of s causing long QT (E1784K) and Brugada (R1512W and R1432G) syndromes. *Cardiovasc. Res.* 2000; **46**: 55–65.

28 Rook MB, Bezzina Alshinawi C, Groenewegen WA *et al.* Human *SCN5A* gene mutations alter cardiac sodium channel kinetics and are associated with the Brugada syndrome. *Cardiovasc. Res.* 1999; **44**: 507–17.

29 Akai J, Makita N, Sakurada H *et al.* A novel *SCN5A* mutation associated with idiopathic ventricular fibrillation without typical ECG findings of Brugada syndrome. *FEBS Lett.* 2000; **479**: 29–34.

30 Shirai N, Makita N, Sasaki K *et al.* A mutant cardiac sodium channel with multiple biophysical defects associated with overlapping clinical features of Brugada syndrome and cardiac conduction disease. *Cardiovasc. Res.* 2002; **53**: 348–354.

31 Van den Berg MP, Wilde AAM, Viersma JW *et al.* Possible bradycardic mode of death and successful pacemaker treatment in a large family with features of long QT syndrome type 3 and Brugada syndrome. *J. Cardiovasc. Electrophysiol.* 2001; **12**: 630–636.

32 Bezzina C, Veldkamp MW, Van den Berg MP *et al.* A single Na+ channel mutation causing both long-QT and Brugada syndromes. *Circ. Res.* 1999; **85**: 1206–1213.

33 Veldkamp MW, Viswanathan PC, Bezzina C *et al.* Two distinct congenital arrhythmias evoked by a multidysfunctional Na(+) channel. *Circ. Res.* 2000; **86**: E91–E97.

34 Rivolta I, Abriel H, Tateyama M *et al.* Inherited Brugada and long QT-3 syndrome mutations of a single residue of the cardiac sodium channel confer distinct channel and clinical phenotypes. *J. Biol. Chem.* 2001; **276/33**: 30 623–30 630.

35 Bezzina CR, Rook MB, Groenewegen WA *et al.* Compound heterozygosity for mutations (W156X and R225W) in *SCN5A* associated with severe cardiac conduction disturbances and degenerative changes in the conduction system. *Circ. Res.* 2003; **92**: 159–168.

36 Wang DW, Viswanathan PC, Balser JR *et al.* Clinical, genetic, and biophysical characterization of *SCN5A* mutations associated with atrioventricular conduction block. *Circulation* 2002; **105**: 341–346.

37 Viswanathan PC, Benson DW, Balser JR. A common *SCN5A* polymorphism modulates the biophysical effects of an *SCN5A* mutation. *J. Clin. Invest.* 2003; **111**: 341–346.

38 Tan HL, Bink-Boelkens MT, Bezzina CR *et al.* A sodium-channel mutation causes isolated cardiac conduction disease. *Nature* 2001; **409**: 1043–1047.

39 Schott JJ, Alshinawi C, Kyndt F *et al.* Cardiac conduction defects associate with mutations in *SCN5A*. *Nature Genet.* 1999; **23**: 20–21.

40 Bezzina CR, Rook MB, Wilde AAM. Cardiac sodium channel and inherited arrhythmia syndromes. *Cardiovasc. Res.* 2000; **49**: 257–271.

41 Brugada R, Brugada J, Antzelevitch C *et al.* Sodium channel blockers identify risk for sudden death in patients with ST-segment elevation and right bundle branch block but structurally normal hearts. *Circulation* 2000; **101**: 510–515.

42 Priori SG, Napolitano C, Schwartz PJ *et al.* The elusive link between LQT3 and Brugada syndrome. The role of flecainide challenge. *Circulation* 2000; **102**: 945–947.

43 Shimizu W, Antzelevitch C, Suyama K *et al.* Effect of sodium channel blockers on ST segment, QRS duration, and corrected QT interval in patients with Brugada syndrome. *J. Cardiovasc. Electrophysiol.* 2000; **11**: 1320–1329.

44 Gasparini M, Priori SG, Mantica M *et al.* Flecainide test in Brugada syndrome: a reproducible but risky tool. *Pacing Clin. Electrophysiol.* 2003; **26**: 338–341.

45 Viswanathan PC, Bezzina CR, George Jr AL *et al.* Gating-dependent mechanisms for flecainide action in *SCN5A*-linked arrhythmia syndromes. *Circulation* 2001; **104**: 1200–1205.

CHAPTER 12

Gender differences in Brugada syndrome

V. Probst, MD, *S. Pattier, J-J. Schott,* PhD, *H. Le Marec,* MD, PhD

Introduction

Brugada syndrome is an inherited arrhythmogenic disease similar to the sudden unexplained nocturnal death syndrome (SUNDS), a disorder described in Southeast Asia. It is an autosomal dominant inherited disease where males represent 50% of the gene carriers and should represent, if the penetrance was complete, 50% of the affected patients. Brugada as well as SUNDS have been linked to mutations in *SCN5A* gene;[1,2] however, it has been confirmed by several groups that it is a heterogeneous inherited disease, as a mutation in *SCN5A* gene is only present in less than 30% of the probands. The presence of families not linked to *SCN5A* and to the second locus identified by the group of London[3] implies that at least two other genes are involved in more than 70% of affected patients.

The male predominance of the disease was apparent since the first reports on Brugada syndrome, even before the description of its genetic background and the identification of *SCN5A* mutations by a candidate gene approach.[2] The male predominance is a common feature of Brugada syndrome and SUNDS, with an 8 to 1 ratio for males compared to females in probands. This male predominance led to the Southeast Asian custom of men dressing in women's clothes at bedtime to fool the evil spirits that were supposed to target males during their sleep.

Cardiac conduction defect (CCD) is another disease allelic to Brugada syndrome and SUNDS.[4,5] The phenotype is different but there are some overlaps between Brugada and CCD phenotypes. In several families with mutations in the *SCN5A* gene, some members develop a Brugada phenotype whereas others develop a CCD phenotype. Moreover, in patients with Brugada syndrome, the main difference between a patient with or without *SCN5A* mutation

is the presence or absence of alteration of conduction.[6] This is not surprising as cardiac conduction defect as well as Brugada syndrome and SUNDS mutations result in a similar loss of function of the protein.[2,5]

Male predominance in Brugada syndrome: clinical evidence from databases

The databases concerning Brugada syndrome have been developed from isolated cases. These isolated cases should be considered as probands of families, and there is a possibility that their clinical characteristics are not representative of all the carriers of the genetic defect. Only familial studies could provide more complete information concerning the penetrance of the disease, its severity, and the variability of the phenotype, but these studies are still limited. Probably because of the lack of sufficient familial studies, the information concerning the effects of gender and genetic defects on the variability of the phenotype of Brugada syndrome are still poor.

The prevalence of the disease is higher in males

Although it is an autosomal dominant inherited disease, a common feature of Brugada syndrome and SUNDS is the large male predominance of the disease. Most of the data published so far concern probands with an 8 to 1 ratio for males compared to females (Table 12.1). In the series of 130 probands described by the group of Priori,[7] 85% were males and in our own series of 73 probands, 81% were males. These data are similar to those of the initial combined experience of Amsterdam, Munster, and Nantes (76% men versus 24% women)[6] and to the 334 patients presented by the group of Brugada

Table 12.1 Summary of the sex ratio in 3 databases. The number of probands is identified in the series of Priori and Nantes, not in the series of Brugada. The series of Priori and Nantes concern only patients who have been screened for *SCN5A* mutations.

	Affected	Male versus female	Probands	Male versus female
Priori	200	152/48	130	110/20
Brugada	334	255/79	?	?
Nantes	122	77/45	73	59/14

(76% versus 24%) where probands and familial cases were not differentiated.[8] As probands were mainly identified because of symptoms or typical ECG patterns it can be concluded that, independently of the type of genetic defect, there is a large male predominance in typical Brugada syndrome. Indeed, in our experience, within the 73 probands that have been genotyped, 49 patients, with a large male predominance (42 men versus 7 women), had a typical ECG (type 1 pattern).

The severity of the disease is higher in males

The initial data concerning the Brugada syndrome were obtained from symptomatic patients, where most of them had a history of sudden death or syncope. Adult males were at higher risk of sudden death in Brugada syndrome and SUNDS. This male predominance that revealed the severity of the disease in males has not changed with the development of databases.

In a series published by the group of Brugada[8] within the 334 affected patients in the database (255 men versus 79 women), 85% of the symptomatic patients were male. Seventy-one had a history of sudden death, with a large predominance of men (61 men versus 10 women), 73 had a history of syncope, with the same male predominance (59 men versus 14 women), whereas 190 were asymptomatic with a lower proportion of men (135 men versus 55 women). In this series the authors concluded that the group with the lowest risk (no risk) was the group of women with normal ECG at baseline.

In the series published by the group of Priori,[7] 200 patients screened for *SCN5A* mutation were in their database (152 men versus 48 women), including 130 probands. A history of cardiac arrest was present in 22 patients, with a large male predominance (20 men versus 2 women).

In our database, within the 122 affected patients that have been genotyped, including 73 probands, 29 were symptomatic with a history of syncope or aborted sudden death. Within these symptomatic patients, the male predominance was similar to the previous studies (23 men versus 6 women).

Clearly the disease is more severe in males. Male sex is the highest risk factor in Brugada syndrome.

Role of the genetic defect and gender in the expression of the disease

There is a large variability in the phenotype—it can vary from typical ECG pattern associated with syncope or sudden death, to absence of any ECG and clinical abnormalities.[9] Furthermore, at least for patients with mutations in *SCN5A* gene, some of the carriers may develop cardiac conduction defect instead of Brugada syndrome.

The penetrance is incomplete and the phenotype is highly variable, but little information is available concerning the role of gender according to the genetic status. The lack of information is mainly due to the fact that some patients included in the databases are not genotyped and that familial studies are rare.

A major problem is the absence of a gold standard for characterization of each patient. The genetic defect could represent the gold standard; however, more than 70% of patients with Brugada syndrome have a normal *SCN5A* gene and the other causative genes are unknown. In patients with the *SCN5A* mutation, furthermore, the penetrance is incomplete and the phenotype is highly variable, with a large spectrum of ECG anomalies from typical Brugada syndrome to cardiac conduction defect.

There are two, unsatisfying, ways to present and analyze data from genotyped patients. The first is to analyze patients with an *SCN5A* mutation and patients without an *SCN5A* mutation separately. The second is to analyze all the patients according to the presence or absence of a Brugada phenotype.

The only data published are from the group of Priori.[7] Eighty-four patients (28 probands and 56 family members) were carriers of an *SCN5A* mutation. No data concerning the ECG at baseline are available, but 46 have had a pharmacologic provocative testing. Within these 46 patients, 13 (3 men, 10 women) were silent carriers with normal ECG at baseline and negative flecainide test. They have calculated the global penetrance to be 71% but they did not provide data for the penetrance according to sex.

In our database, all patients with a typical ECG aspect of Brugada (type 1) at baseline or after a pharmacologic provocative test (flecainide or ajmaline) were included as affected patients. In all patients included, the *SCN5A* gene was screened for mutations using the d-HPLC technique.

Within the 122 patients with positive ECG, 36 were carriers of an *SCN5A* mutation (Table 12.2) whereas 86 had no mutation in the *SCN5A* gene.

Within the 36 carriers of a *SCN5A* mutation (19 men and 17 women), 11 men (58%) and 7 women (41%) had a positive ECG at baseline. However,

Table 12.2 *SCN5A* mutation identified in patients with Brugada syndrome included in the Nantes database.

Mutation	Effect	Type
C673T	R225W	ms
G1078A	D356N	ms
T1106A	M369K	ms
C1603T	R535X	ns
G2254A	G752R	ms
G2314A	D772N	ms
G3622T	E1200X	ns
G3656A	S1219N	ms
3816delG		se or ns
T3682C	Y1228H	ms
G3823A	D1275N	ms
IVS21+1G>		se
IVS22+2T>C		se
T4079G	F1360C	ms
G4222A	G1408R	ms
G4295T	S1382I	ms
C5015A	S1672Y	ms
5356–5357delCT	fs	del

ms, missense mutation; ns, non-sense; se, splice error; del, deletion; fs, frameshift.

within the 86 *SCN5A*-negative patients (58 men and 28 women), 34 men (58%) and 1 woman (3%) had a positive ECG at baseline. So, whatever the true penetrance of the disease in non-*SCN5A* Brugada syndrome, it is clear that the penetrance is very low at baseline in females.

In five families linked to *SCN5A*, we were able to perform a familial study in at least three generations with a baseline ECG (and pharmacologic testing in most of the cases) and a genotype. Forty-eight (30 women, 18 men) were carriers of a mutation. Most of the mutated patients (80%) accepted a pharmacologic testing. Figure 12.1 shows an example of a familial study.

Within the 30 women, 9 (30%) had a positive Brugada aspect after pharmacologic testing (1 had a history of sudden death), 14 (47%) had only cardiac conduction defect and the ajmaline test was negative (performed in 12), and 7 (23%) had a normal ECG.

Within the 18 males, 9 (50%) had a positive Brugada aspect (5 had a history of syncope or sudden death), 8 (45%) had only cardiac conduction defect and a negative ajmaline test, and 1 (5%) had a normal ECG.

In these families, the penetrance of Brugada was 50% in male, 30% in female and the most frequent ECG abnormality was cardiac conduction defect. Finally, 23% of women and 5% of men had strictly normal ECGs.

The large male predominance of the disease, the wide spectrum of phenotype, and the low penetrance emphasizes the major role of modulating factors, in particular those depending on sex, in the expression of the disease.

Cellular bases for male predominance of Brugada syndrome phenotype

Clinical data clearly show that male predominance is not the result of a familial trait but a major clinical characteristic of Brugada syndromes. This sex-linked difference is much more pronounced than the female predominance of QT duration in long QT syndromes.[10] Both Brugada with or without *SCN5A* mutation display a male predominance. This observation suggests that strong, sex-linked, modulating factors are mainly independent of the genetic defect leading to Brugada syndrome but are dependent on the general cardiac characteristics of males revealed by the genetic defect.

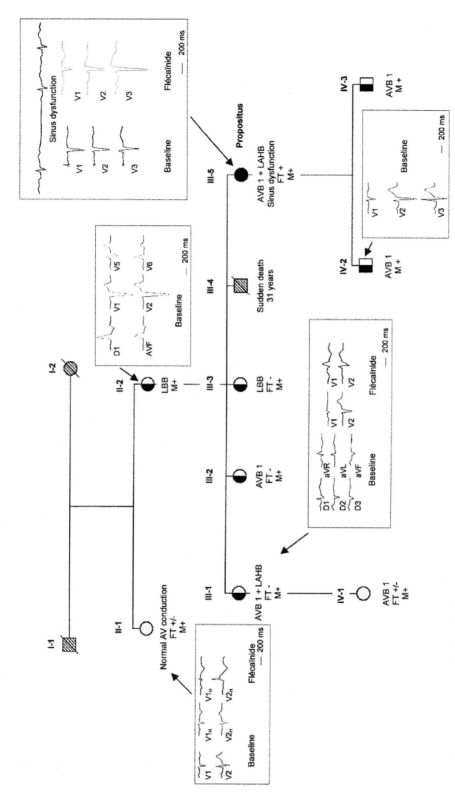

Figure 12.1 Two pedigrees of families affected by a *SCN5A* mutation. Empty symbols (circles indicate females, and squares, males) depict unaffected members, filled symbols depict Brugada syndrome phenotype and half-filled symbols depict the cardiac conduction defect phenotype, M+ means that the patient is carrier of the mutation, FT means flecainide test. These two examples show that the expression of *SCN5A* mutations is highly variable from normal phenotype to cardiac conduction defect and/or Brugada phenotype.

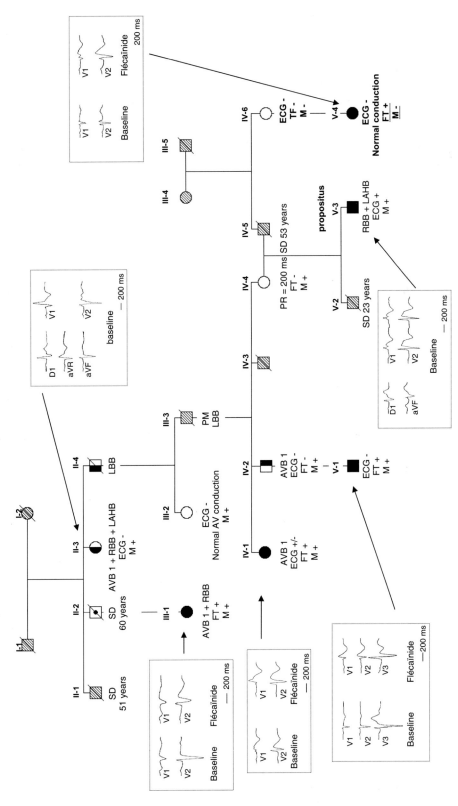

Figure 12.1 *Continued*

The cellular mechanisms underlying Brugada syndrome have been mainly studied by the group of Antzelevitch.[11,12] The cellular basis of Brugada syndrome is the result of their extensive work on the cellular heterogeneity of the ventricular myocardium.[13] They have proposed that the accentuation of the epicardial action potential notch and an eventual loss of the epicardial action potential dome (all-or-none repolarization at the end of phase 1) should result in ST segment elevation and phase 2 reentry. These modifications of epicardial action potential could be dependent on a reduction of inward currents (I_{Na} or I_{Ca}) or an increase of outward currents ($I_{to}, I_{K-ATP}, I_{Kr}, I_{Ks} \ldots$). I_{to} is much greater in the right than in the left ventricular epicardium, especially in the right ventricular outflow track; this could explain the right ventricular aspect of repolarization abnormalities and makes the presence of a prominent I_{to}-mediated notch a prerequisite for the disease.

The understanding of the cellular basis for male predominance of Brugada syndrome has largely benefited from the work of the group of Antzelevitch.[14] They have studied the main characteristics of the action potential from slices of right and left ventricle of adult male or female dogs.

Figure 12.2 shows that while phase 0 (representing sodium current) are similar, phase 1 amplitude is significantly smaller in males versus females. This sex difference in the notch of the epicardial action potential is abolished by 2 mmol/L of 4-aminopyridine, a blocker of I_{to}. These action potential differences are present only in epicardial cells from the right ventricle; in particular, phase 1 is similar in male and female epicardial cells from the left ventricle, as shown in Fig. 12.3.

The cardiac cellular sexual differences are localized in the right ventricle in accordance with the hypothesis about the role of the large cellular heterogeneity of the right ventricle in development of the electrocardiographic aspect of the Brugada syndrome. In arterially perfused right ventricular wedge preparations, pinacidil has been used to increase the repolarization heterogeneity of ventricular wall (Fig. 12.4). Probably because of the difference in amplitude of phase 1, the action potential duration was dramatically shortened in male epicardial cells and phase 2 reentry was inducible in males but not in females.

The main differences in male versus female right ventricular epicardial I_{to} seem to be the major causes of gender differences in Brugada syndrome.

This hypothesis was confirmed using a patch-clamp technique in isolated epicardial cells. It was demonstrated that no sex differences were observed in left ventricular epicardial cells whereas I_{to} density

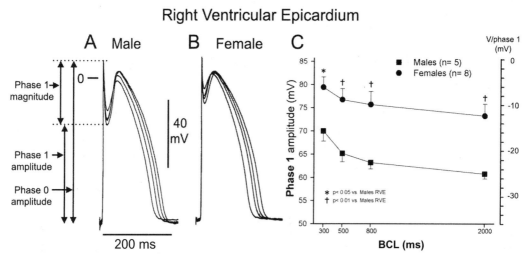

Figure 12.2 Transmembrane action potentials recorded from isolated canine RV epicardial male (**A**) and female (**B**). Pacing cycle length (BCL) 300, 500, 800, and 2000 ms. (**C**) Rate dependence of phase 1 amplitude and voltage at end of phase 1 (V/phase 1, mV) in males (solid squares) versus females (solid circles). Reproduced from Di Diego et al.[14] with the permission of the American Heart Association.

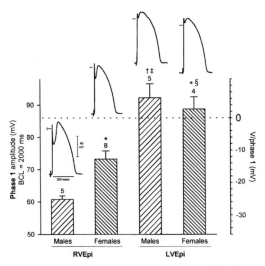

Figure 12.3 Phase 1 amplitude and voltage at end of phase 1 (V/phase 1) of epicardial action potentials recorded from male and female tissue slices from RV (RVEpi) and LV (LVEpi) of canine hearts (BCL = 2000 ms). Insets: representative action potentials from respective tissues. $*p < 0.01$ versus male RVEpi; $\dagger p < 0.001$ versus males RVEpi; $\ddagger p < 0.01$ versus female RVEpi; $\S p < 0.05$ versus female RVEpi. Reproduced from Di Diego et al.[14] with the permission of the American Heart Association.

is smaller and inactivation kinetics more rapid in epicardial cells isolated from female than male right ventricle, leading to a 62% reduction of I_{to} in females compared to males.

Molecular basis for male predominance of Brugada syndrome phenotype

The group of Antzelevitch have provided strong evidence for the role of I_{to} in sex-linked differences of Brugada syndrome. These sex differences could depend on many factors, for example the number of functional channels or regulatory proteins.

The transient Ca^{2+}-independent outward K^+ current (I_{to}) is mainly dependent on Kv4.3 channel activity.[15] Nothing is known concerning the expression of Kv4.3 in epicardial cells from right or left ventricles of males or females. However, it as been shown that in rat myometrium Kv4.3 is downregulated at the end of pregnancy secondary to a rise in estrogen levels.[16] These results suggest that sex-linked differences in Brugada syndrome could be

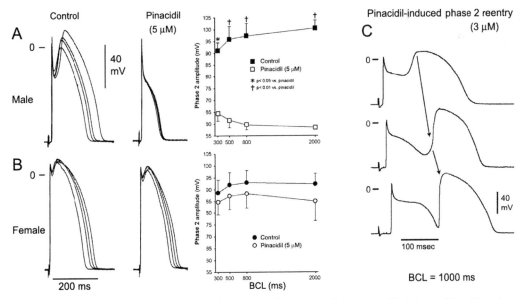

Figure 12.4 Pinacidil induces phase 2 reentry in male, but not female, RV epicardium. Each panel shows superimposed action potentials recorded at pacing cycle length of 300, 500, 800, and 2000 ms in absence (control) and presence of pinacidil (5 μmol/L, 45 min) in male (**A**) and female (**B**) RV epicardial tissue slices. Graphs at the right show rate dependence of phase 2 amplitude (peak plateau) in males versus females before (solid squares) and after pinacidil (open squares). (**C**) Pinacidil (3 μmol/L)-induced phase 2 reentry in male RV epicardium at a pacing cycle length of 1000 ms. Reproduced from Di Diego et al.[14] with the permission of the American Heart Association.

attributed to modification in gene expression of Kv4.3 via sex hormones.

Conclusion

Despite an autosomal dominant transmission, the Brugada syndrome displays a strong male predominance. This male predominance concerns not only the penetrance of the disease but also its severity, the disease being much more dangerous in men than in women.

The male predominance seems to be due to an accentuation of the ventricular cellular heterogeneity of the right ventricular outflow track, largely mediated by a prominent I_{to} current in males. These cellular differences could be good targets for the development of new therapeutic strategies in the Brugada syndrome.

References

1 Chen Q, Kirsch GE, Zhang D *et al.* Genetic basis and molecular mechanism for idiopathic ventricular fibrillation. *Nature* 1998; **392**: 293.

2 Vatta M, Dumaine R, Varghese G *et al.* Genetic and biophysical basis of sudden unexplained nocturnal death syndrome (SUNDS), a disease allelic to Brugada syndrome. *Hum. Mol. Genet.* 2002; **11**: 337–345.

3 Weiss R, Barmada MM, Nguyen T *et al.* Clinical and molecular heterogeneity in the Brugada syndrome: a novel gene locus on chromosome 3. *Circulation* 2002; **105**: 707–713.

4 Schott JJ, Alshinawi C, Kyndt F *et al.* Cardiac conduction defects associate with mutations in *SCN5A*. *Nature Genet.* 1999; **23**: 20–21.

5 Probst V, Kyndt F, Potet F *et al.* Haploinsufficiency in combination with aging causes *SCN5A*-linked hereditary Lenegre disease. *J. Am. Coll. Cardiol.* 2003; **41**: 643–652.

6 Smits JP, Eckardt L, Probst V *et al.* Genotype–phenotype relationship in Brugada syndrome: electrocardiographic features differentiate *SCN5A*-related patients from non-*SCN5A*-related patients. *J. Am. Coll. Cardiol.* 2002; **40**: 350–356.

7 Priori SG, Napolitano C, Gasparini M *et al.* Natural history of Brugada syndrome: insights for risk stratification and management. *Circulation* 2002; **105**: 1342–1347.

8 Brugada J, Brugada R, Antzelevitch C *et al.* Long-term follow-up of individuals with the electrocardiographic pattern of right bundle-branch block and ST-segment elevation in precordial leads V1 to V3. *Circulation* 2002; **105**: 73–78.

9 Wilde AA, Antzelevitch C, Borggrefe M *et al.* Study Group on the Molecular Basis of Arrhythmias of the European Society of Cardiology. Proposed diagnostic criteria for the Brugada syndrome: consensus report. *Circulation* 2002; **106**: 2514–2519.

10 Zareba W, Moss AJ, Locati EH *et al.* International Long QT Syndrome Registry. Modulating effects of age and gender on the clinical course of long QT syndrome by genotype. *J. Am. Coll. Cardiol.* 2003; **42**: 103–109.

11 Yan GX, Antzelevitch C. Cellular basis for the Brugada syndrome and other mechanisms of arrhythmogenesis associated with ST-segment elevation. *Circulation* 1999; **100**: 1660–1666.

12 Antzelevitch C, Shimizu W, Yan GX *et al.* The M cell: its contribution to the ECG and to normal and abnormal electrical function of the heart. *J. Cardiovasc. Electrophysiol.* 1999; **10**: 1124–1152.

13 Antzelevitch C. The Brugada syndrome: ionic basis and arrhythmia mechanisms. *J. Cardiovasc. Electrophysiol.* 2001; **12**: 268–272.

14 Di Diego JM, Cordeiro JM, Goodrow RJ *et al.* Ionic and cellular basis for the predominance of the Brugada syndrome phenotype in males. *Circulation* 2002; **106**: 2004–2011.

15 Hoppe UC, Marban E, Johns DC. Molecular dissection of cardiac repolarization by in vivo Kv4.3 gene transfer. *J. Clin. Invest.* 2000; **105**: 1077–1084.

16 Song M, Helguera G, Eghbali M *et al.* Remodeling of Kv4.3 potassium channel gene expression under the control of sex hormones. *J. Biol. Chem.* 2001; **276**: 31 883–31 890.

CHAPTER 13

Predisposing factors

K. Nademanee, MD, *G. Veerakul*, MD, *M. Schwab*, MD

Summary

Ventricular fibrillation (VF) in patients with the Brugada syndrome has unique clinical characteristics.

1 VF is almost always triggered by a very short coupled PVC (premature ventricular contraction), even though most Brugada patients rarely have PVCs on their 24 hour Holter recording.

2 The majority of VF episodes occur at night during sleep.

3 VF episodes are commonly self-terminating, so Brugada patients may present with symptoms of syncope, seizure, or sleep disturbances with agonal respiration; whereas sustained VF episodes present with cardiac arrests or sudden death.

Mutations of the *SCN5A* sodium channel gene result in the net loss of sodium current, and are the primary genetic defect underlying the arrhythmia substrate of these patients. However, only 10–20% of the patients with the Brugada ECG pattern had the *SCN5A* gene mutation, while the majority of the Brugada patients did not yet have any identifiable genetic defect. Conversely, many patients who were found to have the *SCN5A* gene mutation did not have the overt Brugada ECG marker or arrhythmia symptoms. The clinical spectrum of the Brugada patients ranges from asymptomatic to sudden cardiac death. Patients may have the late onset of VF despite having had an abnormal ECG pattern for decades. Clearly there must be modulating and precipitating factors that influence the clinical presentations and outcomes of the Brugada syndrome patients.

Predisposing factors such as changes in autonomic nervous system activity, hypokalemia, body temperature, or a host of clinical conditions, can affect the arrhythmia and the clinical outcomes in many ways:

1 modifying the VF substrates

2 affecting the gene expression of the ion channel defects

3 affecting the triggering PVCs and the initiating process of VF and

4 influencing the sustaining process of the VF episodes.

Although data related to the precipitating factors in patients with the Brugada syndrome are scarce, there are specific clinical settings and certain environments that could lead to clinical events in these patients. Any modulating factor that causes further reduction of I_{Na} (i.e., sodium channel blockers), will contribute to arrhythmogenesis in the Brugada syndrome. Similarly, any agent or condition which promotes the increase in I_{to} by other mechanisms, such as inhibiting I_{Ca} (e.g., verapamil) or by activating $I_{K\text{-}ATP}$ (e.g., pinacidil), could provoke VF in the Brugada syndrome patients. The purpose of this review is to discuss what we have learned about the predisposing factors over the past decade since the discovery of the syndrome.

Introduction

Although it has been a century since the electrocardiogram was invented, it was but a decade ago that an abnormal ECG of the RBBB pattern and the ST elevation over the right precordial leads was first linked, by Brugada and Brugada, to primary ventricular fibrillation and sudden cardiac death in victims with structurally normal hearts.[1] Recognized as the Brugada syndrome, this clinical entity has drawn attention from cardiologists, electrophysiologists, and physicians worldwide.[2] The syndrome is fascinating to arrhythmia scholars, whose research has advanced our understanding and through which we have learned that the Brugada syndrome affects mainly only males and is a familial disease with an autosomal dominant mode of transmission and has incomplete penetrance.[2,3] Shortly after the syndrome was described by the Brugada, Chen *et al.* first discovered the mutation of sodium channel gene *SCN5A* as the underlying genetic defect of the syndrome,[4] leading to the identification of many more mutations. Unfortunately, only 10–30% of patients diagnosed with the Brugada pattern have the *SCN5A* mutation, leaving the remaining majority with no identified abnormal gene mutation.[5] Conversely, many patients who had the *SCN5A* mutation did not exhibit the abnormal ECG marker.[2] Curiously, the clinical characteristics and ECG pattern of the Brugada syndrome are similar to those of sudden unexplained death syndrome (SUDS) in Southeast Asia.[6] A recent study demonstrates that both syndromes are genetically and functionally the same disorder.[7] The Brugada ECG patterns can wax and wane and can be unmasked by sodium channel blockers.[8] We have made significant progress in understanding the syndrome, and we know that asymptomatic patients with the Brugada ECG pattern have a much better prognosis than those who are symptomatic.[9,10] Nevertheless we are still in the dark about the precipitating factors that induce spontaneous VF episodes in symptomatic patients and why there are not more VF occurrences in asymptomatic patients. Although there is little data related to the modulating factors, we discuss (below) our experiences (largely from SUDS patients in Thailand), which hopefully will shed light on some predisposing factors for ventricular fibrillation and the spectrum of clinical events in Brugada syndrome.

Mode of VF onset

One of the most consistent features of Brugada syndrome is that a short-coupled PVC almost always causes the VF initiation. Figure 13.1 shows an example of VF onset from a SUDS patient from Thailand who had a typical Brugada ECG pattern. The two VF episodes were initiated by PVCs with a short coupling interval at 310 and 320 ms respectively, right at the peak of the T waves, compared to a longer coupling interval PVC approximately 360 ms (asterisk at the lower panel) that fell on the down-slope of the T wave initiating only a couplet. Strangely, this patient had no PVCs during the monitoring period prior to the occurrence of these two VF episodes; once PVCs appeared, they immediately triggered VF. In contrast, patients with ischemic

heart disease and poor left ventricular function tend to have frequent PVCs throughout the 24-hour recordings but they rarely precipitate VF. From this, one can hypothesize that PVCs and VF in the Brugada syndrome are interrelated with respect to arrhythmogenesis, with one triggering the other. In contrast PVC and VF occurrence in patients with ischemic heart disease are not necessarily connected with respect to their arrhythmogenesis. The above case illustrates the typical mode of VF onset in the Brugada patients.

Using the data of 64 VF episodes from 19 patients who had multiple VF episodes detected and successfully treated by an ICD, we found that the mean coupling interval of the PVC that initiated VF was 330 ± 60 ms (Fig. 13.2). The mean cycle length of the preceding sinus beats before the onset of VF was 790 ± 124 ms; no sudden change in heart rate or cycle length prior to the VF onset. The prematurity index, defined as the coupling interval divided by the basic cycle length, was 0.4 ± 0.06. The prematurity index of the PVCs that initiated VF in our patients was short and comparable to that in idiopathic VF observed by Viskin *et al.*[11] The QT index, defined as the coupling interval divided by the actual QT, was 0.89 ± 0.1 and similar to that reported by Viskin *et al.*

This observation of the mode of VF onset fits nicely with the proposed arrhythmia mechanisms of the Brugada syndrome by Antzelevitch.[12] Yan and Antzelevitch used a right ventricular wedge preparation to show that the heterogeneous loss of the action potential dome of the epicardium led to a marked dispersion of the repolarization in the epicardium and transmurally as well.[13] The loss of the action potential dome created not only a large transmural gradient that was responsible for the ST elevation, identical to that observed in the Brugada ECG pattern type 1, but also gave rise to phase 2 reentrant extrasystole that was short-coupled and triggered VF. Using this model, Antzelevitch contends that a prerequisite for phase 2 reentry and the VF substrate is the presence of the Brugada ECG pattern showing the coved type ST elevation and deep negative T wave.[12]

Indeed, several studies show that patients with a spontaneously occurring Brugada ECG marker have a worse prognosis with more symptomatic episodes and cardiac arrests than those whose Brugada patterns have to be unmasked by sodium channel blockers.[8,9] The coved type ECG pattern is

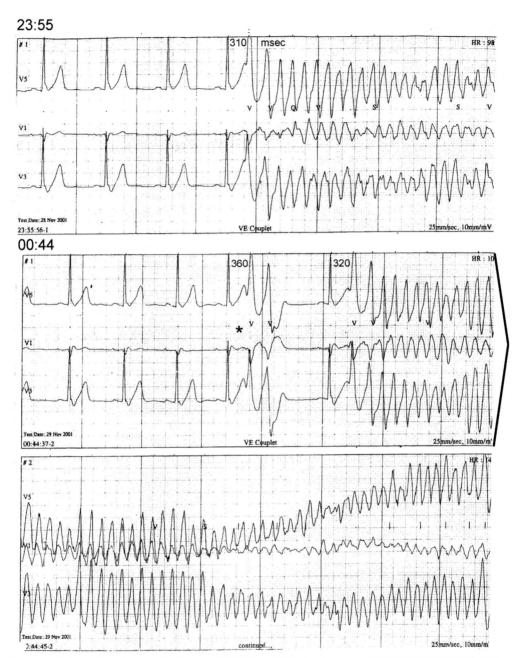

Figure 13.1 Holter tracings show two short-coupled PVC-induced VF during sleep around midnight and relatively longer PVC (asterisk) induced (merely just a couplet).

also associated with a worse prognosis than the saddleback pattern.[14] Therefore, one can speculate that any modulating factors that promote the significant heterogeneous loss of the epicardial dome will precipitate phase 2 reentry and enhance the Brugada substrate for VF. In addition to sodium channel blockers, vagotonic agents,[15] alpha adrenergic agonists,[15] tricyclic antidepressants,[16–19] antihistamine,[20] and cocaine[21] are examples of precipitating factors that could unmask the Brugada syndrome or accentuate ST elevation in patients with the syndrome.

Self-terminated VF episodes versus sustained VF episodes

One of the striking phenomena in the Brugada syndrome is that some patients could have sympto-matic attacks (e.g., syncope, seizure) for years and never have a cardiac arrest.[22] Such patients were commonly misdiagnosed and treated as vasovagal syncope or Grand mal seizure. Similarly, SUDS patients in Thailand, whose clinical presentations are agonal respiration at night or laborious breathing, could have symptoms for years before being diagnosed with the Brugada syndrome.[23] Since VF is the only arrhythmia associated with the Brugada syndrome, the VF episodes in these patients are quite commonly self-terminating, contradicting the conventional wisdom that VF episodes are equivalent to death. Indeed, the growing numbers of patients with this syndrome have taught us that VF in patients with a structurally normal heart, unlike those with ischemic heart disease, often spontaneously reverts back to sinus rhythm. Figure 13.3 shows an example of one of the many asymptomatic non-sustained VF episodes in SUDS patients who have the coved type Brugada ECG pattern. This patient also has multiple sustained episodes treated successfully with ICD. Interestingly, before the ICD implantation, patients were symptomatic for a couple of years with the symptoms of struggling during sleep and difficulty breathing at night. These symptoms correlated well with VF episodes detected by the ICD and the patient had frequent self-terminated VF episodes without dying; he was quite fortunate to be treated with ICD before anything catastrophic occurred.

The question then arises, why are some VF episodes sustained and lead to sudden death or cardiac arrests? What are the predisposing and precipitating factors that modulate the substrate resulting in the perpetuation of the VF? Our line up of likely culprits includes the autonomic nervous system, hypokalemia, factors that enhance loss of the sodium channel function, and changes in the repolarization (see below).

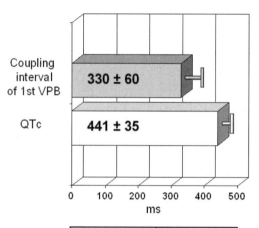

Cycle length (ms)	790 ± 124
QT index (ms)	0.89 ± 0.1
Prematurity index (ms)	0.4 ± 0.6

Figure 13.2 Characteristics of the onset of ventricular fibrillation. Mode of onset of VF analyzed from 64 VF episodes. Coupling interval (mean ± SD) is the interval from the last sinus beat to the first PVC. QTc (mean ± SD) is calculated from the preceding sinus beats. Cycle length (mean ± SD) is measure from the preceding sinus beats. Prematurity index = coupling interval/RR interval. QT index = CI/QT.

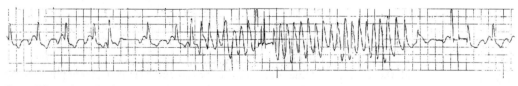

Figure 13.3 An example of spontaneous terminated VF (see text for more details).

Circadian variation of the VF occurrences

Unlike ischemic VF and sudden death in post MI patients, VF and sudden death in the Brugada syndrome usually occurs at rest and at night. Figure 13.4 shows the circadian pattern of 64 VF episodes from our SUDS population who had ICD treatment. Data show that there is a nocturnal increase in VF occurrences that peak around midnight in the SUDS population. The increased incidence of VF at night in this particular syndrome is similar to the arrhythmia pattern of patients with LQT3, whose sudden death rate is common at night and among the highest of the different subsets of long QT syndromes. It is noteworthy that both syndromes share one thing in common: both have abnormal sodium channel *SCN5A* gene mutations.

While it is unknown whether there is an association between sleep or nocturnal factors and the *SCN5A* gene expression, other factors such as circadian variation of sympatho-vagal balance, hormones, and various metabolic factors could very well play a role in the genesis of VF at night in the Brugada syndrome.

Autonomic nervous system

The role of the autonomic nervous system in ventricular arrhythmias has been well established. However, its role in precipitating VF in the Brugada syndrome is more complex. The effect of sympathetic stimulation by isoproterenol infusion, result-

ing in normalization of the Brugada pattern, suggests that sympathetic activity could modify the VF substrate.[24] As mentioned earlier, the presence of the Brugada ECG pattern is probably a prerequisite for the increased risk of sudden cardiac death and the normalization of the ECG pattern is associated with a decreased risk.[12] This concept is strengthened by the fact that some patients with 'VF storms' associated with the Brugada syndrome could be effectively treated with isoproterenol infusion.[25] On the other hand, increased vagal tone could be arrhythmogenic in the Brugada syndrome patients. Increased vagal tone, as well as acute beta-blockade, was found to promote VF induction in the electrophysiology laboratory.[15] Therefore, it is plausible that at night during sleep, when the vagal tone is usually increased and associated with the withdrawal of sympathetic activity, the VF substrate was modulated and more susceptible to arrhythmogenesis of VF. Supporting this supposition is the observation of Litovsky and Antzelevitch who showed that acetylcholine facilitates loss of the action potential dome and in turn accentuates the ST segment elevation.[26]

Kasanuki *et al.* also showed a sudden increase of vagal activity as measured by heart rate variability just before the episodes of VF in a patient with Brugada syndrome.[15] However, Krittayaphong *et al.* studied heart rate variability from 24-hour Holter data of SUDS patients with the Brugada ECG marker, aiming to determine the circadian pattern of sympathetic and parasympathetic activity.[27] Surprisingly, they found decreased heart rate variability at night in SUDS patients when compared to the

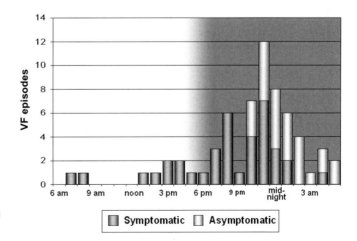

Figure 13.4 A bar graph show distribution of 64 VF episodes detected from ICD interrogation. Note the nocturnal increase of VF episodes around midnight.

control group and suggested that these patients had an abnormal increase in sympathetic activity or a decrease in the vagal tone at night. Although the explanation for the different findings between Kasanuki *et al.* and that of Krittayaphong *et al.* is unknown, it is clear that the sympatho-vagal balance in the Brugada patients plays a significant role in the circadian variation of the VF occurrences in these patients. However, further studies are needed to clearly define and understand the complex interplay between the autonomic nervous system and the arrhythmic mechanisms of the Brugada syndrome.

Wichter *et al.* demonstrated an abnormal ^{123}I-MIBG uptake in 8 (17%) of the 17 Brugada syndrome patients but none in the control group.[28] There was segmental reduction of ^{123}I-MIBG in the inferior and the septal left ventricular wall, indicating presynaptic sympathetic dysfunction (uptake 1). Although this finding is intriguing, it is unclear what role this reduced uptake function plays in the arrhythmogenesis of the Brugada syndrome. In fact, the reduced uptake represents a complex sympathetic–parasympathetic interaction and if there is reduced pre-synaptic reuptake of norepinephrine and epinephrine, then vagal tone may increase at rest. However, at the same time, the postsynaptic adrenergic receptor site may be supersensitive to circulating catecholamine and could have an exaggerated response to the increase in adrenergic activity, i.e., during stress. Thus, it is likely that there are dynamic changes in sympatho-vagal balance in the Brugada syndrome patients and in turn these produce variable effects on the VF substrate in these patients.

Hypokalemia

Hypokalemia has been implicated as a contributing cause for SUDS prevalence in the Northeastern region of Thailand, where potassium deficiency is endemic.[23] Serum potassium in the Northeastern Thailand population is significantly lower than that of the population in Bangkok, which lies in the central part of Thailand where potassium is abundant in food. Hypokalemia is a well-known predisposing factor to ventricular arrhythmias, especially when associated with abnormal repolarization. One can postulate that hypokalemia could worsen the dispersion of repolarization in the Brugada/SUDS patients and in turn precipitate PVCs and cause the

perpetuation of VF. Furthermore, it has been shown that there is commonly a shift of serum potassium into the muscular compartment between midnight and 7 am, decreasing the amount of serum potassium.[29] If this phenomenon indeed occurs in SUDS patients, then it is likely that low serum potassium is a key factor that precipitates VF at night within these patients.

Recently, an interesting case report of a 60-year-old man who had asymptomatic Brugada syndrome, without a family history of sudden cardiac death, showed how hypokalemia could provoke VF leading to syncope/cardiac arrest.[30] This patient initially received steroid treatment for asthma, lowering his serum potassium from 3.8 mmol/L on admission to 3.4 mmol/L and 2.9 mmol/L on the 7th day and 8th day after admission, respectively. Both were associated with unconsciousness and spontaneously terminated VF episodes. This case shares many similarities with our SUDS patients in Thailand and provides a very strong argument that hypokalemia is an important precipitating factor in the Brugada syndrome patients.

Sleep and heavy meal

Since a majority of VF episodes occur at night, the question remains, is a sleep disorder a trigger of VF? Thus far, none of our sleep studies in our SUDS patients found any evidence of sleep disorder, including sleep apnea.

One theory that many SUDS scholars have casually discussed as a possible precipitating factor is eating a heavy meal at dinnertime before retiring to bed. The Thai Ministry of Public Health Report (1990) suggested that a large meal of glutinous rice ('sticky rice') or carbohydrates that was eaten on the night of death precipitated the SUDS attacks.[23] Both carbohydrates and glutinous rice have been shown to shift potassium into cells and in turn lower the amount of serum potassium. A recent study by Nokami *et al.* showed that glucose and insulin could unmask the Brugada ECG marker or accentuate the J junction elevation of the ST segment.[31] They observed a slight decrease in the serum potassium in their study patients but this did not reach statistical significance. Nevertheless, these findings bode well for heavy carbohydrate meals as a precipitating factor for sudden death in SUDS patients.

Body temperature and febrile illness

Dumaine *et al.* discovered the T1620M missense mutation that causes accelerated inactivation of the sodium channel only at the physiologic body temperature but not at room temperature.[32] Identification of this temperature-sensitive gene that precipitates the net loss of sodium current prompted investigators to recognize that a hot climate and body temperature may be important modulating factors. Indeed, several case reports have emerged recently demonstrating that febrile illness could unmask the Brugada syndrome and precipitate VF occurrences.[33–37] We have encountered a case of a young male patient who died suddenly after a spiking fever of 40°C following abdominal surgery. Upon review of the ECG, the patient had the typical Brugada ECG pattern, but the victim had no prior medical problems and had been asymptomatic. Unfortunately, we did not have an opportunity to perform a genetic study to determine whether the patient had T1620M mutation.

The Northeastern part of Thailand where SUDS is prevalent is well known for its hot climate, the temperature reaching as high as 41°C. It is again not clear how much climate influences the victims of SUDS in Thailand, but a study is underway. It is entirely possible that a high temperature or a febrile state could modulate the functional expressions of mutational channels in other genes responsible for the Brugada syndrome. In the meantime, physicians should consider temperature as a cause for arrhythmogenesis of the Brugada syndrome. They should be aware of the association between temperature and the Brugada syndrome during diagnosis and treatment, advising patients to treat febrile states promptly.

Miscellaneous factors

In addition to the above precipitating factors, it is clear that any modulating factors that cause further reduction in I_{Na} will contribute to arrhythmogenesis of the Brugada syndrome (Fig. 13.5 and Table 13.1). Antzelevitch and colleagues believe that a decrease in I_{Na} will result in unopposed I_{to}, allowing greater contribution of I_{to} to phase 1 of the action potential; this thereby produces more negative membrane potential of the phase 1 of the action potential. If the end of the phase 1 negative potential is below the threshold of the I_{Ca}, then all or none repolarization of the action potential will occur, causing the loss of the action potential dome and markedly abbreviating the action potential duration. As mentioned earlier, the loss of an action potential dome is usually heterogeneous, creating transmural and regional dispersion of the repolarization, and provides an excellent substrate for phase 2 reentry that could open a vulnerable window for reentry in precipitating polymorphic VT/VF.

Similarly, any agents or conditions that promote the increase in I_{to} by other mechanisms, such as inhibiting I_{Ca} (e.g., verapamil) or by activating I_{K-ATP} (e.g., pinacidil), could provoke VF in the Brugada syndrome patients.

Patients with the Brugada syndrome could have

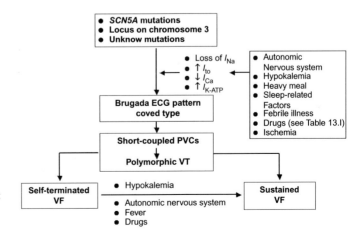

Figure 13.5 Proposed pathophysiologic mechanisms of Brugada syndrome with respect to predisposing factors.

Table 13.1 A list of agents or drugs that could precipitate Brugada syndrome.

Agent or drug	Reference
Antiarrhythmic drugs	
• class Ia (except quinidine) and class Ic antiarrhythmic drugs	
• (?) calcium antagonist	
Tricyclic depressant	15–18
Antihistamine	19
Anesthetic agents	37
Cocaine	20
Vagotonic agents	14, 23
α-agonists	14, 23

other concomitant diseases that could precipitate VF occurrence. For example, vasospastic angina could cause ischemia, a well-known cause of phase 2 reentry, in tandem with the Brugada substrate this can clearly precipitate VF.[38] As research in the syndrome continues at a rapid pace, we will learn more about factors that contribute to the genesis of VF and clinical presentations of the syndrome. Undoubtedly, this will lead to better protection and treatment of our Brugada syndrome patients.

Summary and conclusions

The Brugada syndrome is a fascinating clinical entity that has a dynamic interplay between a plethora of predisposing factors (i.e., autonomic nervous system, antiarrhythmic drugs, hypokalemia, and fever) and the well-established ion-channelopathy. Just like the other arrhythmic syndromes that came before, WPW or long QT syndromes, we now know that the Brugada syndrome has various precipitating factors that could modulate the electrophysiologic substrates and could trigger malignant arrhythmias. The syndrome provides us with an excellent arrhythmia model for arrhythmogenesis of VF via the mechanisms by which the loss of sodium-channel function and the balance between outward and inward currents play a significant role in marked dispersion of the repolarization and phase 2 reentry. Future research will further our understanding of the pathophysiologic mechanisms of the syndrome, genetics of the ionic channel, and precipitating factors.

References

1 Brugada P, Brugada J. Right bundle branch block, persistent ST segment elevation and sudden cardiac death: a distinct clinical and electrocardiographic syndrome: a multicenter report. *J. Am. Coll. Cardiol.* 1992; **20**: 1391–1396.

2 Antzelevitch C, Brugada P, Brugada J, Brugada R, Towbin JA, Nademanee K. Brugada syndrome, 1992–2002 An historical perspective. *J. Am. Coll. Cardiol.* 2003; **41**(10): 1665–1671.

3 Antzelevitch C, Brugada P, Brugada J, Brugada R, Nademanee K, Towbin JA. *The Brugada Syndrome.* 1999. Armonk, NY: Futura Publishing Company, Inc.

4 Chen Q, Kirsch GE, Zhang D *et al.* Genetic basis and molecular mechanisms for idiopathic ventricular fibrillation. *Nature* 1998; **392**: 293–296.

5 Wilde A, Antzelevith C, Borggrefe M *et al.* Proposed criteria of the Brugada syndrome. *Eur. Heart J.* 2002; **23**: 1648–1654.

6 Nademanee K, Veerakul G, Nimmannit S *et al.* Arrhythmogenic marker for the sudden unexplained death syndrome in Thai men. *Circulation* 1997; **96**: 2595–2600.

7 Vatta M, Dumaine R, Varghese G *et al.* Genetic and biophysical basis of sudden unexplained nocturnal death syndrome (SUNDS), a disease allelic to Brugada syndrome. *Hum. Mol. Genet.* 2002; **11**: 337–345.

8 Brugada R, Brugada J, Antzelevitch C *et al.* Sodium channel blockers identify risk for sudden death in patients with ST-segment elevation and right bundle branch block but structurally normal hearts. *Circulation* 2000; **101**: 510–515.

9 Priori SG, Napolitano C, Gasparini M *et al.* Natural history of Brugada syndrome: insights for risk stratification and management. *Circulation* 2002; **105**: 1342–1347.

10 Brugada J, Brugada R, Antzelevitch C, Towbin J, Nademanee K, Brugada P. Long-term follow-up of individuals with the electrocardiographic pattern of right bundle-branch block and ST-segment elevation in precordial leads V(1) to V(3). *Circulation* 2002; **105**: 73–78.

11 Viskin S, Lesh MD, Eldar M *et al.* Mode of onset of malignant ventricular arrhythmias in idiopathic ventricular fibrillation. *J. Cardiovasc. Electrophysiol.* 1997; **8**: 1115–1120.

12 Antzelevitch C. The Brugada syndrome: ionic basis and arrhythmia mechanisms. *J. Cardiovasc. Electrophysiol.* 2001; **12**: 268–272.

13 Yan GX, Antzelevitch C. Cellular basis for the Brugada Syndrome and other mechanisms of arrhythmogenesis associated with ST segment elevation. *Circulation* 1999; **100**: 1660–1666.

14 Atarashi H, Ogawa S, Harumi K, Sugimoto T, Inoue H. Three-year follow-up of patients with right bundle branch block and ST segment elevation in the right precordial

leads: Japanese Registry of Brugada Syndrome. *JACC* 2001; **37**: 1916–1920.

15 Kasanuki H, Ohnishi S, Ohtuka M *et al.* Idiopathic ventricular fibrillation induced with vagal activity in patients without obvious heart disease. *Circulation* 1997; **95**: 2277–2285.

16 Babaliaros VC, Hurst JW. Tricyclic antidepressants and the Brugada syndrome: an example of Brugada waves appearing after the administration of desipramine. *Clin. Cardiol.* 2002; **25**: 395–398.

17 Goldgran-Toledano D, Sideris G, Kevorkian JP. Overdose of cyclic antidepressants and the Brugada syndrome. *N. Engl. J. Med.* 2002; **346**: 1591–1592.

18 Rouleau F, Asfar P, Boulet S *et al.* Transient ST segment elevation in right precordial leads induced by psychotropic drugs: relationship to the Brugada syndrome. *J. Cardiovasc. Electrophysiol.* 2001; **12**: 61–65.

19 Tada H, Sticherling C, Oral H, Morady F. Brugada syndrome mimicked by tricyclic antidepressant overdose. *J. Cardiovasc. Electrophysiol.* 2001; **12**: 275.

20 Pastor A, Nunez A, Cantale C, Cosio FG. Asymptomatic brugada syndrome case unmasked during dimenhydrinate infusion. *J. Cardiovasc. Electrophysiol.* 2001; **12**: 1192–1194.

21 Ortega-Carnicer J, Bertos-Polo J, Gutierrez-Tirado C. Aborted sudden death, transient Brugada pattern, and wide QRS dysrrhythmias after massive cocaine ingestion. *J. Electrocardiol.* 2001; **34**: 345–349.

22 Bjerregaard P, Gussak I, Kotar SL *et al.* Recurrent syncope in a patient with prominent J-wave. *Am. Heart J.* 1994; **127**: 1426–1430.

23 Nimannnit S, Malasit P, Chaovakul V, Susaengrat W, Vasuvattakul S, Nilwaranangkur S. Pathogenesis of unexplained nocturnal death and endemic distal renal tubular acidosis. *Lancet* 1991; **338**: 930–932.

24 Miyazaki T, Mitamura H, Miyoshi S, Soejima K, Aizawa Y, Ogawa S. Autonomic and antiarrhythmic drug modulation of ST segment elevation in patients with Brugada syndrome. *J. Am. Coll. Cardiol.* 1996; **27**: 1061–1070.

25 Tanaka H, Kinoshita O, Uchikawa S *et al.* Successful prevention of recurrent ventricular fibrillation by intravenous isoproterenol in a patient with Brugada syndrome. *Pacing Clin. Electrophysiol.* 2001; **24**: 1293–1294.

26 Litovsky SH, Antzelevitch C: Differences in the electrophysiologic response of canine ventricular subendocar-

dium and subepicardium to acetylcholine and isoproterenol. A direct effect of acetylcholine in ventricular myocardium. *Circ. Res.* 1990; **67**: 615–627.

27 Krittayaphong R, Veerakul G, Bhuripanyo K, Jirasirirojanakorn K, Nademanee K. Heart rate variability in patients with sudden unexpected cardiac arrest in Thailand. *Am. J. Cardiol.* 2003; **91**: 77–81.

28 Wichter T, Matheja P, Eckardt L *et al.* Cardiac autnomic dysfunction in Brugada syndrome. *Circulation* 2002; **105**: 702–706.

29 Andres R. Cader G, Goldman P, Zeirler K. Net potassium movement between resting muscle and plasma in man in the basal state and during the night. *J. Clin. Invest.* 1957; **36**: 723–729.

30 Araki J, Konno T, Itoh H, Ino H, Shimizu M. Brugada syndrome with ventricular tachycardia and fibrillation related to hypokalemia. *Circ. J.* 2003; **67** (1): 93–95.

31 Nogami A, Nakao M, Kubota S *et al.* Enhancement of J-ST-segment elevation by the glucose and insulin test in Brugada syndrome. *Pacing Clin. Electrophysiol.* 2003; **26**(1 Pt 2): 332–337.

32 Dumaine R, Towbin JA, Brugada P *et al.* Ionic mechanisms responsible for the electrocardiographic phenotype of the Brugada syndrome are temperature dependent. *Circ. Res.* 1999; **85**: 803–809.

33 Antzelevitch, C, Brugada, R. Fever and the Brugada syndrome. *Pacing Clin. Electrophysiol.* 2002; **25**: 1537–1539.

34 Morita H, Nagase S, Kusano K, Ohe T. Spontaneous T wave alternans and premature ventricular contractions during febrile illness in a patient with Brugada syndrome. *J. Cardiovasc. Electrophysiol.* 2002; **13**(8): 816–818.

35 Saura D, Garcia-Alberola A, Carrillo P, Pascual D, Martinez-Sanchez J, Valdes M. Brugada-like electrocardiographic pattern induced by fever. *Pacing Clin. Electrophysiol.* 2002; **25**(5): 856–859.

36 Porres JM, Brugada J, Urbistondo V, Garcia F, Reviejo K, Marco P. Fever unmasking the Brugada syndrome. *Pacing Clin. Electrophysiol.* 2002; **25**: 1646–1648.

37 Kum LCC, Fung JWH, Sanderson JE. Brugada syndrome unmasked by febrile illness. *Pacing Clin. Electrophysiol.* 2002; **25**: 1660–1661.

38 Chinushi M, Kuroe Y, Ito E, Tagawa M, Aizawa Y. Vasospastic angina accompanied by Brugada-type electrocardiographic abnormalities. *J. Cardiovasc. Electrophysiol.* 2001; **12**(1): 108–111.

CHAPTER 14

Acquired forms of Brugada syndrome

W. Shimizu, MD, PhD

Summary

Experimental studies have suggested that an intrinsically prominent transient outward current (I_{to})-mediated action potential (AP) notch and a subsequent loss of AP dome in the epicardium, but not in the endocardium of the right ventricular outflow tract (RVOT), give rise to a transmural voltage gradient, resulting in ST segment elevation in leads V_1–V_3 and induction of subsequent ventricular fibrillation (VF) due to the mechanism of phase 2 reentry. Because the maintenance of the AP dome is determined by the balance of currents active at the end of phase 1 of the AP, any interventions that increase outward currents (e.g., I_{to}, adenosine triphosphate sensitive potassium current [$I_{K\text{-}ATP}$], slow and fast activating components of delayed rectifier potassium current [I_{Ks}, I_{Kr}]) or decrease inward currents (e.g., L-type calcium current [$I_{Ca\text{-}L}$], fast sodium current [I_{Na}]) at the end of phase 1 of the AP can accentuate or unmask ST segment elevation, similar to that found in Brugada syndrome. A number of drugs and conditions, which cause an outward shift in current active at the end of phase 1, have been reported to induce transient Brugada-like ST segment elevation. This is the so-called 'acquired' form of Brugada syndrome similar to the 'acquired' form of long QT syndrome (LQTS).

Among antiarrhythmic drugs, class IC drugs (flecainide, pilsicainide, propafenone) most effectively amplify or unmask ST segment elevation secondary to their strong effect to block fast I_{Na}, and are used as a diagnostic tool in latent Brugada syndrome with transient or no spontaneous ST segment elevation. Class IA antiarrhythmic drugs (ajmaline, procainamide, disopyramide, cibenzoline, etc.), which exhibit less use-dependent blocking of fast I_{Na} due to faster dissociation of the drug for the Na^+ channels, show weaker ST segment elevation than class IC drugs. In contrast, class IB drugs (mexiletine, lidocaine, etc.) have little or no effect on fast I_{Na} at moderate and slow heart rates, resulting in their inability to cause an ST segment elevation. Other antiarrhythmic drugs such as $I_{Ca\text{-}L}$ blockers (verapamil, etc.) and β-blockers would be expected to unmask ST segment elevation and possibly to induce VF as a result of their ability to inhibit $I_{Ca\text{-}L}$. Several psychotropic drugs including tricyclic antidepressants (amitriptyline, nortriptyline, desipramine, clomipramine, etc.), tetracyclic antidepressants (maprotiline, etc.), phenothiazines (perphenazine, cyamemazine, etc.), and selective serotonin reuptake inhibitors (fluoxetine, etc.) have been reported to unmask Brugada-like ST segment elevation, secondary to block of fast I_{Na} associated with overdoses of these drugs. A sedating, first-generation histaminic H1 receptor antagonist (dimenhydrinate) and cocaine intoxication have also been shown to unmask the Brugada syndrome.

Electrolyte abnormalities, such as hyperkalemia and hypercalcemia, have been reported to be associated with ST segment elevation in the right precordial leads such as in Brugada syndrome.

Acute myocardial infarction or ischemia due to

vasospasm involving the RVOT mimics ST segment elevation similar to that in Brugada syndrome. This effect is secondary to the depression of I_{Ca-L} and the activation of I_{K-ATP} during ischemia, and suggests that patients with congenital and possibly 'acquired' forms of Brugada syndrome may be at a higher risk for ischemia-related sudden cardiac death.

The increased insulin level induced by glucose is reported to amplify or unmask ST segment elevation in Brugada patients mainly due to an increase in an outward current by activating Na^+/K^+ pump, which may be linked to circadian or day-to-day variation of ST segment elevation.

A number of reports have demonstrated that febrile state (hyperthermia) unmasked Brugada-like ST segment elevation and provoked VF as a result of a reduced I_{Na} at high temperature. On the other hand, a prominent J wave associated with ST segment elevation, which is referred to as an Osborn wave, has long been described in hypothermic states due to accidental exposure to cold, probably due to augmented I_{to}.

A mechanical compression of the RVOT by a mediastinal tumor or haemopericardium is reported to produce a Brugada-like ST segment elevation probably as a result of pressure-induced changes in ion channel current in the epicardium of the RVOT.

The genetic background in patients with this 'acquired' form of Brugada syndrome is unclear. However, mutations in *SCN5A* or other candidate genes will likely be identified in the future, like those in congenital LQTS genes in some patients with the 'acquired' form of LQTS.

This is all summarized in Table 14.1.

Introduction

Brugada syndrome is characterized by ST segment elevation in the right precordial leads (V_1–V_3) and an episode of ventricular fibrillation (VF) in the absence of structural heart disease.[1–12] The incidence of Brugada syndrome is higher in Asian countries, including Thailand and Japan, than in the U.S. and European countries, in which more than 80% of those afflicted are adult males.[13–20] Two specific types of ST segment elevation are observed in this syndrome; coved type and saddleback type. Coved type ST segment elevation is of particular impor-

tance in relation to a higher incidence of VF and sudden cardiac death.[8,10,11,14]

Genetic studies have so far identified only one gene mutation linked to Brugada syndrome on *SCN5A*, the gene that encodes for the α subunit of the Na^+ channel.[21,22] The *SCN5A* mutations linked to Brugada syndrome have been reported to result in a reduction in the availability of Na^+ current [I_{Na}] (loss of function). The reduced I_{Na} are secondary to (1) failure of the Na^+ channel to express; (2) a shift in the voltage- and time-dependence of I_{Na} activation, inactivation, or reactivation; (3) entry of the channel into an intermediate inactivation state from which it recovers more slowly; and/or (4) acceleration of the inactivation of the Na^+ channel.

Recent experimental studies have suggested that an intrinsically prominent transient outward current (I_{to})-mediated action potential (AP) notch and a subsequent loss of AP dome in the epicardium, but not in the endocardium of the right ventricular outflow tract (RVOT), give rise to a transmural voltage gradient, resulting in the ST segment elevation in leads V_1–V_3 and the induction of subsequent VF due to the mechanism of phase 2 reentry.[23–25] The maintenance of the AP dome is determined by the balance of currents active at the end of phase 1 of the AP (principally I_{to} and L-type calcium current [I_{Ca-L}]). Therefore, any interventions that increase outward currents (e.g., I_{to}, adenosine triphosphate sensitive potassium current [I_{K-ATP}], slow and fast activating components of delayed rectifier potassium current [I_{Ks}, I_{Kr}]) or decrease inward currents (e.g., I_{Ca-L}, fast I_{Na}) at the end of phase 1 of the AP can accentuate ST segment elevation, as found in Brugada patients (Fig. 14.1).

The ST segment elevation is dynamic, waxing and waning day-to-day even in patients with Brugada syndrome.[26,27] The ST segment elevation is also reported to be modulated by several drugs (mainly antiarrhythmic drugs) and autonomic agents.[13] Among them, class IC antiarrhythmic drugs most effectively amplify or unmask ST segment elevation secondary to their strong effect of blocking fast I_{Na}, and are used as a diagnostic tool in latent Brugada syndrome with transient or no spontaneous ST segment elevation.[28–35] Moreover, several drugs and conditions which cause an outward shift in current active at the end of phase 1 described above are reported to induce transient ST segment elevation like

Table 14.1 Acquired forms of Brugada syndrome.

Drug-induced	
I Antiarrhythmic drugs	
1 Na⁺ channel blockers	Class IC drugs (flecainide[28,29,31,32,35], pilsicainide[30,34], propafenone[33])
	Class IA drugs (ajmaline[32,36], procainamide[13,32], disopyramide[13,18], cibenzoline[37])
2 Ca²⁺ channel blockers	Verapamil
3 β blockers	Propranolol etc.
II Antianginal drugs	
1 Ca²⁺ channel blockers	Nefedipine, diltiazem
2 Nitrate	Isosorbide dinitrate, nitroglycerine[26]
3 K⁺ channel openers	Nicorandil
III Psychotropic drugs	
1 Tricyclic antidepressants	Amitriptyline[40,41], nortriptyline[42], desipramine[43], clomipramine[44], etc.
2 Tetracyclic antidepressants	Maprotiline[40]
3 Phenothiazine	Perphenazine[40], cyamemazine[41]
4 Selective serotonin reuptake inhibitors	Fluoxetine[41]
IV Other drugs	
1 Histaminic H1 receptor antagonists	Dimenhydrinate[45]
2 Cocaine intoxication[46,47]	
3 Alcohol intoxication	
Electrolyte abnormalities	Hyperkalemia[48–50]
	Hypercalcemia[51,52]
Acute ischemia	Right ventricular infarction/ischemia[53–55]
	Vasospatic angina[56–59]
Increased insulin level[60,61]	
Hyperthermia (febrile state)[62–68]	
Hypothermia[71,72]	
Mechanical compression of right ventricular outflow tract	Mediastinal tumor[73], haemopericardium[74] etc.

that in Brugada syndrome. This is described by some as an 'acquired' form of Brugada syndrome similar to the 'acquired' form of long QT syndrome (LQTS). In this chapter, we review all known causes of a Brugada-like pattern in the ECG.

Drug-induced Brugada syndrome

Antiarrhythmic drugs
Na⁺ channel blockers
Class IC antiarrhythmic drugs (flecainide, pilsicainide, propafenone) produce the most pronounced ST segment elevation, thus they most effectively unmask latent Brugada syndrome as a di-

agnostic tool.[28–35] In other words, class IC drugs most easily induce the 'acquired' form of Brugada syndrome. This effect is secondary to strong use-dependent blocking of fast I_{Na} with class IC drugs due to their slow dissociation from the Na⁺ channels. Among the class IC drugs, pilsicainide, a pure class IC drug developed in Japan, is thought to more strongly induce ST segment elevation than flecainide, which is widely used throughout the world and mildly blocks I_{to}[34] (Fig. 14.2). Therefore, pilsicainide may have the potential to produce false positive result on drug challenge test to unmask latent Brugada syndrome. Class IA antiarrhythmic drugs (ajmaline, procainamide, disopyramide, cibenzoline, etc.), which exhibit less use-dependent block of fast I_{Na} due to faster dissociation of the drug for the Na$^+$ channels, show a weaker ST segment elevation than class IC drugs[13,31,32,36,37] (Figs 14.3A,B). Among the class IA drugs, the weaker accentuation of the ST segment elevation produced by disopyra-

mide is likely due to its modest action to block I_{to} as well as its smaller effect on fast I_{Na}.[31,38] In contrast, quinidine, another class IA drug generally normalizes ST segment elevation owing to its relatively strong I_{to} blocking effect, and is proposed as a pharmacologic treatment for the Brugada syndrome.[39] Class IB drugs (mexiletine, lidocaine, etc.) dissociate from the Na$^+$ channel rapidly and therefore block fast I_{Na} principally at rapid rates. At moderate and slow heart rates, class IB drugs have little or no effect on fast I_{Na}, and thus are unable to cause ST segment elevation[31] (Fig. 14.3C).

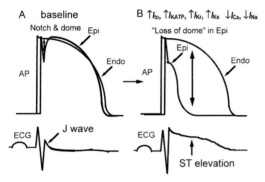

Figure 14.1 Cellular mechanism of ST segment elevation in 'acquired' form of Brugada syndrome. (A) An intrinsically prominent transient outward current (I_{to})-mediated action potential (AP) notch in the epicardium (Epi), but not in the endocardium (Endo), gives rise to a transmural voltage gradient, underlying J wave under baseline condition. (B) Because the loss of the AP dome is produced by an outward shift of currents active at the end of phase 1 of the AP, any interventions that increase outward currents (e.g., I_{to}, adenosine triphosphate sensitive potassium current [I_{K-ATP}], slow and fast activating components of delayed rectifier potassium current [I_{Ks}, I_{Kr}]) or decrease inward currents (e.g., L-type calcium current [I_{Ca-L}], fast sodium current [I_{Na}]) can accentuate ST segment elevation.

Ca^{2+} channel blockers

Verapamil, an I_{Ca-L} blocker, is usually used as a first line of therapy to terminate or prevent paroxysmal supraventricular tachycardia due to accessory pathway or atrioventricular dual pathway. Figure 14.4 illustrates the 'acquired' form of Brugada syndrome induced by intravenous verapamil in a patient with atrio-ventricular nodal reentrant tachycardia (AVNRT) (Fig. 14.4A). In this case, intravenous administration of 10 mg verapamil successfully terminated AVNRT, but unmasked prominent coved and saddleback ST segment elevation in leads V$_1$ and V$_2$ (Fig. 14.4B), which disappeared after washout of verapamil (Fig. 14.4C).

β-blockers

β-blockers are also widely used as antiarrhythmic drugs or as a first line of therapy for vasovagal syn-

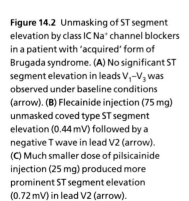

Figure 14.2 Unmasking of ST segment elevation by class IC Na$^+$ channel blockers in a patient with 'acquired' form of Brugada syndrome. (A) No significant ST segment elevation in leads V$_1$–V$_3$ was observed under baseline conditions (arrow). (B) Flecainide injection (75 mg) unmasked coved type ST segment elevation (0.44 mV) followed by a negative T wave in lead V2 (arrow). (C) Much smaller dose of pilsicainide injection (25 mg) produced more prominent ST segment elevation (0.72 mV) in lead V2 (arrow).

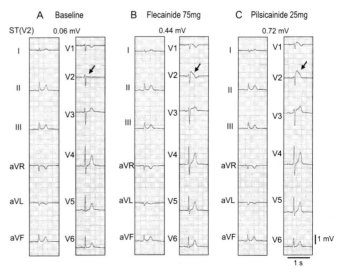

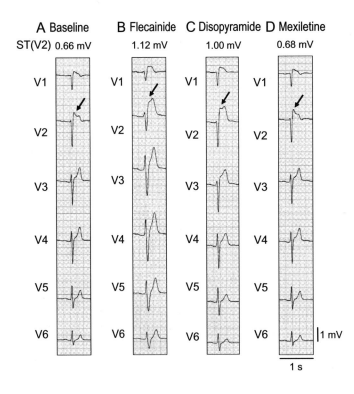

Figure 14.3 Six precordial leads ECG in a patient with diagnosed Brugada syndrome (**A**) under baseline conditions, (**B**) after 100 mg flecainide injection (class IC drug), (**C**) after 100 mg disopyramide injection (class IA drug), and (**D**) after 125 mg mexiletine injection (class IB drug). Saddleback type ST segment elevation was seen in lead V_2 (0.66 mV) under baseline conditions (**A**, arrow). Flecainide more markedly accentuated the ST segment elevation (1.12 mV) than disopyramide (1.00 mV) (**B** and **C**, arrows), while mexiletine had no effect on the ST segment elevation (0.68 mV) (**D**, arrow).

cope. The administration of β-blockers would be expected to accentuate ST segment elevation and possibly to induce VF as a result of inhibiting I_{Ca-L}, if the patients were affected with the 'acquired' form of Brugada syndrome. This must be always taken into account in the use of β-blockers for any arrhythmia or vasovagal syncope.

Antianginal drugs

The first line of therapy for ischemic heart diseases is Ca^{2+} antagonists (nefedipine, diltiazem, etc.) or nitrates which also have a blocking action of I_{Ca-L}. An I_{K-ATP} opener, nicorandil is another choice of therapy. All of these antianginal drugs would be expected to provoke ST segment elevation in patients with the 'acquired' form of Brugada syndrome.[26] Acute ischemia itself involving the RVOT region may be a risk factor for the 'acquired' form of Brugada syndrome, which will be discussed later.

Psychotropic drugs

Brugada-like ST segment elevation has been reported to be unmasked by use of several psychotropic drugs including tricyclic antidepressants (amitriptyline, nortriptyline, desipramine, clomipramine, etc.), tetracyclic antidepressants (maprotiline, etc.), and phenothiazines (perphenazine, cyamemazine, etc.) (Fig. 14.5).[40–44] This effect is likely to be secondary to block of fast I_{Na}, usually associated with overdose. The selective serotonin reuptake inhibitors (SSRIs), such as fluoxetine, are reported to produce ST segment elevation, probably as a result of their effect to depress fast I_{Na} and I_{Ca-L}.[41]

Other drugs

Dimenhydrinate, a sedating, first-generation histaminic H1 receptor antagonist, commonly used as an antiemetic, is reported to produce Brugada-like ST segment elevation.[45] Dimenhydrinate exhibits an anticholinergic action and Na^+ channel blocking effect; the predominance of the latter effect may cause the ST segment elevation.

ST segment elevation is also reported to be provoked by cocaine intoxication, mainly due to its fast I_{Na} blocking effect.[46,47]

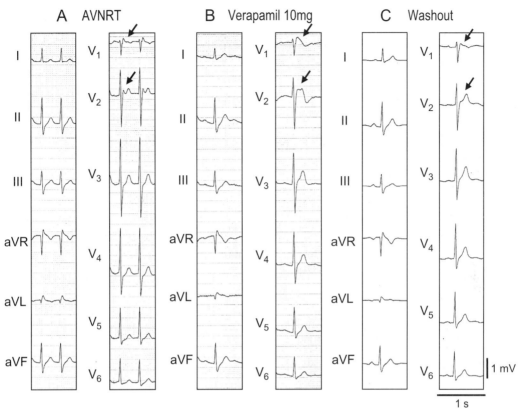

Figure 14.4 (**A**) Verapamil-induced ST segment elevation in a patient with 'acquired' form of Brugada syndrome. Intravenous administration of 10 mg verapamil, an I_{Ca-L} blocker, was used to terminate atrio-ventricular nodal reentrant tachycardia (AVNRT). The prominent coved and saddle-back type ST segment elevation was unmasked in leads V_1 and V_2 after successful termination of AVNRT (**B**, arrows), and disappeared after washout of verapamil (**C**, arrows).

Electrolyte abnormalities

Severe hyperkalemia in patients with renal failure has been reported to be associated with ST segment elevation in the right precordial leads like that in Brugada syndrome.[48–50] Hypercalcemia also has been reported to cause Brugada-like ST segment elevation in the right precordial leads.[51,52]

Acute ischemia

Right ventricular infarction/ischemia

Acute myocardial infarction (AMI) or ischemia of the right ventricle involving the RVOT is reported to mimic ST segment elevation similar to that in Brugada syndrome.[53–55] Figure 14.6 illustrates transient

Brugada-like ST segment elevation during acute occlusion of the RV branch in a patient with inferior AMI. The 12 lead electrocardiogram (ECG) on admission showed ST segment elevation in leads II, III, and aVF indicating inferior AMI (Fig. 14.6A), and 99% stenosis of segment 1 of the right coronary artery (RCA) was revealed by an emergency coronary angiography. Transiently acute occlusion of the RV branch supplying the RVOT region during subsequent angioplasty induced a coved type ST segment elevation in leads V_1–V_3 (Fig. 14.6B), which recovered following spontaneous re-canalization of the RV branch (Fig. 14.6C). Brugada-like ST elevation induced by acute ischemia involving the RVOT region is a result of the depression of I_{Ca-L} and the activation of I_{K-ATP} during ischemia.

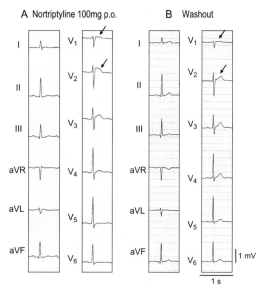

A Nortriptyline 100mg p.o.   B Washout

Figure 14.5 Nortriptyline-induced ST segment elevation in a patient with 'acquired' form of Brugada syndrome. (**A**) The coved type ST segment elevation was observed in leads V_1 and V_2 during oral nortriptyline (100 mg/day), a tricyclic antidepressant (arrows). (**B**) The ST segment elevation disappeared after washout of nortriptyline (arrows).

Vasospastic angina

Along the same lines as the above, vasospasm of the coronary artery supplying the RVOT region would be expected to mimic Brugada-like ST segment elevation. On the other hand, several reports have demonstrated the combination of Brugada syndrome and vasospastic angina in a single patient.[56–58] We recently evaluated systematically the frequency of induced coronary spasm in patients with diagnosed Brugada syndrome.[59] We also examined the hypothesis that the decrease of I_{Ca-L} and the activation of I_{K-ATP} in the RVOT region secondary to ischemia or vagomimetic action induced by intraright coronary injection of acetylcholine (ACh) and/or ergonovine maleate (EM) may enhance ST segment elevation and induce VF. Coronary spasm was induced in 3 (11%) of 27 Brugada patients, suggesting that coronary spasm was not rare in Brugada syndrome. Brugada-like ST segment elevation was augmented by 11 (33%) of the 33 right coronary injections [ACh: 6/11 (55%), EM: 5/22 (23%)] without any induction of coronary spasm, but not by any left coronary injections (Fig. 14.7). VF was induced by 3 (9%) of the 33 right coronary injections [ACh:

2/11 (18%), EM: 1/22 (5%)] but not by any left coronary injections. These results support the hypothesis that mild ischemia and vagal influences act in an additive fashion or synergistically with the substrate responsible for Brugada syndrome to elevate the ST segment and precipitate VF. Our data also suggest that congenital and possibly 'acquired' forms of Brugada syndrome may place a patient at higher risk for ischemia-related sudden cardiac death.

Insulin level

The increased insulin level induced by glucose is suggested to amplify or unmask ST segment elevation in patients with diagnosed Brugada syndrome.[60,61] This effect may contribute to circadian or day-to-day variation in the degree of ST segment elevation in this syndrome.[27] Insulin increases outward current by activating Na^+/K^+ pump and stimulates I_{Ca-L}; the former predominates and contributes to ST segment elevation.

Hyperthermia (febrile state)

A number of reports have demonstrated that febrile state can unmask Brugada-like ST segment elevation and provoke VF.[62–68] Dumaine et al. suggested that accelerated inactivation of the Na^+ channel with the T1620M missense mutation was observed at physiological temperatures, but not at room temperature, and was further exaggerated at temperatures above the physiological range.[69] Baroudi et al. demonstrated that the Na^+ channel involving the T1620M/R1342W double mutation failed to express when the HEK cells were cultured at physiologic versus cold temperatures.[70] These effects of the mutant Na^+ channel result in a reduced I_{Na} at high temperature, and would be expected to accentuate or unmask Brugada-like ST segment elevation during a febrile state.

Hypothermia

A prominent J wave associated with ST segment elevation, which is referred to as an Osborn wave, has long been described in hypothermic states due to accidental exposures to cold.[71,72] Figure 14.8 illustrates serial ECG changes during a hypothermic state in a patient with an accidental exposure to cold.

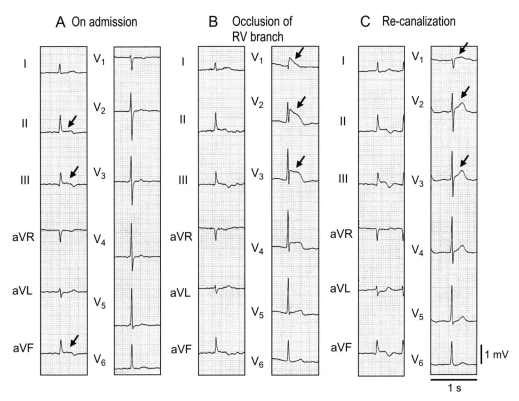

Figure 14.6 Transient Brugada-like ST segment elevation induced by acute occlusion of the right ventricular (RV) branch in a patient with inferior acute myocardial infarction (AMI). (**A**) The 12 lead ECG on admission showed ST segment elevation in leads II, III, and aVF indicating inferior AMI (arrows). (**B**) Transiently acute occlusion of the RV branch supplying the RV outflow tract during angioplasty produced coved type ST segment elevation in leads V_1–V_3 (arrows), (**C**) which recovered following spontaneous re-canalization of the RV branch (arrows).

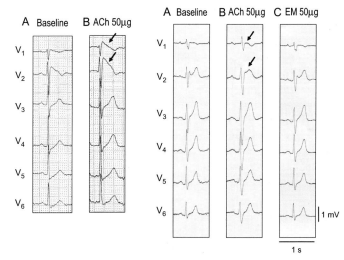

Figure 14.7 Six precordial leads ECG under baseline conditions (**A**), after injection of 50 μg acetylcholine (ACh) into the right coronary artery (**B**), and after injection of 50 μg ergonovine maleate (EM) into the right coronary artery (**C**) in two patients with diagnosed Brugada syndrome. Injection of ACh augmented the ST segment elevation in leads V_1 and V_2 in both cases (**B**, arrows), while injection of EM did not change the ST segment elevation (right panel, **C**).

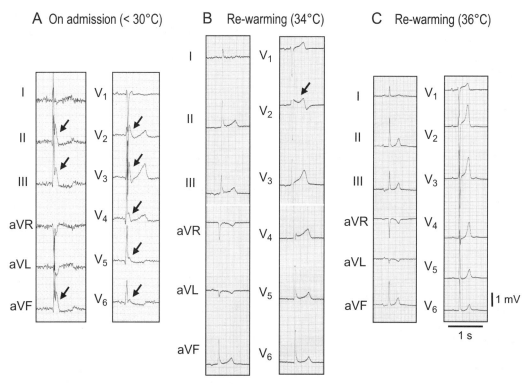

Figure 14.8 Hypothermia-induced prominent J wave and Brugada-like ST segment elevation in a patient with accidental exposure to cold. (**A**) Prominent J waves in leads II, III, aVF, V_2–V_6 were seen on admission when his rectal temperature was less than 30°C (arrows). (**B**) As the body temperature rose with re-warming (34°C), a saddleback type ST segment elevation mimicking Brugada syndrome was transiently observed in lead V_2 (arrow). (**C**) The ST segment elevation finally disappeared as the body temperature rose further (36°C).

Prominent J waves were recorded in leads II, III, aVF, V_2 to V_6 on admission when his rectal temperature was less than 30°C (Fig. 14.8A). As the body temperature rose with re-warming (34°C), a saddleback type ST segment elevation mimicking Brugada syndrome was transiently observed in lead V_2 (Fig. 14.8B), which disappeared later as the body temperature rose further (36°C) (Fig. 14.8C). The Brugada-like ST segment elevation induced by low temperature is probably due to augmented I_{to}.

Mechanical compression of the RVOT

Unmasking of Brugada-like ST segment elevation due to mechanical compression of the RVOT by a mediastinal tumor or hemopericardium was reported.[73,74] This effect is most likely a result of an affect of the impact on multiple ion channel currents leading to an outward shift of net current active during the early phases of the epicardial AP in the RVOT.

Genetic background in 'acquired' form of Brugada syndrome

Mutations in genes (*KCNQ1*, *KCNH2*, and *SCN5A*) causing congenital form of LQTS have been identified in patients with 'acquired' forms of LQTS.[75] Thus, some patients with the 'acquired' form of LQTS are believed to have a genetic predisposition or subclinical ('forme fruste') form of congenital LQTS. A subclinical form of the Brugada syndrome may similarly predispose to the development of 'acquired' forms of the Brugada syndrome or Brugada-like ST segment elevation, as a consequence of polymorphisms or other mutations in *SCN5A* or other genes.

Acknowledgment

I am grateful to Drs Takashi Noda, Miki Yokokawa, and Shiro Kamakura for helpful suggestions and technical assistance.

Dr Shimizu was supported in part by the Vehicle Racing Commemorative Foundation, Kanahara Ichiro Memorial Foundation, Mochida Memorial Foundation, Health Sciences Research Grants from the Ministry of Health, Labour and Welfare, and Research Grant for Cardiovascular Diseases (15C-6) from the Ministry of Health, Labour and Welfare, Japan.

References

1 Brugada P, Brugada J. Right bundle branch block, persistent ST segment elevation and sudden cardiac death: a distinct clinical and electrocardiographic syndrome: a multicenter report. *J. Am. Coll. Cardiol.* 1992; **20**: 1391–1396.

2 Brugada J, Brugada P. Further characterization of the syndrome of right bundle branch block, ST segment elevation, and sudden cardiac death. *J. Cardiovasc. Electrophysiol.* 1997; **8**: 325–331.

3 Brugada J, Brugada R, Brugada P. Right bundle-branch block and ST-segment elevation in leads V_1 through V_3. A marker for sudden death in patients without demonstrable structural heart disease. *Circulation* 1998; **97**: 457–460.

4 Antzelevitch C. The Brugada syndrome. *J. Cardiovasc. Electrophysiol.* 1998; **9**: 513–516.

5 Gussak I, Antzelevitch C, Bjerregaard P et al. The Brugada syndrome: clinical, electrophysiological and genetic aspects. *J. Am. Coll. Cardiol.* 1999; **33**: 5–15.

6 Alings M, Wilde A. 'Brugada' syndrome: clinical data and suggested pathophysiological mechanism. *Circulation* 1999; **99**: 666–673.

7 Antzelevitch C, Brugada P, Brugada J et al. The Brugada syndrome. In: Camm J ed. *Clinical Approaches to Tachyarrhythmias.* Armonk, NY: Futura Publishing Company, Inc. 1999: 1–99.

8 Wilde AA, Antzelevitch C, Borggrefe M et al. Study Group on the Molecular Basis of Arrhythmias of the European Society of Cardiology: Proposed diagnostic criteria for the Brugada syndrome: consensus report. *Circulation* 2002; **106**: 2514–2519.

9 Antzelevitch C, Brugada P, Brugada J et al. Brugada syndrome. A decade of progress. *Circ. Res.* 2002; **91**: 1114–1118.

10 Priori SG, Napolitano C, Gasparini M et al. Natural history of Brugada syndrome: insights for risk stratification and management. *Circulation* 2002; **105**: 1342–1347.

11 Brugada J, Brugada R, Antzelevitch C et al. Long-term follow-up of individuals with the electrocardiographic pattern of right bundle-branch block and ST-segment elevation in precordial leads V1 to V3. *Circulation* 2002; **105**: 73–78.

12 Antzelevitch C, Brugada P, Brugada J et al. Brugada syndrome: 1992–2002: a historical perspective. *J. Am. Coll. Cardiol.* 2003; **41**: 1665–1671.

13 Miyazaki T, Mitamura H, Miyoshi S et al. Autonomic and antiarrhythmic drug modulation of ST segment elevation in patients with Brugada syndrome. *J. Am. Coll. Cardiol.* 1996; **27**: 1061–1070.

14 Atarashi H, Ogawa S, Harumi K et al. Characteristics of patients with right bundle branch block and ST-segment elevation in right precordial leads. *Am. J. Cardiol.* 1996; **78**: 581–583.

15 Kasanuki H, Ohnishi S, Ohtuka M et al. Idiopathic ventricular fibrillation induced with vagal activity in patients without obvious heart disease. *Circulation* 1997; **95**: 2277–2285.

16 Nademanee K: Sudden unexplained death syndrome in southeast Asia. *Am. J. Cardiol.* 1997; **79**(6A): 10–11.

17 Nademanee K, Veerakul G, Nimmannit S et al. Arrhythmogenic marker for the sudden unexplained death syndrome in Thai men. *Circulation* 1997; **96**: 2595–2600.

18 Shimizu W, Matsuo K, Takagi M et al. Body surface distribution and response to drugs of ST segment elevation in the Brugada syndrome: clinical implication of 87-leads body surface potential mapping and its application to 12-leads electrocardiograms. *J. Cardiovasc. Electrophysiol.* 2000; **11**: 396–404.

19 Matsuo K, Akahoshi M, Nakashima E et al. The prevalence, incidence and prognostic value of the Brugada-type electrocardiogram: a population-based study of four decades. *J. Am. Coll. Cardiol.* 2001; **38**: 765–770.

20 Kanda M, Shimizu W, Matsuo K et al. Electrophysiologic characteristics and implication of induced ventricular fibrillation in symptomatic patients with Brugada syndrome. *J. Am. Coll. Cardiol.* 2002; **39**: 1799–1805.

21 Chen Q, Kirsch GE, Zhang D et al. Genetic basis and molecular mechanisms for idiopathic ventricular fibrillation. *Nature* 1998; **392**: 293–296.

22 Vatta M, Dumaine R, Varghese G et al. Genetic and biophysical basis of sudden unexplained nocturnal death syndrome (SUNDS), a disease allelic to Brugada syndrome. *Hum. Mol. Genet.* 2002; **11**: 337–345.

23 Yan GX, Antzelevitch C. Cellular basis for the electrocardiographic J wave. *Circulation* 1996; **93**: 372–379.

24 Yan GX, Antzelevitch C. Cellular basis for the Brugada syndrome and other mechanisms of arrhythmogenesis associated with ST segment elevation. *Circulation* 1999; **100**: 1660–1666.

25 Antzelevitch C, Yan GX, Shimizu W et al. Electrical hetero-

geneity, the ECG, and cardiac arrhythmias. In: Zipes DP, Jalife J, eds. *Cardiac Electrophysiology: From Cell to Bedside.* Philadelphia: W.B. Saunders Co., 1999: 222–238.

26 Matsuo K, Shimizu W, Kurita T *et al.* Dynamic changes of 12-lead electrocardiograms in a patient with Brugada syndrome. *J. Cardiovasc. Electrophysiol.* 1998; **9**: 508–512.

27 Matsuo K, Kurita T, Inagaki M *et al.* The circadian pattern of the development of ventricular fibrillation in patients with Brugada syndrome. *Eur. Heart J.* 1999; **20**: 465–470.

28 Krishnan SC, Josephson ME. ST segment elevation induced by class IC antiarrhythmic agents: underlying electrophysiologic mechanisms and insights into drug-induced proarrhythmia. *J. Cardiovasc. Electrophysiol.* 1998; **9**: 1167–1172.

29 Fujiki A, Usui M, Nagasawa H *et al.* ST segment elevation in the right precordial leads induced with class IC antiarrhythmic drugs: insights into the mechanism of Brugada syndrome. *J. Cardiovasc. Electrophysiol.* 1999; **10**: 214–218.

30 Takenaka S, Emori T, Koyama S *et al.* Asymptomatic form of Brugada syndrome. *Pacing Clin. Electrophysiol.* 1999; **22**: 1261–1263.

31 Shimizu W, Antzelevitch C, Suyama K *et al.* Effect of sodium channel blockers on ST segment, QRS duration, and corrected QT interval in patients with Brugada syndrome. *J. Cardiovasc. Electrophysiol.* 2000; **11**: 1320–1329.

32 Brugada R,. Brugada J,. Antzelevitch C *et al.* Sodium channel blockers identify risk for sudden death in patients with ST-segment elevation and right bundle branch block but structurally normal hearts. *Circulation* 2000; **101**: 510–515.

33 Matana A, Goldner V, Stanic K *et al.* Unmasking effect of propafenone on the concealed form of the Brugada phenomenon. *Pacing Clin. Electrophysiol.* 2000; **23**: 416–418.

34 Shimizu W, Aiba T, Kurita T *et al.* Paradoxical abbreviation of repolarization in epicardium of the right ventricular outflow tract during augmentation of Brugada-type ST segment elevation. *J. Cardiovasc. Electrophysiol.* 2001; **12**: 1418–1421.

35 Gasparini M, Priori SG, Mantica M *et al.* Flecainide test in Brugada syndrome: a reproducible but risky tool. *Pacing Clin. Electrophysiol.* 2003; **26**: 338–341.

36 Rolf S, Bruns HJ, Wichter T *et al.* The ajmaline challenge in Brugada syndrome: diagnostic impact, safety, and recommended protocol. *Eur. Heart J.* 2003; **24**: 1104–1112.

37 Tada H, Nogami A, Shimizu W *et al.* ST-segment and T-wave alternans in a patient with Brugada syndrome. *Pacing Clin. Electrophysiol.* 2000; **23**: 413–415.

38 Virag L, Varro A, Papp C. Effect of disopyramide on potassium currents in rabbit ventricular myocytes. *Naunyn-Schmied. Arch. Pharmacol.* 1998; **357**: 268–275.

39 Alings M, Dekker L, Sadee A *et al.* Quinidine induced electrocardiographic normalization in two patients with Brugada syndrome. *Pacing Clin. Electrophysiol.* 2001; **24**: 1420–1422.

40 Bolognesi R, Tsialtas D, Vasini P *et al.* Abnormal ventricular repolarization mimicking myocardial infarction after heterocyclic antidepressant overdose. *Am. J. Cardiol.* 1997; **79**: 242–245.

41 Rouleau F, Asfar P, Boulet S *et al.* Transient ST segment elevation in right precordial leads induced by psychotropic drugs: relationship to the Brugada syndrome. *J. Cardiovasc. Electrophysiol.* 2001; **12**: 61–65.

42 Tada H, Sticherling C, Oral H *et al.* Brugada syndrome mimicked by tricyclic antidepressant overdose. *J. Cardiovasc. Electrophysiol.* 2001; **12**: 275.

43 Babaliaros VC, Hurst JW. Tricyclic antidepressants and the Brugada syndrome: an example of Brugada waves appearing after the administration of desipramine. *Clin. Cardiol.* 2002; **25**: 395–398.

44 Goldgran-Toledano D, Sideris G, Kevorkian JP. Overdose of cyclic antidepressants and the Brugada syndrome. *N. Engl. J. Med.* 2002; **346**: 1591–1592.

45 Pastor A, Nunez A, Cantale C *et al.* Asymptomatic Brugada syndrome case unmasked during dimenhydrinate infusion. *J. Cardiovasc. Electrophysiol.* 2001; **12**: 1192–1194.

46 Ortega-Carnicer J, Bertos-Polo J, Gutierrez-Tirado C. Aborted sudden death, transient Brugada pattern, and wide QRS dysrrhythmias after massive cocaine ingestion. *J. Electrocardiol.* 2001; **34**: 345–349.

47 Littmann L, Monroe MH, Svenson RH. Brugada-type electrocardiographic pattern induced by cocaine. *Mayo Clin. Proc.* 2000; **75**: 845–849.

48 Myers GB. Other QRS-T patterns that may be mistaken for myocardial infarction. IV. Alterations in blood potassium; myocardial ischemia; subepicardial myocarditis; distortion associated with arrhythmias. *Circulation* 1950; **2**: 75–93.

49 Merrill JP, Levine HD, Somerville W *et al.* Clinical recognition and treatment of acute potassium intoxication. *Ann. Intern. Med.* 1950; **33**: 797–830.

50 Ortega-Carnicer J, Benezet J, Ruiz-Lorenzo F *et al.* Transient Brugada-type electrocardiographic abnormalities in renal failure reversed by dialysis. *Resuscitation* 2002; **55**: 215–219.

51 Douglas PS, Carmichael KA, Palevsky PM. Exreme hypercalcemia and electrocardiographic changes. *Am. J. Cardiol.* 1984; **54**: 674–675.

52 Sridharan MR, Horan LG. Electrocardiographic J wave of hypercalcemia. *Am. J. Cardiol.* 1984; **54**: 672–673.

53 Kataoka H. Electrocardiographic patterns of the Brugada syndrome in right ventricular infarction/ischemia. *Am. J. Cardiol.* 2000; **86**: 1056.

54 Kataoka H, Kanzaki K, Mikuriya Y. Massive ST-segment elevation in precordial and inferior leads in right ventricular myocardial infarction. *J. Electrocardiol.* 1988; **21**: 115–120.

55 Indik JH, Ott P, Butman SM. Syncope with ST-segment abnormalities resembling Brugada syndrome due to reversible myocardial ischemia. *Pacing Clin. Electrophysiol.* 2002; **25**: 1270–1273.

56 Chinushi M, Kuroe Y, Ito E *et al.* Vasospastic angina accompanied by Brugada-type electrocardiographic abnormalities. *J. Cardiovasc. Electrophysiol.* 2001; **12**: 108–111.

57 Itoh E, Suzuki K, Tanabe Y. A case of vasospastic angina presenting Brugada-type ECG abnormalities. *Jpn. Circ. J.* 1999; **63**: 493–495.

58 Imazio M, Ghisio A, Coda L *et al.* Brugada syndrome: a case report of an unusual association with vasospastic angina and coronary myocardial bridging. *Pacing Clin. Electrophysiol.* 2002; **25**: 513–515.

59 Noda T, Shimizu W, Taguchi A *et al.* ST segment elevation and ventricular fibrillation without coronary spasm by intra coronary injection of acetylcholine and/or ergonovine maleate in patients with Brugada syndrome. *J. Am. Coll. Cardiol.* 2002; **40**: 1841–1847.

60 Nishizaki M, Sakurada H, Ashikaga T *et al.* Effects of glucose-induced insulin secretion on ST segment elevation in the Brugada syndrome. *J. Cardiovasc. Electrophysiol.* 2003; **14**: 243–249.

61 Nogami A, Nakao M, Kubota S *et al.* Enhancement of J-ST-segment elevation by the glucose and insulin test in Brugada syndrome. *Pacing Clin. Electrophysiol.* 2003; **26**: 332–337.

62 Antzelevitch C, Brugada R. Fever and Brugada syndrome. *Pacing Clin. Electrophysiol.* 2002; **25**: 1537–1539.

63 Saura D, Garcia-Alberola A, Carrillo P *et al.* Brugada-like electrocardiographic pattern induced by fever. *Pacing Clin. Electrophysiol.* 2002; **25**: 856–859.

64 Porres JM, Brugada J, Urbistondo V *et al.* Fever unmasking the Brugada syndrome. *Pacing Clin. Electrophysiol.* 2002; **25**: 1646–1648.

65 Mok NS, Priori SG, Napolitano C *et al.* A newly characterized *SCN5A* mutation underlying Brugada syndrome unmasked by hyperthermia. *J. Cardiovasc. Electrophysiol.* 2003; **14**: 407–411.

66 Morita H, Nagase S, Kusano K *et al.* Spontaneous T wave alternans and premature ventricular contractions during febrile illness in a patient with Brugada syndrome. *J. Cardiovasc. Electrophysiol.* 2002; **13**: 816–818.

67 Kum LC, Fung JW, Sanderson JE. Brugada syndrome unmasked by febrile illness. *Pacing Clin. Electrophysiol.* 2002; **25**: 1660–1661.

68 Ortega-Carnicer J, Benezet J, Ceres F. Fever-induced ST-segment elevation and T-wave alternans in a patient with Brugada syndrome. *Resuscitation* 2003; **57**: 315–317.

69 Dumaine R, Towbin JA, Brugada P *et al.* Ionic mechanisms responsible for the electrocardiographic phenotype of the Brugada syndrome are temperature dependent. *Circ. Res.* 1999; **85**: 803–809.

70 Baroudi G, Acharfi S, Larouche C *et al.* Expression and intracellular localization of an *SCN5A* double mutant R1232W/T1620M implicated in Brugada syndrome. *Circ. Res.* 2002; **90**: E11–E16.

71 Osborn JJ. Experimental hypothermia: respiratory and blood pH changes in relation to cardiac function. *Am. J. Physiol.* 1953; **175**: 389–398.

72 Noda T, Shimizu W, Tanaka K, *et al.* Prominent J wave and ST segment elevation: serial electrocardiographic changes in accidental hypothermia. *J. Cardiovasc. Electrophysiol.* 2003; **14**: 223.

73 Tarin N, Farre J, Rubio JM *et al.* Brugada-like electro cardiographic pattern in a patient with a mediastinal tumor. *Pacing Clin. Electrophysiol.* 1999; **22**: 1264–1266.

74 Tomcsanyi J, Simor T, Papp L. Haemopericardium and Brugada-like ECG pattern in rheumatoid arthritis. *Heart* 2002; **87**: 234.

75 Donger C D, Denjoy I, Berthet M *et al. KVLQT1* C-terminal missense mutation causes a forme fruste long-QT syndrome. *Circulation* 1997; **96**: 2778–2781.

CHAPTER 15

Atrial tachyarrhythmias in Brugada syndrome

M. Borggrefe, MD, PhD, *R. Schimpf*, MD, *F. Gaita*, MD, *L. Eckardt*, MD, *C. Wolpert*, MD

Introduction

Atrial fibrillation and other supraventricular tachycardias represent a common disorder that constitutes a relevant cause of mortality, morbidity, and economic consequences such as repetitive hospitalizations. Furthermore, atrial fibrillation and atrial flutter account for a relevant 2–15% risk of stroke.[1] The prevalence of atrial fibrillation and atrial flutter is estimated between 0.5 and 2% in the general population and increases with age.[2,3] The real frequency of atrial fibrillation in the population may significantly be underestimated, as approximately 30–50% of episodes are asymptomatic, remain under-detected, and are eventually diagnosed after occurrence of complications such as an embolic stroke.[4]

The main risk factor for the development of atrial fibrillation is a structural heart disease such as coronary artery disease, dilated and hypertrophic cardiomyopathies, or valvular heart disease.[5] Nevertheless, still 5–30% of patients with atrial fibrillation suffer from lone atrial fibrillation without any signs of a structural disease.[6] Lone atrial fibrillation frequently affects young and middle-aged patients.

However, in recent years new insights into the genetic basis of arrhythmias have revealed genetic defects in patients with familial atrial fibrillation.[7,8] Furthermore, inherited diseases such as the long QT syndrome, the short QT syndrome, and the Brugada syndrome, which constitute a risk factor for sudden arrhythmogenic death, have only recently been recognized to be linked to ion channel diseases. These latter syndromes are also associated with supraventricular arrhythmias.[9–13]

Patients with long QT syndrome may exhibit 'atrial torsade', as investigated by Kirchhof *et al.*[9] In 2000 Gussak *et al.*[10] demonstrated that the new entity short QT syndrome is related to familial atrial fibrillation, which was recently confirmed by further families with an additional frequent occurrence of familial sudden death.[10–12]

The initial report on the Brugada syndrome described two out of eight affected individuals with paroxysmal atrial fibrillation.[13] Notably, one patient was suffering from episodes of atrial fibrillation soon after birth, preceding syncopal episodes in young childhood.

Brugada syndrome and atrial fibrillation

The first report by Brugada on the Brugada syndrome already revealed that 2 out of the 8 affected individuals had a history of atrial fibrillation.[13] Eckardt *et al.* reported a low prevalence of atrial fibrillation in a group of 35 patients with Brugada syndrome (*n* = 1), but a relevant number (*n* = 10) of supraventricular tachycardias.[14]

A group of 30 Japanese patients with a Brugada syndrome revealed a relevant number of individuals (*n* = 9) with additional episodes of atrial fibrillation.[15] In this study not only ventricular arrhythmias but also atrial fibrillation occurred predominantly at night and early in the morning, thus suggesting that an increased vagal tone or decreased sympathetic activity may play an important role in the arrhythmogenesis.

Morita *et al.*[16] studied 18 consecutive patients with a Brugada syndrome and compared the electrophysiological findings to an age- and gender-matched population without evidence of heart disease. Spontaneous atrial fibrillation occurred in 7 of 18 patients with Brugada syndrome but none of the control subjects.[16] The right atrial effective refractory period was not different between the two groups; however, intra-atrial conduction times were significantly increased in patients with Brugada syndrome as compared to the control group. The duration of the local atrial electrogram at the atrial refractory period was prolonged in the affected patients. Atrial fibrillation was inducible in 8 patients with Brugada syndrome but in none of the control subjects. The authors concluded that atrial vulnerability is increased in patients with Brugada syndrome. Furthermore, atrial conduction times which form the electrophysiological basis for the spontaneous occurrence and induction of atrial fibrillation are prolonged in Brugada syndrome.

Recently, Bordachar et al.[17] compared 59 patients with Brugada syndrome to an age-matched control group. Atrial fibrillation was diagnosed in 11 out of 59 patients and none in the control group.[17] Furthermore, inducibility of ventricular tachycardia/ventricular fibrillation was significantly related to the history of atrial fibrillation. Patients with a spontaneous positive electrocardiogram had a higher probability of spontaneous atrial fibrillation as compared to patients with drug-induced typical Brugada ECG pattern. Patients with a HV interval >55 ms had significantly more atrial arrhythmic events as compared to patients with a normal HV interval. Finally, the data revealed a significantly higher incidence of inappropriate therapies due to episodes of atrial fibrillation in patients in whom an implantable cardioverter/defibrillator was implanted.

A recent multicenter study conducted at the University hospitals in Turin, Muenster, and Mannheim included 115 patients with Brugada syndrome. Eleven patients revealed episodes of atrial fibrillation and another two patients presented with atrial flutter (n = 13, 11%). During invasive electrophysiologic study, atrial fibrillation was inducible in 9 patients (Fig. 15.1).

Taking the current published observations into account, the overall prevalence of atrial fibrillation in patients with Brugada syndrome is approximately 16% (Table 15.1).

Clinical presentation and therapy of atrial fibrillation in Brugada syndrome

The clinical presentation of atrial fibrillation in patients with Brugada syndrome is usually benign, with relatively infrequent attacks. Furthermore, Morita et al.[16] assessed the ventricular response during atrial fibrillation. They could show that the ventricular rate is relatively slow, which may account for the low severity of symptoms. Therefore atrial fibrillation in Brugada syndrome may be potentially underestimated. Specific pharmacologic therapy of atrial fibrillation in asymptomatic patients or mildly symptomatic patients with Brugada syndrome is generally not indicated. In the rare event of clinically relevant symptomatic atrial fibrillation episodes, or in patients after occurrence of inappropriate shock therapies due to atrial fibrillation, pharmacologic therapy for rhythm control is problematic. Most antiarrhythmic drugs either slow heart rate or may potentially increase transmural dispersion of conduction and refractoriness and thereby promote the risk of ventricular fibrillation in Brugada syndrome patients. Probably, treatment with digitalis or a calcium antagonist may be safe for rate control. Rhythm control may be achieved by quinidine, which may be also be useful in suppressing recurrent ventricular fibrillation episodes by blocking I_{to}-current.[18] Quinidine has been shown to normalize the Brugada ECG pattern in some patients.[19] Other antiarrhythmics such as amiodarone, flecainide, procainamide, and ajmaline for acute conversion may facilitate the occurrence of ventricular fibrillation and should thereby only be advised in patients in whom an ICD is already implanted. β-blockers, including sotalol, may increase episodes of ventricular fibrillation by slowing the heart rate and promoting transmural dispersion of repolarization and refractoriness. Episodes of intrinsic slow heart rate have been linked to the occurrence of sudden death in Brugada syndrome. In 1997, Nademanee et al.[20] reported that among 27 Thai men referred for aborted cases of what is known in Thailand as *Lai Tai* ('death during sleep'), as many as 16 patients had the ECG pattern of Brugada syndrome.[20]

Other supraventricular tachycardias in patients with the Brugada syndrome

The first detailed report on the association of supraventricular tachycardia and Brugada syndrome was provided by Eckardt et al.[14] (Fig. 15.2).

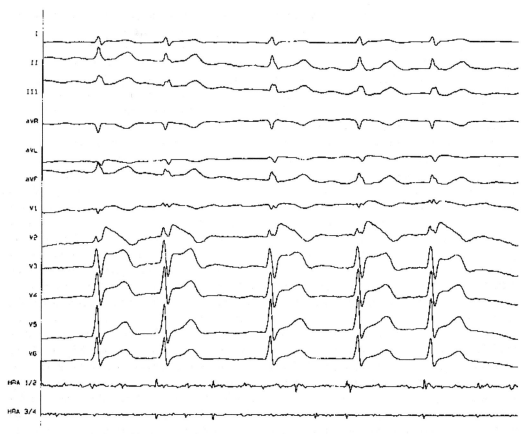

Figure 15.1 Brugada syndrome and atrial fibrillation. 35-year-old male with history of episodes of spontaneous atrial fibrillation and *SCN5A* mutation. Induction of persisting atrial fibrillation during electrophysiologic stimulation.

Table 15.1 Frequency of spontaneous atrial fibrillation in patients with Brugada syndrome. Summarizing the cited studies, approximately 16% of patients with Brugada syndrome present with additional episodes of atrial fibrillation.

Study	Number of patients	Percentage
Brugada 1992[13]	2/8 patients	25%
Eckhardt 2001[14]	1/35 patients (10 with SVT)	3%
Itoh 2001[15]	9/30	30%
Morita 2002[16]	7/18	39%
Bordachar 2004[17]	11/59	19%
Multicenter study (see text)	13/115	11%
Total	43/265	16.2%

These authors studied 35 consecutive patients with Brugada syndrome, of whom 26 had a cardiac arrest or syncope and 9 were asymptomatic.[14] All patients underwent electrophysiologic study including an atrial and ventricular stimulation protocol. Of all patients, 10 were found to have supraventricular tacharrhythmias in addition to Brugada syndrome. These 10 patients presented with aborted sudden cardiac death ($n = 3$) and/or family history of sudden death ($n = 4$), syncope ($n = 4$) or primary with a

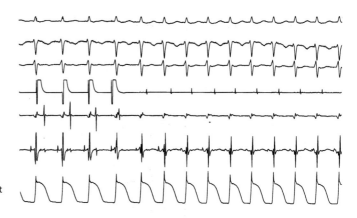

Figure 15.2 Brugada syndrome and AV nodal reentrant tachycardia. 52-year-old female with history of episodes of supraventricular tachycardias and positive family history of sudden cardiac death. Induction of AV-nodal reentrant tachycardia at electrophysiologic study and successful radiofrequency catheter ablation. Furthermore, ventricular fibrillation could be induced at programmed ventricular stimulation (not shown).

Brugada typical ECG, positive family history and palpitations ($n = 2$). In 6 patients AV nodal reentrant tachycardia (AVNRT) was easily and reproducibly inducible. Two patients had clinically documented and inducible episodes of atrial tachycardia (in addition to an AV nodal reentrant tachycardia) and another patient had spontaneous paroxysmal atrial fibrillation. Further two patients with AV nodal reentrant tachycardia and one patient with an accessory pathway underwent successful catheter ablation.

In an extended analysis of 115 consecutive patients with Brugada syndrome diagnosed at the University hospitals in Turin, Muenster, and Mannheim, overall 8 patients presented with an AV nodal reentry tachycardia, 2 patients with accessory pathways with antegrade conduction and 3 patients with ectopic atrial tachycardias (Schimpf et al. in preparation).

The overall incidence of AVNRT in an unselected population is not well documented. Paroxysmal supraventricular tachycardias in the general population are rare. A systematic epidemiologic survey by Orejanrena et al.[21] estimated a low frequency of supraventricular tachycardias which account for approximately 0.25% in the population. Thus, in the present group of 115 patients with Brugada syndrome less than one patient would be expected to have a supraventricular tachycardia. However, in this patient population 26 out of 115 patients with a Brugada syndrome (23%) had supraventricular tachycardias (mean age 45 ± 12 years, male $n = 82$, female $n = 33$). As palpitations or syncope may have been the leading symptoms attracting medical attention in some patients with Brugada syndrome, a referral bias in the series can not be excluded. However, in the majority of cases AVNRT was only detected in the diagnostic work-up of suspected Brugada syndrome. The pathophysiology of AVNRT in Brugada syndrome is not understood. One might speculate that a genetically determined local atrial conduction block in the tissue around the AV node may lead to the occurrence of AVNRT. Whether there is an electrophysiological basis for an association of the Brugada syndrome with atrial fibrillation and further supraventricular tachycardias still remains to be systematically examined in larger patient groups.

The incidence of atrial fibrillation in patients with AVNRT and atrioventricular reentrant tachycardia (AVRT) is ranging between 12 and 22%.[22] In patients with only AVNRT the incidence of atrial fibrillation has been reported to be up to 18% and thus being significantly higher in patients with paroxysmal supraventricular arrhythmias compared to an age-matched control group.[23] This may underline a potential primary abnormality of the atria facilitating a reentry circuit.[24] Radiofrequency ablation may reduce the attacks of atrial fibrillation, but recurrence rates of 33% without relapse of conduction via the accessory pathway/slow pathway are reported.[25]

In rare but clinically relevant cases, patients with antegrade conducting accessory pathways typical right precordial ST segment elevations may be concealed. Additional history of syncopes or ventricular tachyarrhythmias which can not be explained by a short refractory period of the accessory pathway should encourage further evaluation, including intravenous drug testing in the case of suspicious precordial resting ECG (Fig. 15.3).[14,26,27]

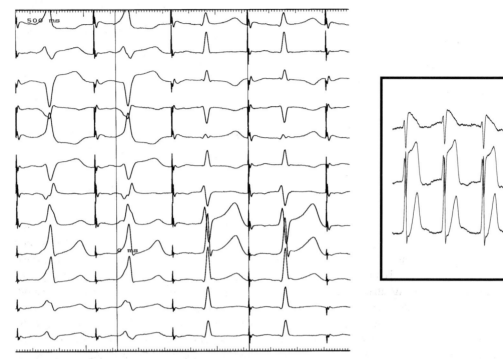

Figure 15.3 Brugada syndrome and Wolff–Parkinson–White syndrome; 30-year-old male with history of resuscitation due to ventricular fibrillation. During electrophysiologic stimulation an parahisian accessory pathway was identified. During programmed atrial stimulation demonstration of antegrade block of the accessory pathway and nodal conduction at cycle length of 500 ms, thus reducing the probability of fast conducted atrial fibrillation as the reason for resuscitation due to ventricular fibrillation.[27] Ajmaline testing revealed typical Brugada syndrome (box).

The therapy of choice in patients with the Brugada syndrome and supraventricular tachyarrhythmias such as AVNRT or accessory pathways is radiofrequency catheter ablation. Because regular supraventricular tachycardias may interfere with ICD detection algorithm leading to inappropriate ICD interventions, the curative approach is the treatment of choice in this condition.

Conclusions

Approximately every 5th patient with a Brugada syndrome may suffer from associated supraventricular tachyarrhythmias. In approximately 16% of patients with Brugada syndrome, episodes of atrial fibrillation can be clinically documented. The possible association of Brugada syndrome and supraventricular tachycardias underlines the importance of a complete electrophysiologic study, including programmed atrial and ventricular stimulation during the diagnostic work-up.

Conversely, in patients with supraventricular tachycardias and a history of syncope or sudden cardiac death, Brugada syndrome should be considered as an additional disorder if there still remains doubt whether the supraventricular arrhythmia is fully responsible for the clinical event.

Finally, the clinical relevance of atrial arrhythmias in patients with Brugada syndrome in whom an ICD is indicated for primary or secondary prophylaxis has to be considered as they could potentially contribute to inappropriate ICD therapies and thus significantly reducing patient compliance and impairing quality of life.

References

1 Feinberg WM, Blackshear JL, Laupacis A, Kronmal R, Hart

RG. Prevalence, age distribution, and gender of patients with atrial fibrillation: analysis and implications. *Arch. Intern. Med.* 1995; **155**: 469–473.

2 Stroke Prevention in Atrial Fibrillation Investigators. Adjusted-dose warfarin versus low-intensity, fixed-dose warfarin plus aspirin for high-risk patients with atrial fibrillation: stroke prevention in atrial fibrillation III randomised clinical trial. *Lancet* 1996; **348**: 633–638.

3 Atrial Fibrillation Investigators. The efficacy of aspirin in patients with atrial fibrillation: analysis of pooled data from three randomized trials. *Arch. Intern. Med.* 1997; **157**: 1237–1240.

4 Roche F, Gaspoz JM, Da Costa A *et al.* Frequent and prolonged asymptomatic episodes of paroxysmal atrial fibrillation revealed by automatic long-term event recorders in patients with a negative 24-hour holter. *Pacing Clin. Electrophysiol.* 2002; **25**: 1587–1593.

5 ACC/AHA/ESC guidelines for the management of patients with atrial fibrillation. *Eur. Heart J.* 2001; **22**: 1852–1923.

6 Kannel WB, Abbott RD, Savage DD *et al.* Epidemiologic features of chronic atrial fibrillation: the Framingham Study. *N. Engl. J. Med.* 1982; **306**: 1018–1022.

7 Brugada R, Tapscott T, Czermuszewickz G *et al.* Identification of a genetic locus for familial atrial fibrillation. *N. Engl. J. Med.* 1997; **336**: 905–911.

8 Chen YH, Xu SJ, Bendahhou S *et al.* KCNQ1 gain-of-function mutation in familial atrial fibrillation. *Science* 2003; **299**: 251–254.

9 Kirchhoff P, Eckardt L, Franz MR *et al.* Further evidence for prolonged atrial action potential durations and polymorphic atrial tachyarrhythmias in patients with long QT syndrome. *Eur. Heart J.* 2003; **24**: 244 (Abstract).

10 Gussak I, Brugada P, Brugada J *et al.* Idiopathic short QT interval: a new clinical syndrome? *Cardiology* 2000; **94**: 99–102.

11 Gaita F, Giustetto C, Bianchi F *et al.* Short QT syndrome: a familial cause of sudden death. *Circulation* 2003; **108**: 965–970.

12 Brugada R, Hong K, Dumaine R *et al.* Sudden death associated with short QT syndrome linked to mutations in HERG. *Circulation* 2004; **109**: r151–r156.

13 Brugada P, Brugada J. Right bundle branch block, persistent ST segment elevation and sudden cardiac death: a distinct clinical and electrocardiographic syndrome: a multicenter report. *J. Am. Coll. Cardiol.* 1992; **20**: 1391–1396.

14 Eckardt L, Kirchhof P, Loh P *et al.* Brugada syndrome and supraventricular tachyarrhythmias: a novel association? *J. Cardiovasc. Electrophysiol.* 2001; **12**: 680–685.

15 Itoh H, Shimizu M, Ino H *et al.* Arrhythmias in patients with Brugada-type electrocardiographic findings. *Jpn. Circ. J.* 2001; **65**: 483–486.

16 Morita H, Kusano-Fukushima K, Nagase S *et al.* Atrial fibrillation and atrial vulnerability in patients with Brugada syndrome. *J. Am. Coll. Cardiol.* 2002; **40**: 1437–1444.

17 Bordachar P, Reuter S, Garrigue S *et al.* Incidence, clinical implications and prognosis of atrial arrhythmias in Brugada syndrome. *Eur. Heart J.* 2004; **25**: 879–884.

18 Suzuki H, Torigoe K, Numata O *et al.* Infant case with a malignant form of Brugada syndrome. *J. Cardiovasc. Electrophysiol.* 2000; **11**: 1277–1280.

19 Alings M, Dekker L, Sadee A, Wilde A. Quinidine induced electrocardiographic normalization in two patients with Brugada syndrome. *Pacing Clin. Electrophysiol.* 2001; **24**: 1420–1422.

20 Nademanee K, Veerakul G, Nimmannit S *et al.* Arrhythmogenic marker for the sudden unexplained death syndrome in Thai men. *Circulation* 1997; **21**: 2595–2600.

21 Orejarena LA, Vidaillet H, DeStefano F *et al.* Paroxysmal supraventricular tachycardia in the general population. *J. Am. Coll. Cardiol.* 1998; **31**: 150–157.

22 Roark SF, McCarthy EA, Lee KL *et al.* Observation on the occurrence of atrial fibrillation in paroxysmal supraventricular tachycardia. *Am. J. Cardiol.* 1986; **57**: 571–575.

23 Hurwitz JL, German LD, Packer DL *et al.* Occurrence of atrial fibrillation in patients with paroxysmal supraventricular tachycardia due to atrioventricular nodal reentry. *Pacing Clin. Electrophysiol.* 1990; **13**: 705–710.

24 Chen J, Josephson ME. Atrioventricular nodal tachycardia during atrial fibrillation. *J. Cardiovasc. Electrophysiol.* 2000; **11**: 812–815.

25 Weiss R, Knight BP, Bahu M *et al.* Long-term follow-up after radiofrequency ablation of paroxysmal supraventricular tachycardia in patients with tachycardia-induced atrial fibrillation. *Am. J. Cardiol.* 1997; **80**: 1609–1610.

26 Ohkubo K, Watanabe I, Okumura Y *et al.* Wolff–Parkinson–White syndrome concomitant with asymptomatic Brugada syndrome. *Pacing Clin. Electrophysiol.* 2004; **27**: 109–111.

27 Eckardt L, Kirchhof P, Johna R *et al.* Wolff–Parkinson–White syndrome associated with Brugada syndrome. *Pacing Clin. Electrophysiol.* 2001; **24**: 1423–1424.

CHAPTER 16

Prognosis in individuals with Brugada syndrome

J. Brugada, MD, *R. Brugada,* MD, *P. Brugada,* MD, PhD

Introduction

During the last 10 years a large amount of information concerning Brugada syndrome[1] has become available, including genetic,[2–5] basic electrophysiologic,[6–8] epidemiologic,[9,10] diagnostic,[11,12] and prognostic[13–20] aspects of the syndrome. It has become clear that patients with an electrocardiogram diagnostic of Brugada syndrome have a high risk of sudden cardiac death related to the disease.[13–17] However, the prognosis of symptomatic and asymptomatic individuals and the value of clinical variables and some tests such as programmed electrical stimulation to predict prognosis are still a matter of discussion.[13–20] In this chapter we review all information available on the natural history and follow-up and on the prognostic value of clinical and electrocardiographic variables in the largest series of individuals with an electrocardiogram diagnostic of Brugada syndrome.

Patients and methods

Data on 667 individuals with an electrocardiogram diagnostic of Brugada syndrome and no demonstrable structural heart disease were analyzed. The data became available thanks to the collaboration of many centers and physicians around the world (see the end of the chapter for a full list). The electrocardiogram was defined as abnormal if a terminal R' wave, with a J point elevation of at least 0.2 mV, with a slowly descending ST segment in continuation with a flat or negative T wave (coved-type electrocardiogram) appeared spontaneously in leads V_1 to V_3 (Fig. 16.1), as defined in a recent consensus paper.[21] The electrocardiogram was also defined as abnormal when the described electrocardiographic abnormalities became evident after the intravenous administration of an antiarrhythmic drug with sodium-channel blocking properties, such as ajmaline, flecainide, or procainamide.[22]

The abnormal electrocardiogram was identified after an episode of aborted sudden death in 120 of the 667 individuals (Fig. 16.1). In 124 patients the abnormal electrocardiogram was identified after one or multiple episodes of syncope and in 423 individuals during routine electrocardiographic screening or during study because they were family members of patients with the syndrome.

Electrophysiologic study included basal measurements of conduction intervals and programmed ventricular stimulation. The protocol recommended used a single site of stimulation (right ventricular apex), three basic pacing cycles (600, 500, and 430 ms) and induction of 1, 2, and 3 ventricular premature beats down to a minimum of 200 ms. A patient was considered inducible if sustained ventricular arrhythmias (ventricular fibrillation, polymorphic ventricular tachycardia, or monomorphic ventricular tachycardia lasting more than 30 s or requiring emergency intervention) were induced.

Statistical analysis

Data were analyzed using the STATA Statistical Software (StataCorp., 1999, 7.0, College Station, TX). The Fisher exact test or the chi-square test was used

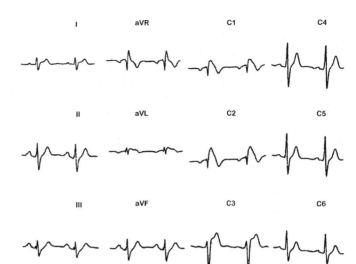

Figure 16.1 Twelve surface lead electrocardiogram showing the typical pattern of right bundle branch block and ST segment elevation in right precordial leads in a patient recovered from sudden cardiac death.

Table 16.1 Clinical characteristics of the patients.

Clinical presentation	Sudden death or ventricular fibrillation	No sudden death or ventricular fibrillation	p
Numbers	164	503	
Male/female	141/23	366/137	0.0001
Age (years)	42 ± 15	43 ± 15	not significant
Spontaneous abnormal electrocardiogram	150	349	0.0001
Family history of sudden cardiac death	70	274	0.03
Inducible/non inducible	95/21	136/241	0.0001

for non-continuous variables. One-way analysis of variance (ANOVA) test was used for comparisons of continuous variables among the different groups. Survival curves were plotted using the Kaplan–Meier method and analyzed by the log-rank test. Cox regression models were used to analyze factors associated to occurrence of events. Those variables that were significant were used in a logistic regression model to predict the probability of having an event. A p value of less than 0.05 (two-tailed) was considered statistically significant. Where applicable, data are presented as mean ± one standard deviation from the mean.

Results

We identified 667 individuals with the abnormal electrocardiogram. Age at diagnosis (first abnormal electrocardiogram ever documented) was 41 ± 15

years (2 to 85 years). There were more males than females (507 versus 160, respectively). In 344 individuals (51.5%) a familial form of the disease was suspected. The electrocardiogram was spontaneously abnormal in 499 cases (75%) and abnormal only after the administration of a class I antiarrhythmic drug in 168. An electrophysiologic study was performed in 493 individuals from whom 231 (47%) had an inducible sustained ventricular arrhythmia during programmed ventricular stimulation.

Natural history

A total of 164 patients presented at least one episode of sudden death or ventricular fibrillation during their lifetime (120 patients before the abnormal electrocardiogram was identified and 44 after the diagnosis). Demographic characteristics and results of the electrophysiologic testing are shown in Table 16.1.

Table 16.2 Probability of sudden death or ventricular fibrillation during lifetime depending on clinical and electrophysiological variables.

	Univariate analysis			Multivariate analysis		
	Hazard ratio	95% CI	p	Hazard ratio	95% CI	p
Inducible	4.76	3.03–7.69	0.0001	3.85	2.38–6.25	0.0001
Non-inducible	1			1		
Basal ECG	3.85	2.17–7.14	0.0001	1.89	1.01–3.70	0.046
AAD ECG	1			1		
Male	2.4	1.56–3.80	0.0001	1.89	1.03–3.45	0.027
Female	1			1		
Family history	1.05	0.69–1.31	0.787			
No family history	1					

Basal ECG, spontaneously abnormal electrocardiogram; AAD ECG, abnormal electrocardiogram only after antiarrhythmic drug administration; CI, confidence intervals.

Using multivariate analysis, inducibility of a sustained ventricular arrhythmia (hazard ratio 3.85, 95% CI 2.38–6.25, $p < 0.0001$), male gender (hazard ratio 1.89, 95% CI 1.03–3.45, $p = 0.027$) and a spontaneously abnormal electrocardiogram (hazard ratio 1.89, 95% CI 1.01–3.70, $p = 0.046$) were predictors of arrhythmia occurrence (Table 16.2).

In Fig. 16.2 the Kaplan–Meier survival curves of the age at which the first arrhythmic event (sudden death or documented ventricular fibrillation) occurred, are plotted depending on gender, inducibility of arrhythmias, and ECG characteristics, respectively.

The probability of having an event was studied using a logistic regression model including different combinations of these predictive factors (Table 16.3). In all categories, male patients had a worse prognosis than female patients. In one extreme, the probability that a male with a spontaneously abnormal electrocardiogram and inducible into a sustained ventricular arrhythmia had an event was 45.1% (95% CI 37.9–52.5%). In the other extreme, the probability that a female with an electrocardiogram abnormal only after antiarrhythmic drug challenge, and non-inducible into sustained ventricular arrhythmias had an event, was only 3% (95% CI 1.3–6.9%).

Follow-up

The individuals in this study were followed-up for a mean of 38 ± 47 months after the diagnosis was made. During that follow-up period 105 patients suffered from new or recurrent sudden cardiac death or from documented ventricular fibrillation. Using multivariate analysis, inducibility of a sustained ventricular arrhythmia (hazard ratio 7.14, 95% CI 2.7–20.0, $p < 0.0001$) and the previous occurrence of aborted sudden death (hazard ratio 3.99, 95% CI 2.09–7.60, $p < 0.0001$) or syncope (Hazard ratio 2.41, 95% CI 1.16–4.99, $p < 0.0001$) were the strongest predictors of events (Table 16.4).

Patients without previous cardiac arrest

A total of 547 individuals with the abnormal electrocardiogram and no previous cardiac arrest were identified. Age at diagnosis (first abnormal electrocardiogram documented) was 41 ± 15 years (2 to 85 years). A predominance of male individuals was observed (408 versus 139). The abnormal electrocardiogram was identified during study of a syncope of unknown origin in 124 patients, during routine electrocardiographic screening in 170 individuals, and during study of family members of patients with the syndrome in 253 individuals.

The electrocardiogram was spontaneously abnormal in 391 cases and abnormal only after the administration of a class I antiarrhythmic drug in 156. During electrophysiologic testing, a sustained ventricular arrhythmia was induced in 163 of 408 individuals. Demographic characteristics and results of

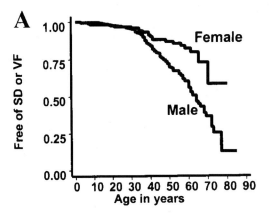

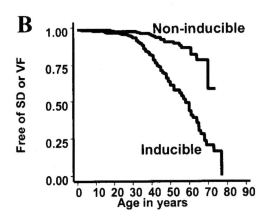

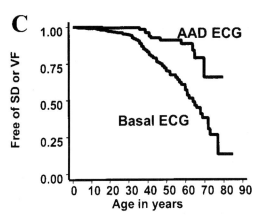

Figure 16.2 Kaplan–Meier survival curve showing age of occurrence of **(A)** a first event (sudden death, SD, or ventricular fibrillation, VF) depending on gender, **(B)** inducibility of ventricular arrhythmias, and **(C)** on the presence of a basal abnormal electrocardiogram (basal ECG) or an electrocardiogram abnormal only after antiarrhythmic drug challenge (AAD ECG).

the electrophysiologic testing are shown in Table 16.5.

Follow-up

The individuals were followed for a mean of 24 ± 33 months after the diagnostic electrocardiogram was recognized. In 44 out of the 547 individuals (8%) an episode of sudden cardiac death or ventricular fibrillation was documented during follow-up (Fig. 16.3).

Using univariate analysis, inducibility of sustained ventricular arrhythmias, the presence of a previous episode of syncope, a basal abnormal electrocardiogram and male gender were predictors of events (Table 16.6). Multivariate analysis identified inducibility of sustained ventricular arrhythmias and a previous history of syncope as predictors of sudden death or ventricular fibrillation.

In Fig. 16.4 the Kaplan–Meier curves of arrhythmic events during follow-up depending on the presence or not of a previous syncopal episode and inducibility of arrhythmias during electrophysiological study are shown.

Using logistic regression analysis of these two variables and the presence or not of a spontaneously abnormal electrocardiogram, eight groups were identified with a risk of sudden death or documented ventricular fibrillation during follow-up varying from 0.5% to 27.2% (Table 16.7). The lowest risk group is an individual with an electrocardiogram diagnostic of Brugada syndrome seen only after drug administration who is not inducible during programmed ventricular stimulation and had no previous symptoms. The highest risk is an individual with a spontaneously abnormal electrocardiogram who is inducible during programmed ventricular stimulation and who has suffered from at least one syncopal episode.

Discussion

This report, based on the largest available series of individuals with an electrocardiogram diagnostic of Brugada syndrome, helps us understand the natural history of the disease. At the same time, analysis of clinical, electrocardiographic, and electrophysiologic data allows us to understand the predictors of prognosis in individuals with such an electrocardiogram.

Table 16.3 Probability of having an event during lifetime.

		Non-inducible at EPS	Inducible at EPS
Male patients	Abnormal ECG after AAD	4.4 (2.0–9.3)	23.4 (12.8–38.8)
	Basal abnormal ECG	11.0 (7.0–16.8)	45.1 (37.9–52.5)
Female patients	Abnormal ECG after AAD	3.0 (1.3–6.9)	17.0 (8.0–32.7)
	Basal abnormal ECG	7.6 (3.8–14.8)	35.5 (21.8–52.1)

EPS, electrophysiologic study; ECG, electrocardiogram; AAD, antiarrhythmic drugs. Data are expressed in percentage (95% confidence intervals). Other abbreviations as in previous tables.

Table 16.4 Probability of sudden death or ventricular fibrillation during follow-up.

	Univariate analysis			Multivariate analysis		
	Hazard ratio	95% CI	p	Hazard ratio	95% CI	p
Inducible	11.1	4.54–25.0	0.0001	7.14	2.7–20.0	0.0001
Non-inducible	1			1		
Basal ECG	3.70	1.75–7.69	0.0001			
AAD ECG	1					
Male	2.94	1.54–5.88	0.0001			
Female	1					
Family history	1.03	0.68–1.55	0.896			
No family history	1					
Asymptomatic	1		0.0001	1		0.0001
Syncope	2.60	1.43–4.76		2.41	1.16–4.99	
Sudden death	6.53	4.08–10.4		3.99	2.09–7.60	
HV < 55 ms	1		0.494			
HV > 55 ms	1.26	0.66–2.40				

Table 16.5 Clinical characteristics of the patients without a previous cardiac arrest.

Number	547
Male	408
Female	139
Age (years)	41 ± 15 (2–85)
Basal abnormal ECG	391
Family history of SCD	302
Inducible	163
Non-inducible	245
History of syncope	124

ECG: electrocardiogram, SCD: sudden cardiac death.

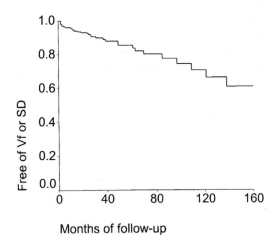

Figure 16.3 Survival curve showing the occurrence of arrhythmic events (sudden cardiac death, SD, or ventricular fibrillation, VF) during follow-up in the group of patients without previous cardiac arrest.

Table 16.6 Probability of sudden death or ventricular fibrillation during follow-up in patients without previous cardiac arrest.

	Univariate analysis			Multivariate analysis		
	Hazard ratio	95% CI	p	Hazard ratio	95% CI	p
Inducible	8.33	2.8–25.0	0.0001	5.88	2.0–16.7	0.0001
Non-inducible	1		1			
Syncope	2.79	1.5–5.1	0.002	2.50	1.2–5.3	0.017
No syncope	1		1			
Basal ECG	7.69	1.9–33.3	0.0001	2.86	0.7–12.3	0.103
AAD ECG	1		1			
Male	5.26	1.6–16.6	0.001			
Female	1					
Family history	1.29	0.7–2.4	0.406			
No family history	1					

Basal ECG; spontaneously abnormal electrocardiogram; AAD ECG, abnormal electrocardiogram only after antiarrhythmic drug administration.

Our data show that:

1 inducibility of a sustained ventricular arrhythmia during programmed ventricular stimulation,

2 male sex,

3 a spontaneous abnormal electrocardiogram, and

4 the previous occurrence of syncope or previous aborted sudden cardiac death are the strongest predictors of outcome.

We analyzed the data in several different ways: Firstly, we tried to understand what the significance is of an electrocardiogram diagnostic of Brugada syndrome independently from the timing of the recording in relation to symptoms or absence of symptoms. In other words, whether this electrocardiogram is or not a marker of sudden arrhythmic death. Secondly, we assessed the value of clinical, electrocardiographic, and electrophysiologic variables to understand their predictive value for arrhythmic events at any time during life, but also after the diagnosis of Brugada syndrome was made. We used the same analysis in the subgroup of patients without a previous history of sudden cardiac death to better understand the prognosis of asymptomatic individuals in whom the abnormal electrocardiogram is detected. The data presented show the following.

1 *An electrocardiogram diagnostic of Brugada syndrome is a marker of sudden arrhythmic death.* Of all the individuals in our series, 25% suffered from sudden death or documented ventricular fibrillation at one or another moment during their life.

With a mean age at the time of diagnosis of 41 years, the incidence of (aborted) sudden death is clearly unexpectedly higher than in a matched general population.

2 *Male sex is a risk factor for sudden death.* For all categories studied, males had a higher risk of (aborted) sudden death as compared to females. This clinical observation has recently been shown to have a pathophysiologic background by the studies of Antzelevitch and coworkers.[7] These authors have elegantly shown that the predominance of the Brugada phenotype in males—and consequently a higher expected incidence of events—is the result of a more prominent I_{to} (the transient outward potassium current) in males than in females.

3 *Inducibility of a sustained ventricular arrhythmia is the strongest marker of prognosis.* Although programmed ventricular stimulation was not performed in all individuals, inducible individuals had an almost four times higher risk of (aborted) sudden death that non-inducible ones.

4 *Familial forms of the disease do not carry a worse prognosis than isolated cases.* A family history of Brugada syndrome did not predict a worse outcome. Data from the present series confirm our previous observations where we reported that a family history of sudden death or a familial form of Brugada syndrome did not carry a poorer prognosis than the isolated forms.[15] These observations have also been confirmed by other reports.[18]

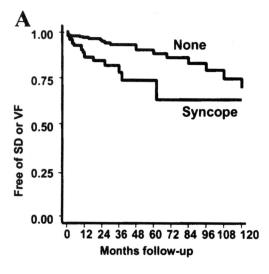

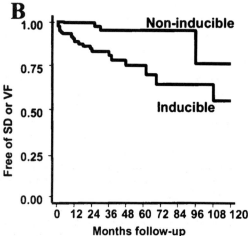

Figure 16.4 Kaplan–Meier analysis of arrhythmic events (sudden cardiac death, SD, or documented ventricular fibrillation, VF) during follow-up.

5 *Individuals with a spontaneously abnormal electrocardiogram have a poorer prognosis than individuals with an abnormal electrocardiogram unmasked only after antiarrhythmic drug challenge.* A spontaneously abnormal electrocardiogram carries almost double the risk of developing an arrhythmic event during lifetime as compared to individuals in whom the electrocardiogram diagnostic of Brugada syndrome was evident only after antiarrhythmic drug challenge. However, there was no power of this variable to predict prognosis after the diagnosis was made. Thus, a spontaneously abnormal electrocardiogram was a marker of an arrhythmic event during lifetime but failed to predict events during follow-up as an isolated variable because other variables (programmed stimulation, male sex) were stronger predictors of outcome.

6 *In patients without a history of previous cardiac arrest the strongest predictor of outcome in patients with an electrocardiogram diagnostic of Brugada syndrome and no previous cardiac arrest is inducibility during programmed ventricular stimulation.* Inducible individuals have an 8 times higher risk of suffering from sudden death or ventricular fibrillation during the subsequent 2 years as compared to non-inducible ones. A spontaneously abnormal electrocardiogram was the second best predictor of outcome with a 7 times higher risk of arrhythmic events as compared to individuals in whom the electrocardiogram was observed only after antiarrhythmic drug challenge. Male sex carries a 5 times higher risk as compared to a female sex. The next best predictor was a previous history of syncope. However, with multivariate analysis, inducibility during programmed ventricular stimulation and a previous history of syncope remained the only predictors of outcome.

Table 16.7 Logistic regression analysis. Probability of events (sudden death or documented ventricular fibrillation) during follow-up in individuals without previous cardiac arrest.

		Non-inducible	*Inducible*
Spontaneously abnormal electrocardiogram	Syncope	4.1% (CI 1.4–11.7%)	27.2% (CI 17.3–40.0%)
	No syncope	1.8% (CI 0.6–5.1%)	14.0% (CI 8.1–23.0%)
Electrocardiogram abnormal only after antiarrhythmic drug challenge	Syncope	1.2% (CI 0.2–6.6%)	9.7% (CI 2.3–33.1%)
	No syncope	0.5% (CI 0.1–2.7%)	4.5% (CI 1.0–17.1%)

The implications of these observations are very relevant for the daily management of individuals with Brugada syndrome and no previous cardiac arrest.

1 Inducibility of a sustained ventricular arrhythmia during programmed ventricular stimulation was the strongest predictor of outcome. The group with inducible ventricular arrhythmias and the *lowest risk* for arrhythmic events was the group without a previous history of syncope and an abnormal electrocardiogram only after the administration of antiarrhythmic drugs. This group had a 4.5% incidence of events during the ensuing 2 years follow-up, an incidence that is clearly too high for a population with a mean age of 41 years. That means that programmed ventricular stimulation must be recommended as a risk stratification method in all patients with an electrocardiogram diagnostic of Brugada syndrome.

2 A previous history of syncope is a risk factor for a poor outcome. Because we deal with a rather young patient population one could argue that the syncopal episodes could be vasovagal in origin and unrelated to arrhythmias caused by the Brugada syndrome. This hypothesis was not tested by systematic tilting test of all individuals with syncope and could represent a limitation in our study. However, the group with previous syncopal episodes had a 1.2 to 4.1% risk of sudden death or documented ventricular fibrillation if non-inducible and a 9.7 to 27.2% risk if inducible. There was thus, an approximate 8 times increase in risk in each category of patients with previous syncope by knowing that individuals were inducible to a sustained ventricular arrhythmia during programmed ventricular stimulation or not.

This research was supported in part and equally by the Ramon Brugada Senior Foundation (Belgium, Spain, USA), the Fundació Privada Clínic per la Recerca (Spain), the Cardiovascular Research and Teaching Institute Aalst (Belgium), and the Mapfre Medicine Foundation (Spain).

References

1 Brugada P, Brugada J. Right bundle branch block, persistent ST segment elevation and sudden cardiac death: a distinct clinical and electrocardiographic syndrome: a multicenter report. *J. Am. Coll. Cardiol.* 1992; **20**: 1391–1396.

2 Chen Q, Kirsch GE, Zhang D *et al.* Genetic basis and molecular mechanisms for idiopathic ventricular fibrillation. *Nature* 1998; **392**: 293–296.

3 Smits JP, Eckardt L, Probst V *et al.* Genotype–phenotype relationship in Brugada syndrome: electrocardiographic features differentiate *SCN5A*-related patients from non-*SCN5A*-related patients. *J. Am. Coll. Cardiol.* 2002; **40**: 350–356.

4 Vatta M, Dumaine R, Valhaus C *et al.* Novel mutations in domain I of *SCN5A* cause Brugada syndrome. *Mol. Genet. Metab.* 2002; **75**: 317–324.

5 Kyndt F, Probst V, Potet F *et al.* Novel *SCN5A* mutation leading either to isolated cardiac conduction defect or Brugada syndrome in a large French family. *Circulation* 2001; **104**: 3081–3086.

6 Yan GX, Antzelevitch C. Cellular basis for the Brugada syndrome and other mechanisms of arrhythmogenesis associated with ST segment elevation. *Circulation* 1999; **100**: 1660–1666.

7 Di Diego JM, Cordeiro JM, Goodrow RJ *et al.* Ionic and cellular basis for the predominance of the Brugada syndrome phenotype in males. *Circulation* 2002; **106**: 2004–2011.

8 Dumaine R, Towbin JA, Brugada P *et al.* Ionic mechanisms responsible for the electrocardiographic phenotype of the Brugada syndrome are temperature dependent. *Circ. Res.* 1999; **85**: 803–809.

9 Miyasaka T, Tsuji H, Yamada K *et al.* Prevalence and mortality of the Brugada-type electrocardiogram in one city in Japan. *J. Am. Coll. Cardiol.* 2001; **38**: 771–774.

10 Hermida J, Lemoine J, Aoun FB, Jarry G, Rey J, Quiret J. Prevalence of the Brugada syndrome in an apparently healthy population. *Am. J. Cardiol.* 2000; **86**: 91–94.

11 Atarashi H, Ogawa S, Harumi K *et al.* Characteristics of patients with right bundle branch block and ST segment elevation in right precordial leads. Idiopathic ventricular fibrillation investigators. *Am. J. Cardiol.* 1996; **78**: 581–583.

12 Shimizu W, Antzelevitch C, Suyama K *et al.* Effects of sodium channel blockers on ST segment, QRS duration, and corrected QT interval in patients with Brugada syndrome. *J. Cardiovasc. Electrophysiol.* 2000; **11**: 1320–1329.

13 Brugada J, Brugada R, Brugada P. Right bundle branch block and ST segment elevation in leads V1 through V3. A marker for sudden death in patients without demonstrable structural heart disease. *Circulation* 1998; **97**: 457–460.

14 Brugada R, Brugada J, Antzelevitch C *et al.* Sodium channel blockers identify risk for sudden death in patients with ST-segment elevation and right bundle branch block but structurally normal hearts. *Circulation* 2000; **101**: 510–515.

15 Brugada J, Brugada R, Antzelevitch C, Towbin J, Nademanee K, Brugada P. Long-term follow-up of indi-

viduals with the electrocardiographic pattern of right bundle-branch block and ST-segment elevation in precordial leads V1 to V3. *Circulation* 2002; **105**: 73–78.

16 Priori SG, Napolitano C, Gasparini M *et al.* Natural history of Brugada syndrome: insights for risk stratification and management. *Circulation* 2002; **105**: 1342–1347.

17 Boveda S, Albenque JP, Baccar H *et al.* Prophylactic value of automatic implantable defibrillators: a case report of a patient with asymptomatic Brugada syndrome. *Arch. Mal Coeur Vaiss* 2001; **94**: 79–84.

18 Takenada S, Kusano KF, Hisamatsu K *et al.* Relatively benign course in asymptomatic patients with Brugada-type electrocardiogram without family history of sudden death. *J. Cardiovasc. Electrophysiol.* 2001; **12**: 2–6.

19 Priori SG, Napolitano C, Gasparini M *et al.* Clinical and genetic heterogeneity of right bundle branch block and ST-segment elevation syndrome. A prospective evaluation of 52 families. *Circulation* 2000; **102**: 2509–2515.

20 Brugada P, Geelen P, Brugada R *et al.* Prognostic value of electrophysiologic investigations in Brugada syndrome. *J. Cardiovasc. Electrophysiol.* 2001; **12**: 1004–1007.

21 Wilde A, Antzelevitch C, Borggrefe M *et al.* Proposed diagnostic criteria for the Brugada syndrome. *Circulation* 2002; **106**: 2514–2518.

22 Miyazaki T, Mitamura H, Miyoshi S, Soejima K, Aizawa Y, Ogawa S. Autonomic and antiarrhythmic drug modulation of ST segment elevation in patients with Brugada syndrome. *J. Am. Coll. Cardiol.* 1996; **27**: 1061–1070.

Physicians and centers

L. Aguinaga, Sanatorio Parque, Tucumán, Argentina

P. Alcaide, Hospital Igualada, Spain

E. Aliot, Centre Hospitalier Universitaire, Nancy, France

J. Alzueta, Hospital Clínico, Málaga, Spain

F. Arribas, M. Lopez Gil, Hospital 12 de Octubre, Madrid, Spain

A. Asso, Hospital Miguel Servet, Zaragoza, Spain

J. Atié, Universidad Federal Rio de Janeiro, Brasil

R. Barba Pichardo, Hospital Juan Ramon Jimenez, Huelva, Spain

X. Beiras, Hospital Xeral Vigo, Spain

I. Blankoff, Centre Hospitalier Universitaire Saint Pierre, Brussels, Belgium

B. Brembilla-Perrot, Centre Hospitalier Universitaire, France

M. Brignole, Ospedali Riuniti, Lavagna, Italy

X. Boada, Hospital de Berga, Spain

A. Bodegas, Hospital de Cruces, Bilbao, Spain

M. Borggrefe, Universitatsklinikum Mannheim, Germany

S. Boveda, Hopitaux de Toulouse, France

J. Brugada, L. Mont, Hospital Clínic, Universitat de Barcelona, Spain

P. Brugada, P. Geleen, OLV Hospital, Aalst, Belgium

C. Bruna, G. Rossetti, A. Vado, Ospedale S. Croce e Carle, Cuneo, Italy

J. Cabrera, J. Farré, Fundación Jimenez Diaz, Madrid, Spain

J.R. Carmona, Hospital de Navarra, Pamplona, Spain

C. Cowan, The General Infirmary, Leeds, Great Britain

F. Dorticós, J. Castro Hevia, Instituto de Cardiología y Cirugía Cardiaca, La Havana, Cuba

J.P. Cebron, Saint Henri Hospital, Nantes, France

K.J. Choi, Asian Medical Center, University of Ulsan, Seul, Corea

L. De Roy, Mont-Godine Hospital, Yvoir, Belgium

P. Della Bella, Università degli Studi di Milano, Italy

P. Denes, Michael Reese Hospital and Medical Center, Chicago, USA

S. Dubner, Clinica Suiza Argentina, Buenos Aires, Argentina

P. Dumoulin, Clinique La Montagne, Centre Ambroise Paré, Paris, France

A. Ebagosti, CHG Martigues, France

L. Eckardt, G. Breithardt, Wilhems-Universitat, Munster, Germany

M. Eldar, Neufeld Cardiac Research Institute, University of Tel-Aviv, Israel

L. Elvas, University Hospital, Coimbra, Portugal

P. Erne, Kantonsspital Luzern, Switzerland

R. Faniel, Brussels, Belgium

I. Fernandez Lozano, Clínica Puerta de Hierro, Madrid, Spain

M. Figueiredo, Ritmocordis, Campinas, Brasil

J. Fisher, Montefiore Medical Center, New York, USA

M. Fromer, Centre Hospitalier Universitaire Vaudois, Lausanne, Switzerland

I. García Bolao, Clinica Universitaria de Navarra, Pamplona, Spain

D. Galley, Centre Hospitalier General, Albi, France

P. Goethals, Hospital St. Jean, Brussels, Belgium

E. Gonzalez, C. Perez Muñoz, Hospital de Jerez de la Frontera, Spain

R. Hauer, University Hospital Utrecht, The Netherlands

M. Helguera, Hospital Italiano, Buenos Aires, Argentina

A. Hernandez Madrid, C. Moro, Hospital Ramon y Cajal, Madrid, Spain

B. Herreros, Hospital Rio Ortega, Valladolid, Spain

M. Jottrand, Hopital Erasme, Brussels, Belgium

W. Kaltenbrunner, Wilhelminenspital, Vienna, Austria

R. Kam, National Heart Centre, Singapore

N.G. Kay, University of Alabama, Birmingham, AL

R. Keegan, Hospital Gutierrez, La Plata, Argentina

G. Kornfeld, Donauspital, Vienna, Austria

C. Lafuente, Hospital General Albacete, Spain

F. Leyva, Good Hope Hospital, Sutton, England

B. Liango, Centre Hospitalier Tubize-Nivelles, France

J. Martinez, F. Picó, Hospital Virgen de la Arrixaca, Murcia, Spain

J.L. Merino, R. Peinado, Hospital Universitario La Paz, Madrid, Spain

J. Metzger, Hopital Cantonal, Geneva, Switzerland

M. McGuire, Royal Prince Alfred Hospital, Camperdown, Australia

A. Moya, Hospital Vall d'Hebrón, Barcelona, Spain

C. Muratore, Sanatorio Mitre, Buenos Aires, Argentina

J. Ollitrault, Hospital Saint Joseph, Paris, France

J. Ormaetxe, Hospital de Basurto, Bilbao, Spain

O. Paredes, Hospital Vera Barros, La Rioja, Argentina

M. Pavón, Hospital Virgen de la Macarena, Sevilla, Spain

B. Pavri, Hospital of the University of Pensilvania, Philadelphia, USA

J. Paylos, Clínica Moncloa, Madrid, Spain

J. Pelegrin, G. Rodrigo, Hospital Clínico Zaragoza, Spain

T. Peter, Cedars Sinai, Los Angeles, CA

D. Pitcher, Hereford Cuntry Hospital, Unkon Walk, USA

J.M. Porres, Hospital Ntra. Sra. Aranzazu, San Sebastian, Spain

D. Potenza, San Giovanni Rotondo, Italy

S. Priori, Salvatore Maugeri Foundation, Molecular Cardiology, Pavia, Italy

F. Provenier, Ziekenhuis Maria Middelares, Gent, Belgium

O. Razali, National Heart Institute, Kuala Lampur, Malaysia

J. Rodriguez, Hospital Virgen de Valme, Sevilla, Spain

M. Rodriguez Serra, Hospital Lluís Alcanyís, Alicante, Spain

J.R. Ruiz, Hospital Santiago Apostol, Miranda de Ebro, Spain

L. Ruiz Valdepeñas, Complejo Hospitalario Ciudad Real, Spain

J. Rubio, Hospital Universitario Valladolid, Spain

X. Sabaté, Hospital Bellvitge, Barcelona, Spain

R. Sanjuan, Hospital Clínico, Valencia, Spain

P. Scanu, CHU Caen, France

E. Sosa, INCOR, Sao Paolo, Brasil

W. Stevenson, Brigham and Women's Hospital, Boston, MA

G. Stix, University of Vienna, Austria

R. Stroobandt, St. Jozef Hospital, Oostende, Belgium

V. Taramasco, CHU Marseille, France

R. Tavernier, J.K. Triedman, Children's Hospital, Boston, MA

L. Tercedor, M. Alvarez, Hospital Virgen de las Nieves, Granada, Spain

H.J. Trappe, Marien Hospital, Herne, Germany, **P. Vanzini**, Asociación Española, Montevideo, Uruguay

A. Vera Almazan, Hospital Carlos Haya, Málaga, Spain

J. Villacastin, J. Almendral, Hospital Gregorio Marañon, Madrid, Spain

M. Wan, W. Siu Hong, Tuen Mun Hospital, Hong Kong

F. Wangüemert, Hospital Ntra. Sra. del Pino, Las Palmas, Spain

T. Wee Siong, Singapore Heart Centre, Singapore

R. Zegarra, Incor Essalud, Lima, Peru

M. Zimmermann, Hopital de la Tour, Meyrin-Geneve, Zwitzerland.

CHAPTER 17

Treatment of Brugada syndrome with an implantable cardioverter defibrillator

P. Brugada, MD, PhD, *E. Bartholomay,* MD, *L. Mont,* MD, *R. Brugada,* MD,
J. Brugada, MD

Summary

- Background. The benefit of the implantable cardioverter defibrillator in a large cohort of patients with Brugada syndrome has not been assessed.
- Methods. Of 690 patients with Brugada syndrome included in a multicentric trial, 258 individuals received an implantable cardioverter defibrillator because of a suspected high risk of sudden arrhythmic death. The stored electrograms were reviewed to assess the efficacy and effectiveness of defibrillation on ventricular fibrillation episodes. Efficacy was defined as the implantable cardioverter defibrillator ability of reversion for each ventricular fibrillation episode. Effectiveness was assessed by the number of patients that had the advantage of appropriate defibrillation for at least one episode of ventricular fibrillation.
- Results. Mean age was 42 ± 13.5 years, there were 210 males (81.3%). A total of 160 patients (62%) were symptomatic before establishing the diagnosis. There were 120 patients (48.4%) with a family history of sudden death and/or a familial Brugada electrocardiographic pattern. A sustained ventricular arrhythmia was induced during the electrophysiologic study in 198 patients (76.7%). During a mean follow-up of 2.5 years (median 2) there were no instances of death. However, 69 patients (26.7%) had at least one appropriate defibrillation of ventricular fibrillation. The efficacy of the implantable cardioverter defibrillator was 100%

and the effectiveness was respectively 14%, 20%, 29%, 38%, 52% at 1, 2, 3, 4, and 5 years of follow-up.
- Conclusion. The implantable cardioverter defibrillator had a 100% efficacy to revert ventricular fibrillation and a high effectiveness in this population of patients with an electrocardiographic pattern of Brugada syndrome.

Introduction

Most patients suffering from sudden arrhythmic death (SAD) have one or another form of structural heart disease, most commonly ischemic heart disease. However, in about 10% of cases the heart is structurally normal.[3] A subgroup of these patients was described in 1992 by Brugada and Brugada with a particular electrocardiographic (ECG) pattern. The ECG shows a right bundle-branch block-like QRS complex and ST segment elevation in leads V_1 through V_3.[4] The genetic nature of this disease was documented shortly thereafter.[5] The follow-up of these patients has shown a high incidence of SAD, a poor response to antiarrhythmic drugs, and a good outcome after the implantation of a cardioverter defibrillator (ICD).[6–8]

The effectiveness of the ICD to reduce mortality in patients with structural heart disease and high risk of SAD has already been demonstrated;[9,10] however, the benefit of the ICD in a large series of patients with Brugada syndrome has not been evaluated.

The objective of this study was to analyze the efficacy and effectiveness of the ICD in a population of patients with the ECG pattern of Brugada syndrome.

Methods

We analyzed the outcome of a cohort of patients with Brugada syndrome included in a multicenter trial (see the list at the end of chapter 16). We focused on the outcome of patients who received an ICD because they were considered to be at high risk for SAD.

Based on the results of previous studies, where the ICD had been shown to be the only effective treatment for SAD prevention in patients with Brugada syndrome,[11] it was considered not ethical to develop a drug or placebo controlled study for this specific population again. The stored ICD electrograms were reviewed to assess the efficacy and effectiveness of the device during spontaneous episodes of ventricular fibrillation (VF).

Definitions

Efficacy was defined as the ability of the ICD to appropriately revert each VF episode.

Effectiveness was assessed by the number of patients that had the advantage of an appropriate defibrillation after implantation of the ICD. Only the first VF episode was considered for analysis.

The presence of structural heart disease was excluded by a complete investigation laboratory analysis, echocardiogram, exercise test, coronary angiography, nuclear magnetic resonance, and endomyocardial biopsies used at the discretion of the treating physician.

The ECG was considered characteristic of Brugada syndrome if a pattern with a prominent coved ST segment elevation in V_1–V_3, displaying a J wave amplitude or ST segment elevation >0.2 mV at its peak was observed.[12]

Patients with clinical suspicion of Brugada syndrome and with a non-diagnostic baseline ECG (normal basal ECG) were submitted to a drug test with intravenous administration of either ajmaline (1 mg/kg body weight over 5 min), flecainide (2 mg/kg body weight over 10 min), or pro-cainamide (1 mg/kg body weight over 10 min). The test was considered positive if a coved ST segment elevation and J wave amplitude of >0.2 mV in lead V_1, and/or V_2, and/or V_3 with or without right bundle branch block became apparent.[12]

Patients with a previous history of syncope, documented sustained ventricular arrhythmias, or aborted SAD were considered symptomatic.

Patients were distributed into two groups according to their family history: sporadic cases or familial. The family history was considered positive when there was a first relative with a Brugada ECG pattern and/or SAD.

An electrophysiological study (EPS) was performed in all patients included in this analysis. The ventricular stimulation protocol included up to three extrastimuli in at least one right ventricular site in all cases. The study was considered positive when a sustained ventricular arrhythmia was induced. Sustained ventricular arrhythmia was defined as any ventricular arrhythmia lasting >30 s, causing syncope, circulatory collapse, or requiring intervention to be terminated.

Statistical analysis

Data were analysed using the SPSS software (version 10.0) package for paired and unpaired data. The time of occurrence of clinical events was analysed using the Kaplan–Meier method. Multivariate Cox regression model analysis was performed to evaluate the statistical significance and independence of predictors of events. A two-tailed value of $p < 0.05$ was considered statistically significant.

Results

Clinical characteristics and indication for ICD implantation

The clinical characteristics of the 258 patients are shown in Table 17.1; 62% patients had suffered from symptoms before the diagnosis, 81 patients (31.3%) had suffered from at least one syncopal episode and 79 (30.7%) had been resuscitated from VF. Of the 258 patients, 198 (76.7%) had an inducible sustained ventricular arrhythmia at EPS.

The indication for ICD implantation was decided by the attending physician. The indications for ICD implantation were:

Table 17.1 Clinical characteristics of 258 individuals with Brugada syndrome.

Variable		
Age (years)		42 ± 13.5
Male (%)		210 (81.3%)
Symptoms	Asymptomatic (%)	98 (38)
	Syncope (%)	81 (31.3)
	Resuscitated SAD (%)	79 (30.7)
Genetic	Positive family history (%)	133 (51.6)
	Sporadic (%)	125 (48.4)
EPS	Positive (%)	198 (76.7)
	Negative (%)	60 (23.3)
Mean follow-up (years)		2.5 (median 2)

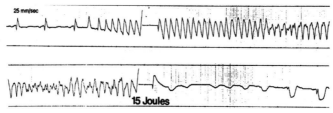

Figure 17.1 A stored electrogram of an ICD with the recording of VF with appropriate defibrillation.

- resuscitated SAD (n = 79, 64 with inducible ventricular arrhythmias),
- syncope (n = 81, 57 with inducible ventricular arrhythmias),
- asymptomatic individuals with a Brugada ECG pattern and inducible ventricular arrhythmias (n = 77),
- asymptomatic individuals with a Brugada ECG pattern, no inducible ventricular arrhythmias but with a familial history of Brugada syndrome and SAD (n = 16),
- asymptomatic individuals with a spontaneous Brugada ECG pattern (n = 5).

Twenty-two patients used an antiarrhythmic drug at one or another time of the follow-up (11 used beta-blockers, 8 quinidine, and 3 amiodarone) without any success to prevent new episodes of VF.

Efficacy and effectiveness of the ICD

The mean follow-up time since implantation of the ICD at analysis was 2.5 years, ranging from 7 months to 8 years (median 2 years). During the follow-up period there were no instances of death. However, 69 patients (26.7%) had an appropriate ICD defibrillation of VF (Fig. 17.1) that could have eventually lead to death if the ICD had not been implanted. The efficacy of the ICD to revert the VF episodes was 100%.

The Kaplan–Meier curve of effectiveness of ICD and the number of events in the first 5 years of follow-up are shown in Fig. 17.2. Most patients presented the first (or recurrent) VF episode during the first year. The effectiveness of the ICD in patients with Brugada syndrome was 14% during the 1st year, 20% at 2 years, 29% at 3 years, 38% at 4 years, and 52% at 5 years of follow-up.

The Kaplan–Meier analysis demonstrated differences in the number of VF events with appropriated defibrillation among the different groups when symptoms were considered (Fig. 17.3). Symptomatic patients had a higher ICD effectiveness compared with asymptomatic patients ($p < 0.001$). The effectiveness in the resuscitated SAD group was 45% in the 1st year, 56% at the 2nd year, and 88% at

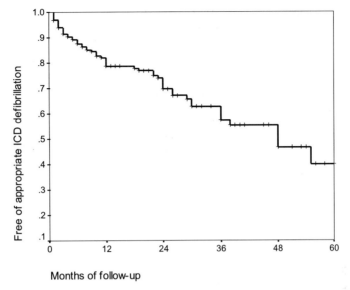

Months of follow-up

Cumulative ventricular events

Follow-up (months)	0	12	24	36	48	60
Number of patients	258	154	101	66	50	35
Cumulative events (%)	0	14	20	29	38	52

Figure 17.2 Kaplan–Meier curve of effectiveness of the ICD in 258 patients with the electrocardiographic pattern of Brugada syndrome. ICD, implantable cardioverter defibrillator.

5 years of follow-up. In the syncope group the effectiveness was 18% in the 1st year, 23% at the 2nd year and 51% at 5 years. The lower effectiveness was observed in patients with a Brugada ECG pattern but no previous symptoms with 4% in the 1st year, 6% at the 2nd year and 37% at 5 years of follow-up.

Cox regression analysis

The variables evaluated in the Cox regression analysis were sex, age, presence of symptoms before diagnosis, characteristics of basal ECG, family history, electrophysiological study results, HV interval, and use of antiarrhythmic drug. Only the presence of symptoms before the diagnosis and the results of the EPS were independently related to VF during follow-up.

Patients previously resuscitated from VF had a hazard ratio (HR) for VF of 3.52 with a 95% confidence intervals (CI) of 1.82–6.82, and those with syncope had a HR of 2.58 (CI 1.25–5.32) when compared to asymptomatic patients. The presence of in-

ducible ventricular arrhythmias during EPS was a risk factor for VF during follow-up ($p = 0.006$). Patients with positive study had a HR for VF of 2.70 (CI 1.22–5.88) compared to patients with a negative study.

Risk stratification

The variables independently associated with VF in the Cox regression analysis were included in the risk stratification.

The presence of symptoms before the diagnosis of Brugada syndrome was the strongest independent predictor of VF during the follow-up. The high association power between the presence of symptoms and VF lowered the stratification capacity of the EPS in this group of patients. Patients with syncope or resuscitated from SAD, even with a negative study, had respectively 17% and 13% VF events during the follow-up.

The results of the EPS were more useful in the asymptomatic group, with a sensitivity and negative

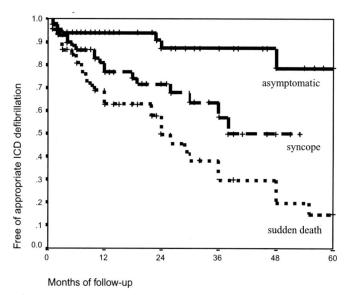

Cumulative ventricular events

	12 months	24 months	36 months	48 months	60 months
Asymptomatic	4%	6%	9%	17%	37%
Syncope	18%	23%	30%	36%	51%
Resuscitated SAD	45%	56%	76%	84%	88%

Figure 17.3 Kaplan–Meier curve of effectiveness of the ICD in 258 patients with electrocardiographic pattern of Brugada syndrome according to symptoms. ICD, implantable cardioverter defibrillator; SAD, sudden arrhythmic death.

predictive value of 100%. In asymptomatic patients with a negative EPS there were no VF episodes during follow-up.

When asymptomatic individuals were separated by considering the results of the basal ECG, none with a normal basal ECG had a VF event during follow-up, even when they had a positive EPS. Sensitivity and negative predictive value of normal ECG among these individuals was 100%.

Eleven asymptomatic individuals (13.2%) with a basal Brugada ECG pattern had a VF event during follow-up. Among these patients the electrophysiologic study could stratify well the risk of VF, with a sensitivity and negative predictive value of 100%.

Based on the results of this study, the use of the algorithm exhibited in Fig. 17.4 to stratify the risk of suffering a VF in patients with Brugada syndrome is recommended.

ICD complications

Most ICD were implanted on the pectoral region and no death occurred during the procedure. Two patients had an infectious complication that required both lead and generator replacement. During follow-up inappropriate shocks were observed in 3 patients (1 sinus tachycardia and 2 atrial fibrillation).

Discussion

The Brugada syndrome was first described in 1992[4] and is believed to be responsible for 4–12% of all SAD and 20–50% of deaths in patients without structural heart disease.[7–13] Thus, there is a high concern in identifying and treating these patients. The inefficacy of antiarrhythmic drugs has been previously described, and today ICD seems to be the only therapeutic option for this disease.[11] We analyzed the outcome in a large series of individuals with a Brugada ECG pattern in whom an ICD was implanted.

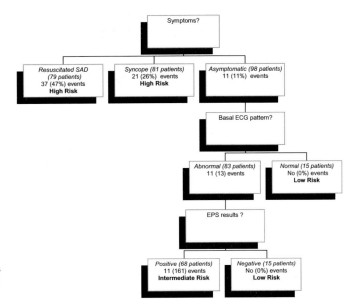

Figure 17.4 Risk stratification of patients with the electrocardiographic pattern of Brugada syndrome.

Population characteristics

The patients that fulfilled our inclusion criteria are not the most typical of Brugada syndrome patients, but rather those with higher risk of SAD. The high risk was assessed by means of the data from previous studies where symptoms and results of EPS were found to be good predictors of outcome.[14-18]

Mean age of 42 years, male sex prevalence (5:1) and 48% having a family history are findings that are in accordance with previous described series.[6,7] The hereditary nature of the syndrome, characterized by an autosomal dominant mode of transmission, is well established.[5] Although a number of candidate genes are considered plausible, thus far the syndrome has been linked to mutation in the gene SCN5A, that encodes for the α subunit of the sodium channel. Only approximately 20% of patients have a mutation in the gene SCN5A. The variability of phenotypic presentation indicates the possibility of various mutations involved, still waiting to be discovered.

ICD implantation was done in this population according to the criteria of the attending physician. However, there was a general agreement in that symptomatic patients have a high risk of VF and that they should be implanted. This is reflected in these series by the high number of symptomatic individuals that were included.

Within the group of asymptomatic patients, the most common group receiving an ICD included patients with a spontaneously abnormal ECG (83 patients, corresponding to 32.1% of the total population). This high implantation rate in asymptomatic individuals with a spontaneously abnormal ECG was the result of previous studies[13,19] that showed a high risk of SAD in this category (8–10% during the 2 first years of follow-up) particularly if inducible during EPS. The follow-up data of these individuals in the present study (16% events during a mean follow-up time of only 2.5 years) confirm the previous results and strengthen the indication of an ICD for this category.

Efficacy and effectiveness of implantable cardioversor-defibrillator

The inefficacy of antiarrhythmic drugs in Brugada syndrome makes it unethical to perform a randomized study of ICD versus drugs.[14-16] Nademanee et al. conducted a randomized clinical trial comparing β-blockers with ICD in patients with unexplained death, in Thailand.[13] 59% of the population had a Brugada ECG pattern. The study was prematurely stopped by the Data Safety Board as a result of the higher mortality in the β-blocker group.

In our study there was no death, despite a high incidence of first or recurrent VF, since all VF episodes were appropriately treated by the ICD, demonstrating a 100% efficacy. The high efficacy of ICD in this population is probably due to the 'pure' arrhythmic disturbance and lack of associated pathologies in this young population.

Effectiveness was defined as the number of patients that had the advantage of an appropriate defibrillation after a VF episode. Kaplan–Meier curves (Fig. 17.3) demonstrated that most events occurred the first year after ICD implantation. Considering that these patients would have died without the ICD, the number of patients needed to be treated by the ICD to save a life would have been 7 after 1 year, 5 in 2 years, and 2 in 5 years of follow-up. Taking into account that we are dealing with young individuals without structural heart disease, these numbers turn out to be even more important.

Risk stratification

The risk of cardiovascular events in asymptomatic individuals with a typical ECG pattern has been previously discussed, with controversial results in different publications.[14–16] The results of EPS are important in the risk stratification of this group. In the present study, the results of the electrophysiological study had a sensitivity and predictive negative value of 100% in asymptomatic patients with an abnormal basal ECG. That is why, based on the use of the ICD during follow-up, that we propose the risk stratification algorithm shown in Fig. 17.4.

Study limitations

A randomized clinical trial is certainly the best model for analysis of the outcome of an intervention. However, data from many publications made it unethical — as far as we are concerned — to use a design such that implantation of the ICD was randomized. Eventually one could test the value of old or new drugs by randomizing the drug in patients implanted with an ICD.

The population included in this study was identified over 33 different centers around the world. Therefore, even trying to collect the data uniformly, measurement bias might have happened. The ventricular stimulation protocol was not uniform in all centers, nor was the programming of the ICD device.

Conclusion

The ICD treatment had a 100% efficacy in reverting

VF episodes in patients with a Brugada ECG pattern. The effectiveness of ICD was also high in this group of patients, especially among symptomatic patients with Brugada syndrome. Both ECG and results of EPS study could be used to screen for ICD indication in individuals with a Brugada ECG pattern. With the available information asymptomatic individuals with normal basal ECG do not seem to expect a benefit from ICD implantation.

Supported by the Ramon Brugada Senior Foundation, The Mapfre Medicine Foundation, and the Fundacio Privada Hospital Clinic, Barcelona.

References

1 Priori S, Alliot E, Blomstrom-Lundqvist *et al*. Task Force on Sudden Cardiac Death of the European Society of Cardiology. *Eur. Heart J*. 2001; **22**: 1374–1450.

2 Eisenberg MS, Mengert TJ. Primary care: cardiac resuscitation. *N. Engl. J. Med*. 2001; **344**; 17.

3 Viskin S, Bellhassen B. Idiopathic ventricular fibrillation. *Am. Heart J*. 1990; **120**: 661–671.

4 Brugada P, Brugada J. Right bundle branch block, persistent ST-segment elevation and sudden cardiac death: a distinct clinical and electrocardiographic syndrome. *J. Am. Coll. Cardiol*. 1992; **20**: 1391–1396.

5 Chen Q, Kirsch GE, Zhang D *et al*. Genetic basis and molecular mechanisms for idiopathic ventricular fibrillation. *Nature* 1998; **392**: 293–296.

6 Brugada J, Brugada R, Brugada P. Right bundle-branch and ST-segment elevation in leads V1 through V3: a marker of sudden death in patients without demonstrable structural heart disease. *Circulation* 1998; **97**: 457–460.

7 Antzelevitch C, Brugada P, Brugada J *et al*. Brugada syndrome: a decade of progress. *Circ. Res*. 2002; **91**: 114–118.

8 Brugada J, Brugada R, Brugada P. Pharmacological and device approach to therapy of inherited cardiac diseases associated with cardiac arrhythmia and sudden death. *J. Electrocardiol*. 2000; **33**(suppl): 41–47.

9 Kuck, K, Cappato R, Siebels J *et al*. Randomized comparison of antiarrhythmic drug therapy and implantable defibrillators in patients resuscitated from cardiac arrest (CASH). *Circulation* 2000; **102**: 748–754.

10 Connoly S, Gent M, Robin S. Canadian Implantable Defibrillator Study (CIDS). A randomized trial of the implantable cardioverter defibrillator against amiodarone. *Circulation* 2000; **101**: 1297–1302.

11 Nademanee K; Veerakul G, Mower M *et al*. Defibrillator versus ß-blockers for unexplained death in Thailand (DEBUT): a randomized clinical trial. *Circulation* 2003; **107**: 2221–2226.

12 Wilde A, Antzelevith C, Borggrefe M *et al*. Proposed crite-

ria of the Brugada syndrome. *Eur. Heart J.* 2002; **23**: 1648–1654.

13 Nademanee K, Veerakul G, Nimmannit S *et al.* Arrhythmogenic marker for sudden death unexplained death syndrome in Thai men. *Circulation* 1997; **96**: 2595–2600.

14 Brugada J, Brugada R, Antzelevitch C *et al.* Long-term follow-up of individuals with the electrocardiographic pattern of right bundle-branch block and ST-segment elevation in precordial leads V1 to V3. *Circulation* 2002; **105**: 73–78.

15 Brugada J, Brugada R, Brugada P. Asymptomatic patients with a Brugada electrocardiogram: are they at risk? *J. Cardiovasc. Electrophysiol.* 2001; **12**: 0–1.

16 Priori S, Napolitano C, Gasparini M *et al.* Natural history of Brugada syndrome. *Circulation* 2002; **105**: 1342–1347.

17 Belhassen B, Viskin S, Fish R *et al.* Effects of electrophysiologic-guided therapy with class IA antiarrhythmic drugs on the long term outcome of patients with idiopathic ventricular fibrillation with an without the Brugada syndrome. *J. Cardiovasc. Electrophysiol.* 1999; **10**: 1301–1312.

18 Brugada P, Geelen P, Brugada R *et al.* Prognostic value of electrophysiologic investigation in Brugada syndrome. *J. Cardiovasc. Electrophysiol.* 2001; **12**: 1004–1007.

CHAPTER 18

Pharmacologic approach to therapy of Brugada syndrome: quinidine as an alternative to ICD therapy?

B. Belhassen, MD, *S. Viskin,* MD

Introduction

In 1992, Pedro and Josep Brugada, two Spanish cardiologist brothers, reported 8 patients with aborted cardiac arrest and no demonstrable heart disease who exhibited in sinus rhythm right bundle branch block (RBBB) with prominent ST segment elevation in precordial leads V_1–V_3.[1] Despite initial controversy about the diagnosis, especially concerning the possibility of a subtle arrhythmogenic right ventricular dysplasia, the repeated lack of right ventricular involvement along with consistent clinical, electrocardiographic (ECG) and electrophysiologic (EP) features convinced the cardiologic community that the Brugada syndrome was actually a new and important cause of sudden cardiac death in ostensibly healthy patients.[2] Since the mid-1990s, an increased awareness among physicians has resulted in a growing number of patients reported worldwide. In 1998, Chen and associates were first to establish that the Brugada syndrome was a genetic disease with an autosomal dominant pattern of transmission.[3] These investigators described mutations, all affecting the cardiac sodium channel *SCN5A* on chromosome 3.[3] The disease appears to be genetically heterogeneous because, at present, *SCN5A* has a proven involvement in only 30% of patients. More recently, a novel gene locus on chromosome 3, distinct from *SCN5A*, has been identified.[4] The genetic pattern of transmission of the disease has lead to the increased detection of asymptomatic patients affected by the disease among families of cardiac arrest survivors.[3–5]

Despite the fact there are still unanswered issues dealing with the clinical and genetic diagnosis of the Brugada syndrome, major advances have been accomplished during the last decade concerning its management. Implantation of an automatic cardioverter-defibrillator (ICD) has been recommended by most electrophysiologists worldwide in symptomatic patients with Brugada syndrome (cardiac arrest survivors, unexplained syncope) as well as in high-risk asymptomatic patients who have inducible ventricular fibrillation (VF) during programmed ventricular stimulation (PVS). Such an attitude is a logical consequence of both the extraordinary efficacy of ICD in terminating VF and the repeated claim of authorities in the field that '*No drug has shown efficacy in the prevention of sudden cardiac death in the Brugada syndrome.*'[6] In fact, while most antiarrhythmic agents (such amiodarone and β blockers) have been found to be ineffective or even deleterious,[7,8] there is preliminary evidence that a few drugs may actually have a beneficial effect on the Brugada syndrome, especially quinidine, a drug we have used routinely for more than two decades in our institution in the management of malignant idiopathic ventricular tachyarrhythmias.

Historical background

The first time we used quinidine for a malignant ventricular arrhythmia in a patient without demonstrable heart disease was in February 1979.[9] The 28-year-old patient had multiple episodes of VF initiated by short-coupled ventricular extrasystoles on a normal QT interval, and required repeated direct current shocks. He did not have any ECG feature suggesting Brugada syndrome. High oral and intravenous doses of amiodarone along with ventricular pacing hardly resulted in arrhythmia control. A recurrent syncopal episode occurred after 1 month of amiodarone therapy (600 mg daily) and prompted us to perform PVS, which showed an easily inducible VF. After addition of oral quinidine (1500 mg daily), VF could no longer be induced. A repeat PVS performed 23.5 years after the first study confirmed the efficacy of that combination. The patient has remained arrhythmia-free during a 24.5 year follow-up period on a combined quinidine–amiodarone therapy.

The positive results observed in this patient led us to systematically use EP-guided therapy with quinidine or other class 1A antiarrhythmic agents (disopyramide, procainamide) in any patient with inducible sustained VF and no obvious heart disease. In 1987, we reported the first series of five patients with aborted cardiac arrest and no heart disease who had inducible VF prevented with class 1A antiarrhythmic agents.[10] One of the patients in these series (patient 3) was a 52-year-old man who collapsed in November 1981 when dancing. After resuscitation from VF, he was found to have some ST-T changes in the right precordial leads along with RBBB (Fig. 18.1). At this time, we did not attribute any significant importance to such findings, especially in the presence of normal coronary anatomy and normal biventricular contraction. The patient had inducible VF at baseline EP study—while on amiodarone therapy—but had only a few repetitive responses after addition of 1500 mg quinidine (Fig. 18.2). Similar VF inducibility (Fig. 18.3) as well as efficacy of quinidine (Fig. 18.4) were found at repeat PVS performed 11 years later. The patient did not have recurrent arrhythmic events on quinidine therapy. He certainly had a Brugada syndrome, a diagnosis that we missed 10 years before the first publication by the Brugada brothers. Finally, in 1999, we reported our experience with EP-guided therapy with class 1A antiarrhythmic drugs (mainly quinidine) on 34 patients with VF and no obvious heart disease, including 5 with Brugada syndrome.[11]

Mechanism of action of quinidine

Basic studies conducted over the past dozen years suggest that the accentuated ST segment elevation associated with the Brugada syndrome is due to a rebalancing of the current active at the end of phase 1, leading to an accentuation of the action potential notch in the right ventricular epicardium.[2,12–14] The

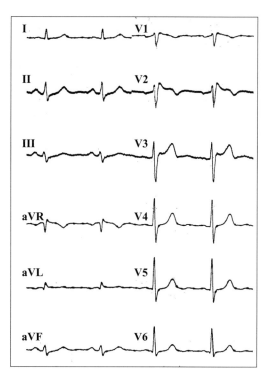

Figure 18.1 ECG in sinus rhythm on no antiarrhythmic medication in a 52-year-old patient resuscitated from out-of-hospital cardiac arrest in November 1981. The diagnosis of Brugada syndrome was not done at this time. Reprinted from Ref. 11 by permission of Futura Publishing Company.

mechanism of the arrhythmias in Brugada syndrome is assumed to be due to electrical inhomogeneity and phase 2 reentry in relation with a prominent transient outward I_{to} current.[12,13] Quinidine, a class 1A antiarrhythmic agent, well known for its depressant effect on the sodium channel current was also found by Antzelevitch and coworkers to strongly inhibit I_{to} in ventricular epicardial cells thus restoring electrical homogeneity and abolishing phase 2 reentrant activity.[12,15]

Quinidine was also found effective in normalizing the ST segment and preventing the development of arrhythmias in experimental models of the Brugada syndrome.[14,15]

In addition, the anticholinergic effect of quinidine might contribute to its antiarrhythmic efficacy in the Brugada syndrome.[16] A cardioselective and ion channel-specific I_{to} blocker does not exist and quinidine is the only agent available worldwide

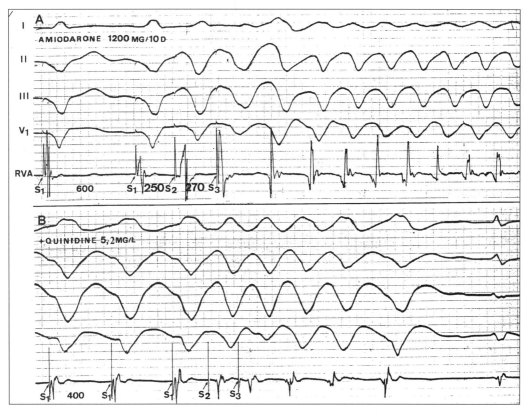

Figure 18.2 This is the same patient as in Fig. 18.1; data from the initial EP studies (November 1981). Shown are ECG leads II, III, V_1, and electrograms from the right ventricular apex (RVA). (**A**) During baseline EP study performed after 10 days of amiodarone therapy (1200 mg/day), sustained polymorphic VT/VF is induced at an 'immediate trial' of double extrastimulation. (**B**) After addition of quinidine bisulfate (1500 mg/day, serum level 5.2 mg/L), only a few repetitive ventricular beats are induced using a protocol that includes up to two extrastimuli and repetition ($n = 10$) of double extrastimulation delivered from the RVA at 3 basic cycle lengths (600, 500, and 400 ms). Reprinted from Ref. 11 by permission of Futura Publishing Company.

capable of exerting significant block of this current. Further discussion of the mechanism of quinidine and other I_{to} blockers in the Brugada syndrome can be found in chapter 5 of this book.

Efficacy of quinidine therapy

At the time of writing the present article (September 2003), and to the best of our knowledge, there have been only a few reported patients with the Brugada syndrome treated with quinidine, most of them originating from our laboratory. Our updated results include 13 symptomatic patients (aborted cardiac arrest, $n = 7$; recurrent unexplained syncope, $n = 5$; palpitations due to exercise-induced ventricular tachycardia, $n = 1$) as well as 9 'asymptomatic',

high-risk patients with the Brugada syndrome and inducible VF (none of these 9 patients had symptoms suggesting an arrhythmic event but 1 of them had typical episodes of vasovagal fainting). All our 22 patients had inducible sustained VF at baseline EP study. Of note is that 3 of the 5 patients that we initially classified as suffering from 'idiopathic VF' in our first publication reporting the EP efficacy of class 1A drugs[10] were later diagnosed as having Brugada syndrome. Our protocol of PVS evolved over the years but included for most patients (studied by 1988), up to triple extrastimuli at two basic cycle lengths (600 and 400 ms) delivered from two right ventricular sites (apex and outflow tract). A special characteristic of our PVS protocol to maximize sensitivity is the use of high stimulus current

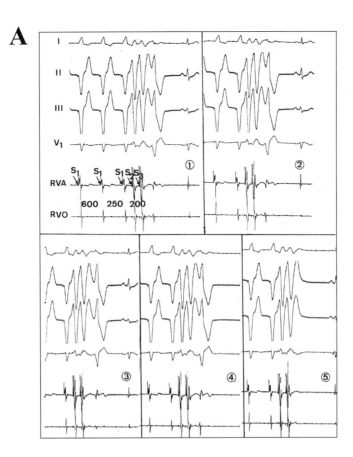

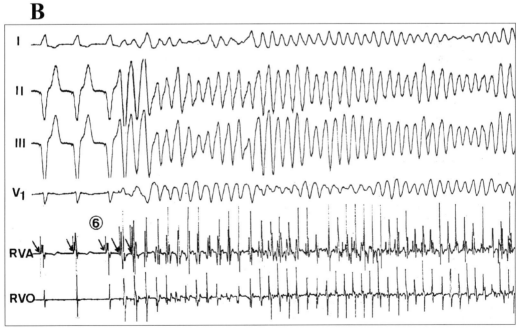

Figure 18.3 This is the same patient as in Fig. 18.1; data from the EP studies performed 11 years later on no antiarrhythmic medication (July 1992). (**A**) Repetition (*n* = 5) of double RVA extrastimulation at the same coupling intervals (600/250/200) induces only a single repetitive ventricular response. (**B**) At the 6th trial using the same coupling interval, sustained polymorphic VT/VF is induced. Reprinted from Ref. 11 by permission of Futura Publishing Company.

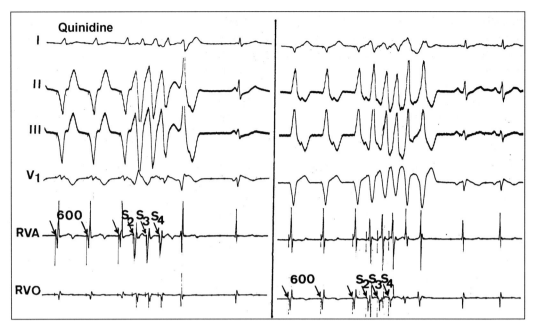

Figure 18.4 This is the same patient as in Fig. 18.1. After administration of quinidine bisulfate (1500 mg/day), VF can no longer be induced using repetition (10 times) of double extrastimulation and repetition (5 times) of triple extrastimulation at the shortest coupling intervals. Note the persistence of the Brugada sign in V_1. Reprinted from Ref. 11 by permission of Futura Publishing Company.

(5 times the diastolic threshold — but never >3 mA) and repetition[17] of the extrastimulation at the shortest coupling intervals (10 times and 5 times for double and triple extrastimulation, respectively). We have used quinidine bisulfate (Quinidurane*, Teva Laboratories) at initial doses of 1500–2000 mg (tailored to achieve a quinidine serum level ≥1.5 mg/l). Sustained VF was defined as a ventricular tachyarrhythmia manifesting a continuously varying morphology with a mean cycle length <200 ms, which required cardioversion for termination or resulted in clinical cardiac arrest before spontaneous termination. Nonsustained ventricular tachycardia (VT) (which was invariably polymorphic) was a VT of ≥6 complexes that was shorter than 30 s in duration and was not associated with loss of consciousness. Arrhythmias were defined as 'non-inducible' when <6 repetitive ventricular complexes were induced.

There were 21 males and 1 female, aged 19 to 80 (37 ± 14) years old at the time of the EP study. All patients but one tolerated quinidine therapy and underwent repeat PVS on that medication. An acute beneficial EP response to quinidine (prevention of

re-induction of sustained VF) was achieved in 19 (90.5%) of the 21 tested patients. Of these 19 responders, no significant ventricular arrhythmias were induced in 16 patients while nonsustained ventricular arrhythmias (lasting from 7 beats to 17 seconds) were induced in 3. The effective dose of quinidine was 1500 mg in all patients except 1 in whom the effective dose was 2000 mg. The quinidine serum levels measured at the time of established drug efficacy during PVS ranged from 1.7 to 5.2 mg/l (2.8 ± 0.9) mg/l. Interestingly, 3 of the 19 patients who responded to a 1500 mg dose of quinidine accepted to undergo a repeat EP evaluation on a lower dose of quinidine (1000 mg). In 1 of these 3 patients, this low quinidine dose was as effective as the high dose. Of the 2 patients who did not respond to a dose of 1500 mg quinidine, repeat EP study was not performed on a higher dose due to achievement of a very high quinidine serum level (8.5 mg/l) in one patient[18] and intolerance to a higher dose of quinidine in the other.

During a follow-up ranging from 1 to 209 months (56 ± 73) on quinidine alone (18 patients), or combined with 200 mg amiodarone (1 patient), none of the patients had a life-threatening arrhythmia documented. Of these 19 patients, 17 remained asymptomatic during quinidine therapy. One patient with previously documented multiple VF episodes controlled for 8 years with 1500 mg quinidine exhibited a syncopal episode compatible with an arrhythmic event. After implantation of an ICD without drug discontinuation, he had a recurrent syncope with no arrhythmia documentation at ICD interrogation. Another patient with typical vasovagal episodes before quinidine therapy had also similar recurrent episodes while on that medication. In the whole group of patients who were treated with quinidine based on the EP results (n = 19), the drug had to be discontinued due to gastrointestinal effects, thrombocytopenia, allergic reaction, or aggravation of sinus node dysfunction in 6 patients (32%)

(after " 1month of therapy in 3 patients). However, no patient developed QT prolongation requiring discontinuation of quinidine therapy. An ICD was implanted in 7 patients due to quinidine-related side effects (6 patients) or patient's wish (1 patient).

Isolated cases of the high efficacy of quinidine in symptomatic patients with the Brugada syndrome have also been reported by others[19,20] and a similarly beneficial effect of disopyramide has been reported in 1 patient.[21] In addition, Alings et al.[22] reported for the first time normalization of right precordial J waves and ST segment elevation following oral administration of quinidine in 2 patients with Brugada syndrome (including one cardiac arrest survivor). We observed similar findings in isolated cases (Fig. 18.5).[23]

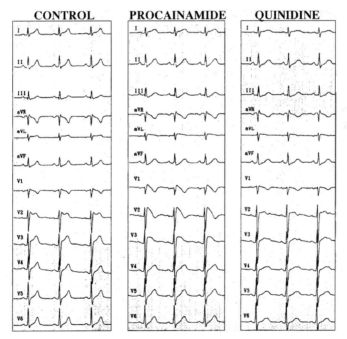

Figure 18.5 Twelve lead ECG tracings in an asymptomatic 26-year-old male with a Brugada sign. (**A**) During control: a 'saddleback-type' ST segment elevation is observed in V₂. (**B**) After intravenous administration of 750 mg procainamide, the 'saddleback-type' ST segment elevation changed into a 'coved-type'. (**C**) A few days after oral administration of quinidine bisulfate (1500 mg/day, serum quinidine level 2.6 mg/L), marked attenuation of the ST segment elevation is noted in right precordial leads. Note that VF could be induced with double ventricular extrastimulation both during control and procainamide infusion; in contrast, only a few repetitive ventricular complexes could be induced during quinidine therapy using an aggressive protocol using quadruple ventricular extrastimulation. This patient has remained asymptomatic during quinidine therapy during a 24-month follow-up period. Reprinted from Ref. 23 by permission of Futura Publishing Company.

Inefficacy of other antiarrhythmic medications

The beneficial results observed with quinidine therapy markedly contrast with those reported with a wide variety of other antiarrhythmic drugs. In a review of the published literature, including 104 symptomatic patients with Brugada syndrome, Alings and Wilde[7] concluded that no particular antiarrhythmic drug seemed useful in preventing new episodes of VF. They found that arrhythmic events recurred in 9 (30%) of 30 patients treated with beta-adrenergic blocker ($n = 9$), amiodarone ($n = 4$), flecainide ($n = 1$), a combination of β-blockers with amiodarone ($n = 15$) or an α-blocker ($n = 1$). More recently, Nademanee and coworkers[8] reported the results of a randomized study of 61 Thai patients with Brugada syndrome who had survived a sudden death episode or had the identifiable ECG pattern. These patients were randomized to either β-blocker or to single chamber ICD. During the 3-year follow-up period of the main trial, there were 4 deaths; all occurred in the β-blocker group. Seven subjects in the ICD arm had recurrent VF, and all were effectively treated by the ICD. On the basis of the main trial results, the Data Safety Monitoring Board stopped the study. In total (both from the pilot study and the main trial), there were 7 deaths (18%) in the β-blocker group and no deaths in the ICD group, but there were a total of 12 ICD patients receiving ICD discharges due to recurrent VF. One could wonder, however, about the clinical importance of this study since β-blocker agents have been reported to worsen the Brugada syndrome.[24]

Quinidine therapy: advantages

Quinidine therapy offers several advantages for patients with Brugada syndrome.

1 In contrast to ICD, which treats the arrhythmic events, this medication is hopefully expected to prevent their occurrence. The patient treated with an effective drug therapy should enjoy a normal life with a substantial reduced rate of hospitalization. Most of our patients are seen at our outpatient clinic every 6 months.

2 The relatively low cost of long-term antiarrhythmic therapy with quinidine makes it available for most medical systems worldwide. In this regard, it is important to note that the Brugada syndrome seems to be more frequent in Southeast Asia,[15] especially in some developing countries where the high cost of ICD therapy is unaffordable.

3 The relative high inducibility rate of VF in patients with symptomatic Brugada syndrome (70% in the large series of Brugada et al.[25]) renders the option of EP-guided therapy with quinidine a very valuable one for most symptomatic patients.

4 Antiarrhythmic therapy may be used as a 'bridge' to ICD. This may be especially suitable in young patients. For example, one of our patients, the only female in the study group, opted for an ICD when she was 42 years old, after 17 years of well-tolerated quinidine therapy. During that period, she had 2 uneventful pregnancies and normal baby deliveries. We can assume that quinidine therapy avoided her the implantation of at least two devices in the abdomen, thoracic surgery for implantation of epicardial patches, and two or three pectoral ICD implantations/replacements. In fact, and contrarily to the latter patient's case, the great majority of our quinidine-treated patients who tolerated the medication refused the ICD therapy option after they have received objective information of the advantages and disadvantages of ICD.

Quinidine therapy: limitations

There are also several limitations to the use of quinidine therapy.

1 EP-guided antiarrhythmic therapy requires baseline inducibility (preferably in a reproducible manner) of sustained ventricular tachyarrhythmias with PVS. Although the inducibility rate observed by Brugada et al.[25] in a large group of symptomatic patients (cardiac arrest survivors and syncope) was relatively high (70%) we believe that it can be further enhanced by the use of a stimulation protocol such as the one used in our laboratory (high stimulus current, repetition of extrastimulation at the shortest coupling intervals as well as pacing from two right ventricular sites).

2 An excellent patient compliance to medications is required. Early detection of patients with low drug compliance may be difficult, especially during the hospitalization period following the cardiac arrest. Late detection (sometimes years after the arrhyth-

mic event) can raise serious problems as we have observed a few patients who refused the ICD therapy option following several uneventful years despite the partial or absent drug therapy.

3 An excellent patient tolerance to medications is imperative. In our experience, which is based on very long follow-up periods for many patients, about one-third of the patients will show drug-related side effects requiring drug discontinuation, with half of them occurring during the first month of treatment.

4 Some data suggest the existence of a mutation resulting in a phenotype combining QT prolongation (LQT3 subtype) and Brugada syndrome.[26] The use of quinidine in patients with the Brugada syndrome who carry such a mutation could have deleterious consequences. In our experience, however, no patient with Brugada syndrome treated with quinidine has developed any abnormal QT prolongation requiring drug discontinuation.

5 Finally, the last limitation of quinidine therapy is that recent years have shown a marked decline in popularity of antiarrhythmic drugs in the medical community after the publication of the CAST results. This is in addition to the fact that quinidine is frequently viewed by many physicians (especially the youngest ones) as an 'old-generation' medication with severe potential proarrhythmic effects, an assumption that was unfounded in patients with normal hearts and normal baseline QT intervals.

ICD therapy: limitations

No one argues about the exceptional efficacy of ICD for terminating VF. Several major limitations do exist, however, regarding the use of ICD.

1 Since the patient is usually left without prophylactic drug therapy, she/he is at risk for recurrent ventricular tachyarrhythmias and subsequent discharges from the device. This may have deleterious consequences, for example, if the arrhythmia occurs while driving or during professionally exposed activities. In contrast, as pointed out above, quinidine therapy is expected to prevent the occurrence of the arrhythmic events.

2 Electrical storms of VF occurring within a few hours are not infrequently observed in the Brugada syndrome.[19,27–29] Arrhythmic storms may lead to multiple ICD discharges with various conse-

quences: need for emergency hospitalization, psychological disorders,[30] proarrhythmia,[31] deleterious effect on cardiac function,[32] electromechanical dissociation,[33] and even death.[34] In contrast, unpublished data by several European electrophysiologists as well as observations in two of our patients (including one who did not undergo EP evaluation), suggest an extraordinary effect of quinidine in the management of these arrhythmic storms.

3 ICD therapy is associated with various complications such as lead dislodgment, device malfunction, device migration, inappropriate device discharges, and vein thrombosis.[35] The risk of early or late infection (pocket, electrode, or both) may reach 4%.[36] Studies of the long-term complications of ICD in patients with Brugada syndrome are not available yet. These patients are estimated to have a normal life expectancy and therefore are expected to undergo multiple device replacements and lead extractions during their life. This is a very important issue, especially for relatively young patients such as those with Brugada syndrome who have a mean age of 35–40 years when studied.[25] The problem is even more crucial in the very young, such as the 6-month-old Japanese infant reported by Suzuki et al.[19] or the 14-month-old girl reported by Priori et al.[37] In such patients, a significant morbidity ought to be expected with ICD over the long-term despite the constant miniaturization of the devices.

4 Dynamic variations in EP phenomena inherent to the Brugada syndrome may also complicate ICD therapy. Stix et al.[38] showed in two of three patients with Brugada syndrome that spontaneous or ajmaline-induced changes in the surface ECG could be paralleled by significant variations in the right ventricular endocardial electrogram that may result in ICD malfunction. In such patients, implantation of a left ventricular epicardial lead for sensing and pacing could be required to avoid inappropriate tachycardia detection.

5 Psychological problems may also affect the ICD patient. For example, some patients (especially the young) may feel vulnerable and fearful of the device in case of frequent appropriate or inappropriate device discharges, repeated hospitalizations, or multiple surgical procedures (ICD implantations and extractions). Others may fear the aesthetic consequences of device implantation or the possible deleterious consequences in their ability to perform sporting activities.

Conclusion

The remarkable efficacy of ICD in preventing sudden death in all high-risk populations including patients with the Brugada syndrome has diminished the urgency of finding a therapeutic alternative. Taking into account the beneficial electrophysiologic and clinical effects of quinidine we observed in our series of patients with the Brugada syndrome as well as its antiarrhythmic efficacy in experimental models observed by Antzelevitch and associates,[14,15] there is a need for further studies of oral quinidine or other I_{to} blockers such as tedisamil in patients with the Brugada syndrome. If others confirm our preliminary results, randomized clinical trials comparing ICD therapy and quinidine could be considered. One of these studies could be a comparison of ICD with EP-guided therapy with quinidine in cardiac arrest survivors and asymptomatic high-risk patients with inducible VF. Another could be a randomized study (placebo versus quinidine) in patients already implanted with an ICD who have been experiencing relatively frequent events. With any of these scenarios, and in contrast to that has been observed in patients with organic heart disease, the long-term prognosis of patients with the Brugada syndrome is expected to be good in both arms and therefore a long study period may be necessary before differences (if any) between the two treatments is detected. At the present time, our policy at the Tel-Aviv Medical Center is to offer the EP drug-responder patients the choice of either ICD or medical therapy following an objective and comprehensive discussion of the advantages and disadvantages of both therapy modes. Patients who prefer the medical therapy option should be recommended to undergo repeat EP testing on medications every 5 years to confirm the initial beneficial results. We believe that there is an important place for antiarrhythmic drug therapy in selected patient populations with the Brugada syndrome such as young patients, or patients who refuse the ICD option or those who suffer from device-related complications. Absolute requirements for this medical option (besides the efficacy of antiarrhythmic therapy at repeat EP study) include an excellent patient tolerance to medications and his/her commitment to long-term pharmacologic therapy.

Since the writing of our article, an important paper dealing with the high efficacy of quinidine in patients with asymptomatic Brugada syndrome was published (Hermida JS, Denjoy I, Clerc J, *et al.* Hydroquinidine therapy in Brugada syndrome. *J. Am. Coll. Cardiol.* 2004; **43**: 1853–1860). In addition, our article summarizing our experience with quinidine in symptomatic and asymptomatic patients with Brugada syndrome is in press (Belhassen B, Glick A, Viskin S. Efficacy of quinidine in high-risk patients with Brugada syndrome. *Circulation* 2004).

References

1 Brugada P, Brugada J. Right bundle branch block, persistent ST-segment elevation and sudden cardiac death. *J. Am. Coll. Cardiol.* 1992; **20**: 1391–1396.

2 Antzelevitch C, Brugada P, Brugada J *et al.* Brugada syndrome: 1992–2002. A historical perspective. *J. Am. Coll. Cardiol.* 2003; **41**: 1665–1671.

3 Chen Q, Kirsh GE, Zhang D *et al.* Genetic basis and molecular mechanism for idiopathic ventricular fibrillation. *Nature* 1998; **392**: 293–296.

4 Weiss R, Barmada M, Nguyen T *et al.* Clinical and molecular heterogeneity in the Brugada syndrome. A novel gene locus on chromosome 3. *Circulation* 2002; **105**: 707–713.

5 Priori SG, Napolitano C, Gasparini M *et al.* The Brugada syndrome: clinical and genetic heterogeneity of right bundle branch block and ST-elevation syndrome. A prospective evaluation of 52 families. *Circulation* 2000; **102**; 2509–2515.

6 Priori SG, Aliot E, Blomstrom-Lundqvist C *et al.* Task Force on sudden cardiac death of the European Society of Cardiology. *Eur. Heart J.* 2001; **22**: 1374–1450.

7 Alings M, Wilde A. 'Brugada syndrome'. Clinical data and suggested pathophysiological mechanism. *Circulation* 1999; **99**: 666–673.

8 Nademanee K, Veerakul G, Mower M *et al.* Defibrillator versus beta-blockers for unexplained death in Thailand (DEBUT): a randomized clinical trial. *Circulation* 2003; **107**: 2221–2226.

9 Belhassen B, Pelleg A, Miller HI *et al.* Serial electrophysiological studies in a young patient with recurrent ventricular fibrillation. *Pacing Clin. Electrophysiol.* 1981; **4**: 92–99.

10 Belhassen B, Shapira I, Shoshani D *et al.* Idiopathic ventricular fibrillation: inducibility and beneficial effects of class I antiarrhythmic agents. *Circulation* 1987; **75**: 809–816.

11 Belhassen B, Viskin S, Fish R *et al.* Effects of electrophysio-

logic-guided therapy with class 1A antiarrhythmic drugs on the long-term outcome of patients with idiopathic ventricular fibrillation with or without the Brugada syndrome. *J. Cardiovasc. Electrophysiol.* 1999; **10**: 1301–1312.

12 Antzelevitch C. The Brugada syndrome. *J. Cardiovasc. Electrophysiol.* 1998; **9**: 513–516.

13 Gussak I, Antzelevitch C, Bjerregaard P *et al.* The Brugada syndrome: clinical, electrophysiological and genetic aspects. *J. Am. Coll. Cardiol.* 1999; **33**: 5–15.

14 Antzelevitch C. The Brugada syndrome: ionic basis and arrhythmia mechanisms. *J. Cardiovasc. Electrophysiol.* 2001; **12**: 268–272.

15 Yan GX, Antzelevitch C. Cellular basis for the Brugada syndrome and other mechanisms of arrhythmogenesis associated with ST-segment elevation. *Circulation* 1999; **100**: 1660–1666.

16 Nakajima T, Kurachi Y, Ito H *et al.* Anticholinergic effects of quinidine, disopyramide, and procainamide in isolated atrial myocytes: mediation by different molecular mechanisms. *Circ. Res.* 1989; **64**: 297–303.

17 Belhassen B, Shapira I, Sheps D *et al.* Programmed ventricular stimulation using up to two extrastimuli and repetition of double extrastimulation for induction of ventricular tachycardia: a new highly sensitive and specific protocol. *Am. J. Cardiol.* 1990; **65**: 615–622.

18 Viskin S, Belhassen B. Clinical problem-solving. When you only live twice. *N. Engl. J. Med.* 1995; **332**: 1221–1225.

19 Suzuki H, Torigoe K, Numata O *et al.* Infant case with a malignant form of Brugada syndrome. *J. Cardiovasc. Electrophysiol.* 2000; **11**: 1277–1280.

20 Garg A, Finneran W, Feld G. Familial sudden cardiac death associated with a terminal QRS abnormality on surface 12-lead electrocardiogram in the index case. *J. Cardiovasc. Electrophysiol.* 1998; **9**: 642–647.

21 Chinushi M, Aizawa Y, Ogawa Y *et al.* Discrepant drug action of disopyramide on ECG abnormalities and induction of ventricular arrhythmias in a patient with Brugada syndrome. *J. Electrocardiol.* 1997; **30**: 133–136.

22 Alings M, Dekker L, Sadee A *et al.* Quinidine induced electrocardiographic normalization in two patients with Brugada syndrome. *Pacing Clin. Electrophysiol.* 2001; **24**: 1420–1422.

23 Belhassen B, Viskin S, Antzelevitch C. The Brugada syndrome: is an implantable cardioverter defibrillator the only therapeutic option? *Pacing Clin. Electrophysiol.* 2002; **25**: 1634–1640.

24 Miyazaki T, Mitamura H, Miyoshi S *et al.* Autonomic and antiarrhythmic drug modulation of ST segment elevation in patients with Brugada syndrome. *J. Am. Coll. Cardiol.* 1996; **27**: 1061–1070.

25 Brugada P, Brugada R, Mont L *et al.* Natural history of Brugada syndrome: the prognostic value of programmed electrical stimulation of the heart. *J. Cardiovasc. Electrophysiol.* 2003; **14**: 455–457.

26 Bezzina C, Veldkamp MW, van Den Berg MP *et al.* A single Na(+) channel mutation causing both long-QT and Brugada syndromes. *Circ. Res.* 1999; **85**: 1206–1213.

27 Chalvidan T, Deharo JC, Dieuzaide P *et al.* Near fatal electrical storm in a patient equipped with an implantable cardioverter-defibrillator for Brugada syndrome. *Pacing Clin. Electrophysiol.* 2000; **23**: 410–412.

28 Nakamura M, Isobe M, Imamura H. Incessant ventricular fibrillation attacks in a patient with Brugada syndrome. *Int. J. Cardiol.* 1998; **64**: 205–206.

29 Tanaka H, Kinoshita O, Uchikawa S *et al.* Successful prevention of recurrent ventricular fibrillation by intravenous isoproterenol in a patient with Brugada syndrome. *Pacing Clin. Electrophysiol.* 2001; **24**: 1293–1294.

30 Hegel MT, Griegel LE, Black C *et al.* Anxiety and depression in patients receiving implanted cardioverter-defibrillators: a longitudinal investigation. *Int. J. Psychiatry* 1997; **27**: 57–69.

31 Pinski SL, Fahy GJ. The proarrhythmic potential of implantable cardioverter-defibrillators. *Circulation* 1995; **92**: 1651–1664.

32 Joglar JA, Kessler DJ, Welch PJ, *et al.* Effects of repeated electrical defibrillations on cardiac troponin I levels. *Am. J. Cardiol.* 1999; **83**: 270–272.

33 Pires LA, Hull ML, Nino CL *et al.* Sudden death in recipients of transvenous implantable cardioverter defibrillator systems. Terminal events, predictors, and potential mechanisms. *J. Cardiovasc. Electrophysiol.* 1999; **10**: 1049–1056.

34 Bigersdotter-Green U, Rosenquist M, Lindemans FW *et al.* Holter documented sudden death in a patient with an implanted defibrillator. *Pacing Clin. Electrophysiol.* 1992; **15**: 1008–1014.

35 Glikson M, Friedman PA. The implantable cardioverter defibrillator. *Lancet* 2001; **357**: 1107–1117.

36 Schwartzman D, Nallamothu N, Callans DJ *et al.* Postoperative lead-related complications in patients with nonthoracotomy defibrillation lead systems. *J. Am. Coll. Cardiol.* 1995; **26**: 776–786.

37 Priori SG, Napolitano C, Giordano U *et al.* Brugada syndrome and sudden cardiac death in children. *Lancet* 2000; **355**: 808–809.

38 Stix G, Bella PD, Carbucicchio C *et al.* Spatial and temporal heterogeneity of depolarization and repolarization may complicate implantable cardioverter defibrillator therapy in Brugada syndrome. *J. Cardiovasc. Electrophysiol.* 2000; **11**: 516–521.

CHAPTER 19

Potential for ablation therapy in patients with Brugada syndrome

L-F. Hsu, MBBS, *et al.*

Introduction

Since its initial description by Brugada in 1992,[1] the inherited syndrome of sudden cardiac death allied with the electrocardiographic (ECG) features of a right bundle branch block pattern and persistent ST segment elevation in precordial leads V_1–V_3 has gained worldwide recognition. The Brugada syndrome is an important cause of mortality, thought to be responsible for 4–12% of all sudden deaths and up to 20% of deaths in patients with structurally normal hearts. The incidence is of the order of 5 per 10 000 and, apart from accidents, it is the leading cause of death in men under the age of 50 years in endemic regions.[2,3] The episodes of sudden death (aborted or otherwise) are caused by fast polymorphic ventricular tachycardia (VT) or ventricular fibrillation (VF), which usually occur without warning.[4]

Though significant progress has been made in the clinical and genetic identification and characterization of the syndrome, relatively little progress has been made on the therapeutic front. Despite the pharmacologic or device therapies tested over the past decade, the implantable cardioverter-defibrillator (ICD) remains the only established effective treatment.[2,5–7] However, the obvious problems with ICDs are their prohibitive cost in many countries and the fact that they deal with established arrhythmias rather than prevent their occurrence. Given the high incidence of recurrent arrhythmias in these patients,[4,8] and that some of them present with arrhythmic storms resulting in multiple ICD shocks, a curative rather than palliative treatment strategy is ultimately needed to further improve prognosis.

Triggers and substrate — from atrium to ventricle

As in the case of atrial fibrillation (AF), our understanding of the mechanisms of VF can be broadly classified into initiation by triggers and maintenance by substrate. The role of triggers, most commonly ectopic beats from the thoracic veins, in the initiation of AF has been well established.[9] Maintenance of AF, independent of the initiating event, has also drawn significant attention to the role of the substrate.[10] Elimination of the triggers and modification of the substrate have both, individually and in combination, been shown to be effective in the long-term cure of AF.

Triggers

Extending this concept to VF, the importance of the initiating triggers in idiopathic VF and their successful catheter ablation has been demonstrated recently.[11,12] These triggering ectopic beats, usually originating from the Purkinje system, and less frequently from the right ventricular outflow tract (RVOT), were amenable to mapping and ablation, with excellent long-term results in various different centers (89% free of recurrent VF without the need for antiarrhythmic drugs). Further applying these observations to patients with repolarization disorders, it was demonstrated that VF associated with the long QT and Brugada syndromes could be initiated by similar triggers, and that these could also be eliminated by focal RF ablation.[13]

These results confirmed early observations regarding the initiation of VF by ectopic beats. These ectopics could be close-coupled, occurring during the vulnerable period of the ventricle, or they could have an apparently normal coupling interval.[14–16] Their initiating role could be due to automaticity, reentry, or triggered activity.[14,17] Though they could be suppressed by pharmacologic or pacing therapies, these are not curative in the long term.

Substrate

Based on the multiple reentrant wavelet hypothesis proposed by Moe, it has now been accepted that the maintenance of VF is similarly due to different forms of reentry or rotors. The role of reentrant wavelets, whether single or multiple, was revealed by computerized mapping of the ventricle during fibrillation,[18] while the concept of rotors, defined as sustained electrical activity rotating around a functional obstacle, has been supported by independent *in vitro* studies.[14,19] However, it is possible that VF is the end-point of a heterogeneous group of electrical disturbances and it may, in fact, not be possible to identify a single mechanism to adequately account for all cases.

Target for ablation

As in AF, while both triggers and substrate may theoretically be the target of catheter ablation strategies, presently published literature on catheter ablation of VF, including isolated case reports, have focused on ablation of triggers.[11–13,20–23] The large mass of ventricular myocardium, the importance of maintaining normal mechanical ventricular function, and the risk of creating other forms of malignant arrhythmias mean that ablation strategies aimed at substrate modification are currently not viable using presently available technology. However, again drawing from observations in AF, it is possible that both triggers and substrate may share a close structural relationship. In the case of AF, the pulmonary veins are not only the triggers, but recent studies have cast light on their role in the maintenance of AF in some patients. Similarly, parts of the cardiac conduction system known to trigger VF, like the Purkinje arborization,[11,12] have also been shown to have a possible role in its maintenance through various mechanisms.[17,24,25] Hence, by ablating an area where the triggering ectopics are found to originate, it is possible additionally to effect substrate modification if the area is implicated in the maintenance of VF as well.

Triggers of VF in the Brugada syndrome

Role of ectopy

Various hypotheses have been advanced with regard to the triggering mechanisms of VF in the Brugada syndrome. A role for the autonomic nervous system had been proposed, with vagal stimulation believed to trigger arrhythmia in some patients,[4] and related observations had suggested that the beginning of VT/VF was bradycardia-dependent.[26] Though these could explain the higher incidence of arrhythmia and sudden death at night in this group of patients, there are many other patients who develop arrhythmias not associated with such factors.

Regardless of mechanism, it is likely that the actual triggers for VF or polymorphic VT in most cases of the Brugada syndrome are ventricular ectopic beats, most of them monomorphic. This was initially observed in isolated cases (Fig. 19.1),[27] and confirmed by studying the stored electrograms in patients with ICDs.[28] In the latter study, 19 patients with the Brugada syndrome implanted with an ICD were followed-up over a mean duration of 14 months, during which spontaneous VF occurred in 7 (37%), with 3 having multiple episodes. Analysis of 33 episodes of VF revealed that 22 episodes (67%) were preceded by isolated ventricular ectopics, which were identical in morphology to the ectopics triggering these episodes. Furthermore, in the 3 patients with multiple episodes, the VF attacks were always triggered by the same respective ectopics.

Location of ectopy

Current observations suggest that ectopy arising in the Brugada syndrome are predominantly of right ventricular origin. Chinushi *et al.* described recurrent episodes of VF in a patient with Brugada syndrome initiated by monomorphic ectopics with a left bundle branch block morphology.[29] This was corroborated by Morita *et al.*,[30] who observed ventricular ectopics in 9 out of 45 patients studied. Eleven ectopic morphologies were observed in these 9 patients, of which 10 were of right ventricular origin (7 RVOT, 2 septal, and 1 from the apex). In addition, induction of VF was found to be site-specific. Of the 17 inducible patients, VF was induced by programmed stimulation at the RVOT in all (100%), at

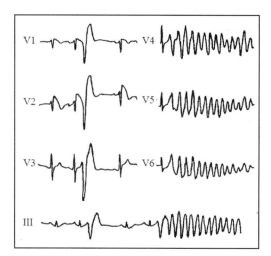

Figure 19.1 ECG recorded at the moment a patient presented with a syncopal episode followed by cardiac arrest. A single ventricular ectopic with left bundle branch block and superior axis morphology is recorded, followed by a second ectopic triggering VF. Modified from Ref. 27, by permission of Blackwell Publishing, Futura Division.

the right ventricular apex in only 2 (12%) and none from the left ventricle. This latter observation supported the initial findings of Kanda et al.,[31] who induced VF using programmed stimulation from the RVOT in 68% compared to 32% from the right ventricular apex. Of note was the ease with which VF could be induced at the RVOT, using just 1 or 2 extrastimuli in most of the patients.

Based on these reports, and on our previous experience with idiopathic VF,[11,12] we devised an ablation strategy targeting these triggers in patients with the Brugada syndrome having recurrent episodes of VF with ICD intervention, the initial results of which have been published recently.[13]

Mapping and ablation procedure

Timing of procedure
In some patients, the triggering ventricular ectopics are persistent even after a long absence of VF episodes, and can be mapped easily. However, as in most cases of idiopathic VF,[12] it is likely that the ectopics are episodic, only appearing just prior to and several days after the onset of VF or polymorphic VT, giving only a narrow time window whereby mapping and ablation can be performed under optimum conditions. Hence the procedures were performed within a few days of the VF episodes.

Electrophysiology study and endocardial mapping
Using a similar technique to that described for idiopathic VF,[12] the electrophysiology study was performed with 2–4 multielectrode catheters. Surface ECG recordings and bipolar intracardiac electrograms were filtered at 30–500 Hz and recorded simultaneously with a polygraph digital system (LabSystem, Bard Electrophysiology, sampling rate 1–4 kHz) or analog system (Midas, sampling rate 10 kHz). High gain amplification (1 mm = 0.1 mV) was used during mapping to clearly identify the potentials. Induction of sustained VF was attempted using 1–3 programmed extrastimuli at the right ventricular apex and (if negative) from the RVOT at twice the diastolic threshold.

The triggers were localized by mapping the earliest electrogram relative to the onset of the ectopic QRS complex. In the case of triggers from the Purkinje system, mapping in sinus rhythm at the distal Purkinje system produced an initial sharp potential (<10 ms in duration) preceding the larger and slower ventricular electrogram by <15 ms. Such a potential preceding ventricular activation during ectopy confirmed that the ectopic beats originated from the Purkinje system.[32]

Radiofrequency ablation
Ablation was performed with conventional 4 mm-tip catheters with a thermocouple, using radiofrequency (RF) energy with a target temperature of 55–60°C and a maximum power of 50 watts. The ectopic focus was targeted first, and after abolition of the ectopics, the lesion was extended to cover a larger area around the focus to minimize recurrence. The duration of ablation thus included time to abolish the ectopic beats and subsequent consolidating applications. Post-ablation, VF induction was attempted again with the same stimulation protocol used at the beginning of the procedure.

Catheter ablation of VF in the Brugada syndrome
Currently, we have performed mapping and catheter ablation of VF in 3 patients with the Brugada syndrome. All of them had presented with an electrical

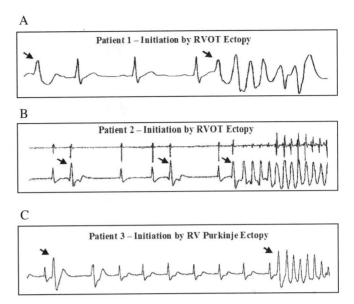

Figure 19.2 Triggering of VF by isolated monomorphic ectopic beats in all three patients who underwent ablation.

storm, with the VF episodes initiated by monomorphic ventricular ectopics (Fig. 19.2), and had received multiple appropriate ICD shocks.

Patient 1

A 35-year-old male patient was diagnosed with the Brugada syndrome in 1998. Of note, he had a documented history of ventricular ectopic beats of RVOT origin (left bundle branch block/inferior axis morphology) with an otherwise normal ECG for 11 years prior to first diagnosis of the Brugada syndrome. Though asymptomatic initially, an ICD was implanted at that time for inducible VF. He presented 4 years after initial diagnosis with an electrical storm, possibly in association with a recent episode of chest infection. Seventeen episodes of VF requiring appropriate ICD discharges were documented. These episodes were triggered by monomorphic RVOT ectopics similar to his usual ones with coupling intervals of 340 ± 20 ms (Fig. 19.2A). The VF episodes only subsided after infusion of low-dose isoproterenol at 0.15 μg/min, with resultant decreased ST segment elevation. Thus stabilized, he was referred for catheter ablation, which was performed a few days later.

During the procedure, the patient continued to have frequent monomorphic ventricular ectopics of RVOT origin (Fig. 19.3). VF was easily and reproducibly induced (Fig. 19.4) by programmed ventricular stimulation with 2 extrastimuli (S1 500, S2 240, S3 220 ms). The triggering ectopic was mapped to the RVOT, with the earliest site 40 ms ahead of the QRS onset on the surface ECG. Ablation at the site resulted in abolition of the ectopics after 2 min, with a further 5 min of RF applied to consolidate the ablation. Post-ablation, VF was no longer inducible with 2 extrastimuli, but was ultimately induced at the RVOT with 3 extrastimuli at short coupling intervals (S1 500, S2 240, S3 220, S4 180 ms). During 10 months of follow-up, interrogation of his ICD revealed no recurrence of ventricular ectopics and no arrhythmic events without antiarrhythmic drugs.

Patient 2

A 36-year-old male patient had an ICD implanted for VF associated with the Brugada syndrome. He had a family history of sudden death, and genetic testing revealed the presence of *SCN5A* channelopathy. Two years after ICD implantation, he presented with 5 episodes of VF in a day, triggered by monomorphic ectopics and appropriately treated by the ICD (Fig. 19.2B). He continued to have frequent monomorphic RVOT ectopics (coupling interval 408 ± 15 ms) between episodes.

During the procedure, VF was easily and reproducibly inducible with 2 extrastimuli (S1 500, S2 240, S3 220). The triggering ectopic was mapped to

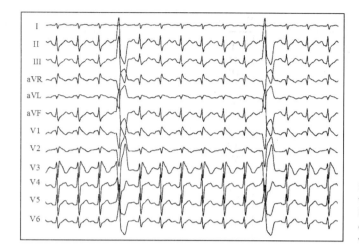

Figure 19.3 Isolated monomorphic ventricular ectopics with left bundle branch block/inferior axis consistent with RVOT origin observed with patient 1.

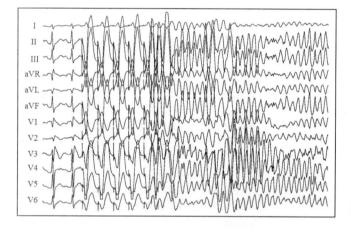

Figure 19.4 Easily inducible VF using two programmed extrastimuli in patient 1 before ablation.

the RVOT, with the earliest site 25 ms before the QRS onset on the surface ECG. Ablation at the site resulted in abolition of the ectopics after 3 min, with a further 7 min of RF applied to consolidate the ablation. Post-ablation, VF was no longer inducible with up to 3 extrastimuli at short coupling intervals down to 180 ms. During 19 months of follow-up, interrogation of his ICD revealed no recurrence of ventricular ectopics and no arrhythmic events without antiarrhythmic drugs.

Patient 3

A 47-year-old female patient with a strong family history of sudden death was diagnosed with the Brugada syndrome (after an ajmaline test) in 1999 after presenting with aborted sudden death from documented VF. She was being investigated for frequent and recurrent episodes of syncope at that time,

always occurring 1–2 days before menstruation, and had a history of multiple spontaneous abortions. Three years after ICD implantation, she had had a total of 21 documented episodes of VF, 14 of them on quinidine therapy, with appropriate ICD intervention. Interestingly, these VF episodes invariably occurred just before menstruation. During these episodes, she was noted to have frequent monomorphic ventricular ectopic beats with left bundle branch block/superior axis morphology (coupling interval 278 ± 29 ms). Interrogation of the ICD revealed that the episodes of VF were triggered by ectopics with a similar morphology to her usual ones (Fig. 19.2C).

During the procedure, VF could not be induced at baseline. The triggering ectopic (Fig. 19.5A) was mapped to the anterior right ventricular Purkinje network. Ablation at this site (Fig. 19.5B) resulted in

A

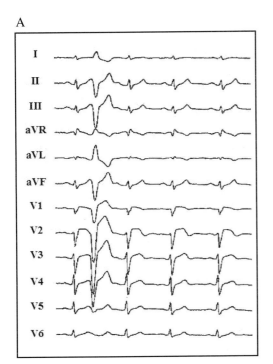

B

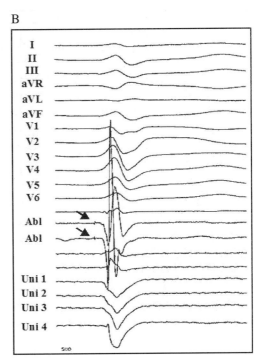

Figure 19.5 (A) Ventricular ectopic in patient 3 demonstrating left bundle branch block/superior axis morphology, later mapped to the anterior Purkinje system. The patient was diagnosed with the Brugada syndrome after an ajmaline test. **(B)** Site of successful ablation, demonstrating the Purkinje activation (arrows) preceding the muscle potential during sinus rhythm. Though the Purkinje potential was very early relative to the muscle potential, suggestive of a more proximal ablation site, no significant intraventricular delay was observed post-ablation.

abolition of the Purkinje potentials and ectopics after 2 min, with a further 8 min of RF applied to consolidate the ablation. Post-ablation, VF was still not inducible with up to 3 extrastimuli at short coupling intervals down to 180 ms. During 7 months of follow-up, interrogation of her ICD revealed no recurrence of ventricular ectopics nor arrhythmic events without antiarrhythmic drugs.

Implications and further observations

Triggers

Though our experience with catheter ablation of VF in the Brugada syndrome is currently limited, the results of ablation are strikingly similar to those achieved with idiopathic VF.[12] As idiopathic VF has been considered not to involve any form of abnormal substrate, while patients with the Brugada syndrome clearly have an abnormal electrophysio-logical substrate despite normal cardiac function and lack of gross structural cardiac abnormalities, these results support the important role of focal triggers in the initiation of VF in multiple substrates. With no recurrence of ectopics or VT/VF over a mean of 12 ± 6 months, these cases also illustrate the potential benefit of catheter ablation of these triggers.

The propensity of the triggering ectopics to originate from the right ventricle, and especially the RVOT, is noteworthy. Antzelevitch *et al.* suggested that the mechanism of ventricular arrhythmias could be phase 2 reentry.[33,34] This predominantly epicardial mechanism is associated with the difference in the action potential duration in the ventricular wall, especially in the region of the RVOT,[33,35,36] and should produce closely coupled ectopic beats, which could then initiate circus movement reentry and hence VF.[37] However, our observations appear contrary to this hypothesis. In the two patients with

RVOT triggers, the coupling intervals of the initiating beats were long (340 ± 20 and 408 ± 15 ms, respectively), while in the third case, the Purkinje source of the initiating beat provides evidence for an endocardial origin as opposed to the epicardial phase 2 reentry. A possible explanation for these apparent discrepancies, derived from an experimental model of the Brugada syndrome, could be that the first reentrant extrasystole (phase 2 reentry) has a very short coupling interval and is buried within the T wave of the previous beat, while the observed ectopic beat is actually the second reentrant extrasystole. In addition, endocardial activation ahead of the extrasystolic R wave was also observed in the same model (Antzelevitch—personal communication). On the other hand, it is also possible that the mechanism producing the triggering beats could be more complex and multifactorial.

Of further interest, in one of the patients with an RVOT trigger, frequent monomorphic ventricular ectopics similar to the triggering beats had been documented many years before, with a normal QRST on the ECGs. The ECG changes of the Brugada syndrome were then noted 11 years after first documentation of the ectopics. This phenomenon was also observed in one of our patients with the long QT syndrome.[13] Though rare cases have been observed in whom the ST segment elevation increased just prior to the onset of polymorphic VT or VF,[4] the existence of potential triggers that were apparently quiescent till the development of ECG evidence of repolarization abnormalities may suggest a complex interaction between triggers and substrate.

Substrate

The existence of an abnormal electrophysiological substrate despite an apparently normal heart in the Brugada syndrome is evidenced by the fact that most of them have inducible polymorphic VT or VF and a positive signal-averaged ECG.[38] In a group of patients with sudden unexplained death syndrome, VF was inducible in 93% of patients with the Brugada pattern on the ECG compared to only 11% in those with a normal ECG.[39]

It is interesting to note that in our two patients with RVOT triggers, VF inducibility was modified after ablation. While VF was reproducibly and easily inducible before ablation with 2 extrastimuli, it could not be induced in one patient after ablation,

while in the other, it was only inducible with 3 extrastimuli at very short coupling intervals (180 ms) from the RVOT. While the implications of this observation are presently unclear, it may suggest an additional role for the RVOT as the substrate. As discussed previously, VF was more frequently and easily induced from the RVOT than other regions of the heart.[30,31] The dispersion of repolarization in the epicardium, as proposed by Antzelevitch,[33–35] and located predominantly at the right ventricle and especially the RVOT region, could provide the substrate for reentrant activity. Hence, for our ablation procedure in these three patients, it may be important not only to eliminate the focus of ectopy, but to further consolidate and extend the lesion to involve a wider area. Whether this approach can result in significant modification of the electrophysiological substrate will require greater patient numbers.

Conclusion

Though catheter ablation of VF is still an emerging technique, the initial experiences with idiopathic VF,[11,12] and latterly with VF secondary to ischemic heart disease and repolarization disorders, including the Brugada syndrome,[13,40,41] have provided important insights into the role of focal triggers from the Purkinje system and RVOT in multiple substrates. In particular, it is eminently applicable to patients having frequent recurrent episodes of VF, which make up an estimated 20% of patients with ICDs,[42] provided the triggers can be localized by mapping. Reducing the incidence of VF with localized ablation may reduce defibrillation requirement and replacement and improve the patients' quality of life.

The excellent long-term results after successful ablation of these triggers have been demonstrated at many centers, with the data-logging capabilities of the ICDs implanted in these patients proving ideal for clinical follow-up. As illustrated by our experience with the Brugada syndrome, successful catheter ablation has relegated the implanted ICDs to a sentinel role. With the development of new catheter designs and mapping technologies, and greater physician experience, catheter ablation of VF, with the ultimate aim of curing such patients at risk of sudden cardiac death, may not be an unrealistic goal in the future.

References

1 Brugada P, Brugada J. Right bundle branch block, persistent ST-segment elevation and sudden cardiac death: a multicenter report. *J. Am. Coll. Cardiol.* 1992; **20**: 1391–1396.

2 Antzelevitch C, Brugada P, Brugada J *et al.* Brugada syndrome: 1992–2002. A historical perspective. *J. Am. Coll. Cardiol.* 2003; **41**: 1665–1671.

3 Antzelevitch C, Brugada P, Brugada J *et al.* Brugada syndrome. A decade of progress. *Circ. Res.* 2002; **91**: 1114–1118.

4 Brugada P, Brugada R, Antzelevitch C *et al.* The Brugada syndrome. In: Santini M, eds. *Non-Pharmacological Treatment of Sudden Death.* Bologna: Arianna Editrice, 2003: 73–93.

5 Brugada J, Brugada R, Brugada P. Pharmacological and device approach to therapy of inherited cardiac diseases associated with cardiac arrhythmias and sudden death. *J. Electrocardiol.* 2000; **33** (Suppl.): 41–47.

6 Brugada P, Brugada R, Brugada J *et al.* Use of the prophylactic implantable cardioverter defibrillator for patients with normal hearts. *Am. J. Cardiol.* 1999; **83**: 98–100D.

7 Brugada J, Brugada R, Brugada P. Right bundle-branch block and ST-segment elevation in leads V1 through V3. A marker for sudden death in patients without demonstrable structural heart disease. *Circulation* 1998; **97**: 457–460.

8 Brugada J, Brugada R, Antzelevitch C *et al.* Long-term follow-up of individuals with the electrocardiographic pattern of right bundle-branch block and ST-segment elevation in precordial leads V1 to V3. *Circulation* 2002; **105**: 73–78.

9 Haissaguerre M, Jais P, Shah DC *et al.* Spontaneous initiation of atrial fibrillation by ectopic beats originating in the pulmonary veins. *N. Engl. J. Med.* 1998; **339**: 659–666.

10 Allesie MA, Boyden PA, Camm AJ *et al.* Pathophysiology and prevention of atrial fibrillation. *Circulation* 2001; **103**: 769–777.

11 Haissaguerre M, Shah DC, Jais P *et al.* Role of Purkinje conducting system in triggering of idiopathic ventricular fibrillation. *Lancet* 2002; **359**: 677–678.

12 Haissaguerre M, Shoda M, Jais P *et al.* Mapping and ablation of idiopathic ventricular fibrillation. *Circulation* 2002; **106**: 962–967.

13 Haissaguerre M, Extramiana F, Hocini M *et al.* Mapping and ablation of ventricular fibrillation associated with long-QT and Brugada syndromes. *Circulation* 2003; **108**: 925–928.

14 Jalife J. Ventricular fibrillation: mechanisms of initiation and maintenance. *Annu. Rev. Physiol.* 2000; **62**: 25–50.

15 Viskin S, Lesh MD, Eldar M *et al.* Mode of onset of malignant ventricular arrhythmias in idiopathic ventricular fibrillation. *J. Cardiovasc. Electrophysiol.* 1997; **8**: 1115–1120.

16 Eisenberg SJ, Scheinman MM, Dullet NK *et al.* Sudden cardiac death and polymorphous ventricular tachycardia in patients with normal QT intervals and normal systolic cardiac function. *Am. J. Cardiol.* 1995; **75**: 687–692.

17 Berenfeld O, Jalife J. Pukinje-muscle reentry as a mechanism of polymorphic ventricular arrhythmias in a 3-dimensional model of the ventricles. *Circ. Res.* 1998; **82**: 1063–1077.

18 Chen PS. Electrode mapping of ventricular fibrillation. In: Zipes DP, Jalife J, eds. *Cardiac Electrophysiology: From Cell to Bedside.* Philadelphia: WB Saunders.

19 Gray RA, Jalife J, Panfilov AV *et al.* Mechanisms of cardiac fibrillation. *Science* 1995; **270**: 1222–1225.

20 Aizawa Y, Tamura M, Chinushi M *et al.* An attempt at electrical catheter ablation of the arrhythmogenic area in idiopathic ventricular fibrillation. *Am. Heart J.* 1992; **123**: 257–260.

21 Ashida K, Kaji Y, Sasaki Y. Abolition of torsade de pointes after radiofrequency catheter ablation at right ventricular outflow tract. *Int. J. Cardiol.* 1997; **59**: 171–175.

22 Kusano KF, Yamamoto M, Emori T *et al.* Successful catheter ablation in a patient with polymorphic ventricular tachycardia. *J. Cardiovasc. Electrophysiol.* 2000; **11**: 682–685.

23 Takatsuki S, Mitamura H, Ogawa S. Catheter ablation of a monofocal premature ventricular complex triggering idiopathic ventricular fibrillation. *Heart* 2001; **86**: e3.

24 Caceres J, Jazayeri M, McKinnie J *et al.* Sustained bundle branch reentry as a mechanism of clinical tachycardia. *Circulation* 1989; **79**: 256–270.

25 Sasyniuk B, Mendez C. A mechanism for reentry in canine ventricular tissue. *Circ. Res.* 1971; **28**: 3–15.

26 Kasanuki H, Ohnishi S, Ohtuka M *et al.* Idiopathic ventricular fibrillation induced with vagal activity in patients without obvious heart disease. *Circulation* 1997; **95**: 2277–2285.

27 Vanzini P, Brugada J. Spontaneous recurrent ventricular fibrillation in a patient with a structurally normal heart. *Pacing Clin. Electrophysiol.* 2000; **23**: 266–267.

28 Kakishita M, Kurita T, Matsuo K *et al.* Mode of onset of ventricular fibrillation in patients with Brugada syndrome detected by implantable cardioverter defibrillator therapy. *J. Am. Coll. Cardiol.* 2000; **36**: 1646–1653.

29 Chinushi M, Washizuka T, Chinushi Y *et al.* Induction of ventricular fibrillation in Brugada syndrome by site-specific right ventricular premature depolarization. *Pacing Clin. Electrophysiol.* 2002; **25**: 1649–1651.

30 Morita H, Kusano KF, Nagase S *et al.* Site-specific arrhythmogenesis in patients with Brugada syndrome. *J. Cardiovasc. Electrophysiol.* 2003; **14**: 373–379.

31 Kanda M, Shimizu W, Matsuo K *et al.* Electrophysiologic characteristics and implications of induced ventricular

fibrillation in symptomatic patients with the Brugada syndrome. *J. Am. Coll. Cardiol.* 2002; **39**: 1799–1805.

32 Nakagawa H, Beckman KJ, McClelland JH *et al.* Radiofrequency catheter ablation of idiopathic left ventricular tachycardia guided by a Purkinje potential. *Circulation* 1993; **88**: 2607–2617.

33 Antzelevitch C, Brugada P, Brugada J *et al.* The Brugada syndrome. In: Camm AJ, eds. *Clinical Approaches to Tachyarrhythmias.* Armonk, NY: Futura Publishing Co., 1999.

34 Antzelevitch C. The Brugada syndrome. *J. Cardiovasc. Electrophysiol.* 1998; **9**: 513–516.

35 Antzelevitch C. Late potentials and the Brugada syndrome. *J. Am. Coll. Cardiol.* 2002; **39**: 1996–1999.

36 Nagase S, Kusano KF, Morita H *et al.* Epicardial electrogram at the right ventricular outflow tract in patients with Brugada syndrome using epicardial lead. *J. Am. Coll. Cardiol.* 2002; **39**: 1992–1995.

37 Lukas A, Antzelevitch C. Phase 2 reentry as a mechanism of initiation of circus movement reentry in canine epicar-dium exposed to simulated ischemia. The antiarrhythmic effects of 4-AP. *Cardiovasc. Res.* 1996; **32**: 593–603.

38 Corrado D, Buja G, Basso C *et al.* What is the Brugada syndrome? *Cardiol. Rev.* 1999; **7**(4): 191–195.

39 Nademanee K, Veerakul G, Nimmannit S *et al.* Arrhythmogenic marker for the sudden unexplained death syndrome in Thai men. *Circulation* 1997; **96**: 2595–2600.

40 Bansch D, Ouyang F, Ernst S *et al.* Drug-refractory incessant ventricular fibrillation during acute myocardial infarction can be cured by radiofrequency ablation. *Pacing Clin. Electrophysiol.* 2003; **26**(II): 944 (Abstract).

41 Haissaguerre M, Weerasooriya R, Walczack F *et al.* Catheter ablation of polymorphic VT or VF in multiple substrates. In: Santini M, eds. *Non-Pharmacological Treatment of Sudden Death.* Bologna: Arianna Editrice, 2003: 237–253.

42 Exner DV, Pinski SL, Wyse DG *et al.* AVID Investigators. Electrical storm presages nonsudden death. *Circulation* 2001; **103**: 2066–2071.

Index

Page numbers in *italics* refer to figures and those in **bold** to tables; but note that figures and tables are only indicated when they are separated from their text references. Index entries are filed in letter-by-letter alphabetical order.